Men's Sexual Health and Fertility

John P. Mulhall • Wayland Hsiao
Editors

Men's Sexual Health and Fertility

A Clinician's Guide

Springer

Editors
John P. Mulhall, MD
Director, Male Sexual and Reproductive Medicine Program
Memorial Sloan-Kettering Cancer Center
New York, NY, USA

Wayland Hsiao, MD
Department of Urology
Kaiser Permanente, Oakland Medical Center
Oakland, CA, USA

ISBN 978-1-4939-0424-2 ISBN 978-1-4939-0425-9 (eBook)
DOI 10.1007/978-1-4939-0425-9
Springer New York Heidelberg Dordrecht London

Library of Congress Control Number: 2014931238

Printed on acid-free paper

Springer is part of Springer Science+Business Media (www.springer.com)

This project is dedicated to our mentors and our trainees. When the answer is not readily apparent in medical research or clinical practice, our mentors give us the tools to shed light into the darkness. True mentorship sparks the torch of curiosity and guides us as we go forth into the unknown and discover new truths. We will never reach the end of the unknown; this is up to our trainees.

Preface

Andrology, the study of all things male, straddles two worlds in our modern medical apparatus: sexual medicine and reproductive medicine. With differing focuses and often-different patient populations, an andrologist has to truly master both disciplines to take care of the whole male. It is our great privilege to bring to you this book, which tries to bridge a gap between sexual medicine and reproductive medicine. While sexual dysfunction is common and its effects on reproduction just as common, reproductive medicine practitioners often disregard male sexual dysfunction in this age of gamete-centric reproduction.

Our idea was to provide a guide and reference for the reproductive medicine practitioner to better understand and treat sexual medicine problems in the infertile couple. To do this, we pulled together some of the youngest and brightest minds in clinical andrology and asked them to not only give us a review of what is known but also tell us what we still need to learn. We hope you will enjoy this book as much as we have enjoyed creating it!

Best regards,

New York, NY — John P. Mulhall
Oakland, CA — Wayland Hsiao

Contents

List of Contributors

Dylan Brock, BA University of Louisville School of Medicine, Louisville, KY, USA

Claire Brookings, MBBS, MRCP Department of Genitourinary Medicine, Lincolnshire Community Health Services NHS Trust, Marson, UK

Seth D. Cohen, MD, MPH Department of Urology, University of California, San Diego, San Diego, CA, USA

Robert C. Dean, MD Walter Reed National Military Medical Center, NCC (Walter Reed) Urology Residency, Bethesda, MD, USA

Nathaly François, MD Division of Urology, Department of Surgery, Southern Illinois University School of Medicine, Springfield, IL, USA

Geoffrey S. Gaunay, MD Department of Urology, Beth Israel Medical Center, A Member of the Mount Sinai Health System, New York, NY, USA

David Goldmeier, MD, FRCP Imperial College Healthcare NHS Trust, Paddington, London, UK

Wayland Hsiao, MD Department of Urology, Kaiser Permanente, Oakland Medical Center, Oakland, CA, USA

Mohit Khera, MD, MBA, MPH Scott Department of Urology, Baylor College of Medicine, Houston, TX, USA

Tobias S. Köhler, MD, MPH, FACS Department of Urology, Southern Illinois University School of Medicine, Springfield, IL, USA

Richard K. Lee, MD, MBA Department of Urology and Public Health, Weill Cornell Medical College, New York, NY, USA

Philip S. Li, MD Department of Urology, Weill Cornell Medical College of Cornell University, Center for Male Reproductive Medicine and Microsurgery, New York, NY, USA

Joseph W. McQuaid, MD Department of Urology, Massachusetts General Hospital, Boston, MA, USA

Akanksha Mehta, MD Department of Urology, Emory University School of Medicine, Atlanta, GA, USA

Mark A. Moyad, MPH, MD Department of Urology, University of Michigan, Ann Arbor, MI, USA

John P. Mulhall, MD Department of Surgery, Section of Urology, Memorial Sloan-Kettering Cancer Center, New York, NY, USA

Christian J. Nelson, PhD Department of Psychiatry and Behavioral Sciences, Memorial Sloan-Kettering Cancer Center, New York, NY, USA

E. Charles Osterberg, MD New York Presbyterian Hospital–Weill Cornell Medical College, New York, NY, USA

Alexander W. Pastuszak, MD, PhD Scott Department of Urology, Baylor College of Medicine, Houston, TX, USA

Raunak D. Patel, BS Department of Surgery, Southern Illinois University School of Medicine, Springfield, IL, USA

Louis M. Revenig, BS Department of Urology, Emory University Hospital, Atlanta, GA, USA

Hossein Sadeghi-Nejad, MD, FACS UMDNJ New Jersey Medical School, Hackensack University Medical Center, Hackensack, NJ, USA

Geraldine Sheu, MD Department of Urology, Emory University Hospital, Atlanta, GA, USA

Alan W. Shindel, MD Department of Urology, University of California, Davis, Sacramento, CA, USA

Vikram Soni, MD Scott Department of Urology, Baylor College of Medicine, Houston, TX, USA

Peter J. Stahl, MD Department of Urology, Columbia University Medical Center, New York, NY, USA

Doron S. Stember, MD Department of Urology, Beth Israel Medical Center, A Member of the Mount Sinai Health System, New York, NY, USA

Cigdem Tanrikut, MD Department of Urology, Massachusetts General Hospital, Boston, MA, USA

Patrick E. Teloken, MD Department of General Surgery, Royal Perth Hospital, Perth, Australia

Landon W. Trost, MD Department of Urology, Mayo Clinic, Rochester, MN, USA

Genevieve Von Thesling-Sweet, MD Department of Urology, University of California, Davis, Sacramento, CA, USA

Daniel H. Williams IV, MD Department of Urology, University of Wisconsin School of Medicine and Public Health, Madison, WI, USA

Chapter 1
Physiology of Erection

Genevieve Von Thesling Sweet and Alan W. Shindel

Introduction and Background

Penile erection is a complex process involving anatomic, vascular, neurologic, hormonal, molecular, and psychological factors [1]. A thorough understanding of erectile anatomy and physiology is essential for fertility specialists as erectile dysfunction (ED) is common in infertile men; it is estimated that some degree of ED is present in 11–28 % of male partners of infertile couples [2–4]. ED and other sexual dysfunctions may pose serious barriers to conception in infertile couples. Aside from compromising a couple's ability to conceive, sexual dysfunction may add to the already substantial psychological toll of an infertility diagnosis [2, 5].

Penile Anatomy

Penile tumescence occurs by the expansion of three chambers of the spongy erectile tissue in the penis (Fig. 1.1) [6]. The paired dorsal corpora cavernosa function as a single unit due to an incomplete septum and extensive vascular communications. Each corpus cavernosum is surrounded by a bilayered collagenous sheath called the tunica albuginea [7]. The tunica provides rigidity and strength to the penis during erection by limiting the degree of corporal expansion and compressing the emissary veins to restrict the outflow of blood from the corporal bodies [6, 8, 9]. The tunica also contains internal fibrous struts that provide additional support. The thickness and strength of the tunica varies over its length; it is weakest on the ventral sides at

A.W. Shindel (✉)
Department of Urology, University of California at Davis, Suite 3500, 4860 Y Street, Sacramento, CA, USA
e-mail: awshindel@ucdavis.edu

J.P. Mulhall and W. Hsiao (eds.), *Men's Sexual Health and Fertility*,
DOI 10.1007/978-1-4939-0425-9_1, © Springer Science+Business Media New York 2014

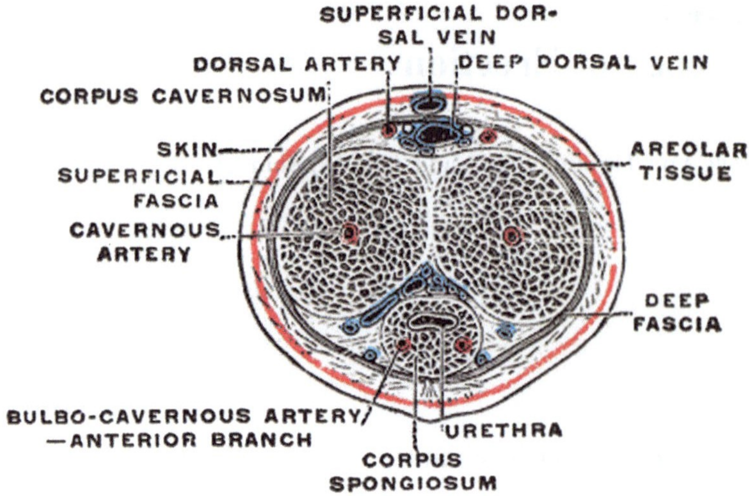

Fig. 1.1 Cross-sectional anatomy of the penis (adapted from Gray's anatomy)

the 5 and 7 o'clock positions and it is in this vicinity that most penile fractures occur [7].

The third erectile chamber of the penis is the ventrally located corpus spongiosum. The corpus spongiosum surrounds the urethra and enlarges distally as the glans penis, the most sensitive portion of the male phallus. The spongiosum lacks a dense tunica sheath and therefore does not become erect in the same fashion as the corpora cavernosa [6]. However, during rigid (maximal) erection the spongiosum and the corpora cavernosa are engorged by contraction of the bulbospongiosus and ischiocavernosus muscles; this forces additional blood into all three erectile chambers [6]. During this phase of the erectile response, intrapenile pressure may exceed systolic blood pressure [6].

All three erectile bodies are surrounded by Buck's fascia. External support of the penis is provided by the fundiform ligament laterally. Medially and dorsally, the suspensory ligament of the penis helps anchor the phallus to the pubic bone [10]. Testosterone appears to play an important role in maintenance of corporal tissue integrity; androgen ablation has been associated with penile tissue atrophy, decreased smooth muscle content, and nerve changes [11]

Vascular Anatomy

The blood supply to the penis is derived from the internal iliac artery via the internal pudendal artery, which gives rise to the common penile artery. The common penile artery also supplies the scrotum and portions of the urethra. The common penile artery bifurcates into the dorsal artery of the penis and the deep penile artery; the latter supplies the corpora cavernosa via the cavernous and helicine arteries [12]. Branches of the deep penile arteries are given off throughout the length of each corporal body and flow in a radial fashion towards the tunica albuginea and the emissary venous network [12]. Variations in this anatomy do exist. Common variants include unilateral arterial dominance and/or the presence of accessory pudendal arteries [13].

The venous outflow from the penis is primarily via the internal pudendal veins. Emissary veins within the cavernous bodies join to form cavernous and crural veins; these veins either lead to the internal pudendal veins or communicate with circumflex veins which converge on the deep dorsal vein of the penis and eventually the periprostatic plexus. Proximal drainage also flows from Santorini's plexus [12, 14]. Drainage of the skin and subcutaneous tissues of the penis is typically via the saphenous veins. Communication occurs between all the venous systems of the penis and can be highly variable between patients [14].

Neural Anatomy

Central Nervous System

The nervous system regulates penile erection at multiple levels and acts to coordinate the overall process of erection and detumescence. Many of the central nervous system effects may relate to sexual drive (libido) more than penile tumescence; however, the intimate relationship between sexual drive and penile erection makes an understanding of these effects relevant when discussing erectile physiology.

Brain Centers Involved in Penile Erection

The brain has a modulatory effect on the spinal pathways of erection and serves to integrate various sensory inputs. Several supraspinal regions have been implicated including the hypothalamus, limbic system, amygdale, thalamus, substantia nigra, periaqueductal gray, and tegmentum. Additional brainstem and medullary centers are also thought to be involved. The paraventricular and preoptic nuclei found near the hypothalamus in the brain are believed to be specifically associated with facilitation of erection [6, 15].

Neurotransmitters and Neurohormonal Regulation of Sexual Function in the Brain

The modulation of sexual function in the brain is affected by a number of neurotransmitters and hormones; these pathways are incompletely understood and therefore will be considered only briefly here.

Dopaminergic, adrenergic, oxytocin, and melanocortin pathways appear to promote sexual function, while the 5-HT serotonin pathway and prolactin generally appear to inhibit sexual function [1, 16, 17]. Oxytocin is a hormone and neurotransmitter that can act centrally or peripherally. The release of oxytocin tends to promote sexual function and orgasm and may influence nitric oxide production [18]. Norepinephrine from locus ceruleus and in the pons and medulla act on the paraventricular and supraoptic nuclei of the hypothalamus and appear to have a positive effect on sexual function [15]. Finally, the melanocortins additionally modulate sexual behavior and, at the level of the spinal cord, possibly erectile function as well [19]. Less clear are the roles of GABA and opioids, both of which appear to oppose erectile response [20].

Androgens appear to play a role in modulating erectile function in the brain. Testosterone receptors are present in the medial preoptic area and paraventricular nucleus and the medial amygdala [21]. Studies in rats have demonstrated that testosterone appears to prime the central neurologic response to dopamine release [22, 23]. Castrated rats very quickly lose the pro-erectogenic effects of dopamine release; the administration of exogenous testosterone prevents this loss of dopamine sensitivity [21, 22]. Testosterone thus appears to bias sensorimotor integration to elicit pro-sexual effects in response to stimulation in the central nervous system, possibly by the production of nitric oxide [22–24].

5-HT is believed to have a central inhibitory effect in the brain on sexual drive by action on the hypothalamus and limbic system [1]. 5-HT may affect spinal reflexes involved with erection, though some supraspinal facilitator effects may exist as well [25]. Prolactin generally decreases sexual arousal, and this is likely via its negative action on dopaminergic activity. Higher serum prolactin levels have been linked to decreased sexual activity and libido [17].

Spinal Cord and Peripheral Nerves

The penis is innervated by somatic and autonomic nerves. The somatic representation is provided by the pudendal nerve, mediating sensation of the penis, and motor control over striated musculature (e.g., contraction of the ischiocavernosus muscle at rigid erection). The somatic motor nerves arise from the ventral horn of S2–S4 [6, 12]. Somatic sensation is derived from highly concentrated free nerve endings and unique structured corpuscular sensory receptors in the corona, glans, and penile skin [26]. These fibers culminate in bundles which eventually converge to form the dorsal nerve of the penis. The dorsal nerve of the penis carries afferent sensory input to the pudendal nerve to enter the spinal cord at the S2–S4 roots at which point they terminate on the spinal neuron tracts [27]. Pain and temperature are carried towards brain via the spinothalamic tract [27]. Complex touch and stimulatory input is carried primarily by the ascending spinoreticular tract, proceeding towards the sensory cortex of the CNS [27]. From there, in conjunction with visual, auditory, and additional sensory inputs, they undergo a more complex processing; it is thought that this process modulates perceptions of arousal and sexual stimulation [21, 27]. Efferent innervations to the pudendal nerve are derived from Onuf's nucleus in the ventral sacral spinal cord, which provides motor input to the perineal striated muscles (bulbospongiosus and ischiocavernosus) important for ejaculation [21].

The autonomic component of the cavernous nerves consists of both sympathetic and parasympathetic fibers. The terminal branches of the cavernous nerves (including sympathetic and parasympathetic fibers) innervate the helicine arteries and trabecular smooth muscle, governing the vascular events of erection [6].

Sympathetic innervation to the vascular smooth muscle of the penis is derived from the sympathetic chain ganglia at the T11-L2 levels [6]. These fibers exit the spinal cord as the superior hypogastric plexus or paravertebral sympathetic chain [21], which sits in close proximity to the aorta and is vulnerable to injury during retroperitoneal surgery [28]. Injury to these nerves may have a very substantial effect on seminal emission during ejaculation [29]. Peripherally, these nerves terminate as the pelvic plexus and cavernous nerves [21]. These fibers also mediate baseline sympathetic tone to the penis by action of adrenergic fibers, which release norepinephrine. This maintains the penis in its flaccid state. Adrenergic tone to the penis may be overridden by inhibition from cortical centers, facilitating penile erection by removing inhibitory sympathetic tone [6].

Pro-erectogenic parasympathetic innervation to the penis is provided by the parasympathetic nuclei of the spinal cord at the S2–4 level [6]. Descending parasympathetic neural pathways involved with erection originate in the interomediolateral nuclei of the sacral spinal cord and course peripherally to form the pelvic nerves and join the cavernous nerves. Along their course, they travel intimately close to the prostate and rectum, making them vulnerable to injury during radical pelvic surgery [30].

The specific contributions of the sympathetic and parasympathetic nerve systems to penile erection explain the variation in erectile response observed in men with spinal cord injuries. Psychogenic erections tend to be preserved in men with lower spinal cord injuries (below T12); these erections appear to be mediated by the central nervous system suppression of sympathetic (vasoconstrictive) tone to the penile circulation [6]. The proposed proximal source of this erectogenic efferent modulation is from the medial preoptic area which in its propagation inhibits the sympathetic pathway and facilitates parasympathetic firing [21]. Reflex erections in response to tactile stimulation may be preserved in men with upper cord lesions (above T12). These erections appear to be mediated by the sacral reflex arc which is not interrupted in men with upper spinal cord lesions [6]. It is apparent that partial preservation of erection is possible in spinal cord injury patients; however, for a complete erectile response it is clear that both the cerebral inhibition of sympathetic stimulation and activation of the parasympathetic response at the level of the sacral spinal cord are required [6].

The Physiology of Penile Erection

Fundamentally, penile erection is a vascular event [6, 8, 9, 12]. There are two components to this vascular process; cavernosal and arterial smooth muscle relaxation/dilation and synergistic restriction of venous outflow [6, 9]. Detumescence occurs following smooth muscle contraction of penile arteries with resultant decreased inflow and drainage of blood trapped within the cavernous spaces [6, 31].

Arterial Dilation

In the flaccid state, there is little blood flow to the penis, and the smooth muscle is in a state of general contraction [6, 31]. Relaxation of the cavernosal arteries increases blood flow 20–40-fold. Within the tunica of the corporal bodies, there are endothelial-lined sinusoids between layers of the trabecular smooth muscle. These lacunar spaces are filled with blood during erection [9].

Venous Occlusion

As the penis expands, pressure increases at the outer circumference of the corpora near the tunica albuginea; this is the primary site of the venous outflow from the corporal bodies. As filling continues, the peripherally located subtunical venous plexus and the emissary veins are compressed between the relatively inelastic outer layer of tunica albuginea and the corporal sinusoids. This veno-occlusive mechanism enhances tumescence by impeding the outflow of blood [8, 9]. This blood-trapping phenomenon accounts for the rise in cavernous pressure seen at full erection, which typically averages around 100 mg Hg in healthy men [6]. Pressure in the corpus spongiosum is usually a third of what is observed in the corpora cavernosa during this phase of erection because the thinner tunica albuginea of the spongiosum does not permit tight coaptation [6].

The vascular component of erection is further enhanced by the bulbocavernosal reflex brought on by repetitive penile stimulation (e.g., intercourse). During this response, the bases of the corporal bodies (crura) are compressed by a strong sustained contraction of the ischiocavernosus and bulbospongiosus muscles. This contraction forces additional blood into the erectile chambers and increases rigidity of the corpus spongiosum and glans penis. This leads to the rigid erection phase in which intrapenile pressure may exceed systolic blood pressure [6].

Molecular Mechanisms of Penile Erection

Smooth Muscle Activity and Calcium Metabolism

Smooth muscle contraction, in penile vasculature and elsewhere, is modulated by the binding of calcium ion to calmodulin. The calcium–calmodulin complex binds to myosin light chain kinase, creating a calcium–calmodulin–myosin light chain kinase complex (MLCK). The formation of this complex triggers phosphorylation of ATP on myosin light chains, providing energy for actin cross bridging and cycling of myosin attachments to actin. The end result is smooth muscle contraction [32].

Thus, intracellular concentrations of calcium play a role in regulating smooth muscle contraction [33]. There are a number of mechanisms by which intracellular levels of calcium are regulated; the most well understood of these are outlined below.

NO/cGMP

The major neurochemical cascade controlling smooth muscle relaxation in the penis is the nitric oxide-cyclic GMP (NO/cGMP) pathway (Fig. 1.2) [34, 35]. NO is generated by cleavage of its precursor 1-arginine by the enzyme nitric oxide synthase (NOS).

NOS is found in the terminals of non-cholinergic, non-adrenergic, nitrergic cavernous nerves (neuronal NOS, nNOS) and in the endothelium (endothelial NOS, eNOS) of vascular structures including the penis [36]. Neuronal-derived NO is thought to initiate erection, while endothelial-derived NO is thought to help maintain it [36, 37]. eNOS activity is modulated in part by release of Acetylcholine (Ach) from parasympathetic nerves; Ach acts on muscarinic receptors in the cavernous tissue and promotes release of nitric oxide from the endothelium via eNOS [36, 38].

In smooth muscle cells, NO activates the membrane bound enzyme guanylyl cyclase which converts GTP to cyclic GMP (cGMP) [36]. cGMP interacts with protein kinase G. Protein kinase G has numerous downstream effects, the most important of which is the activation of various cell and sarcoplasmic reticulum membrane protein and ion channels [6]. Activation of these channels sequesters calcium ions in the sarcoplasmic reticulum and expels calcium ions from the cell [6, 33]. The flow of calcium is tightly linked to the activity of potassium channels

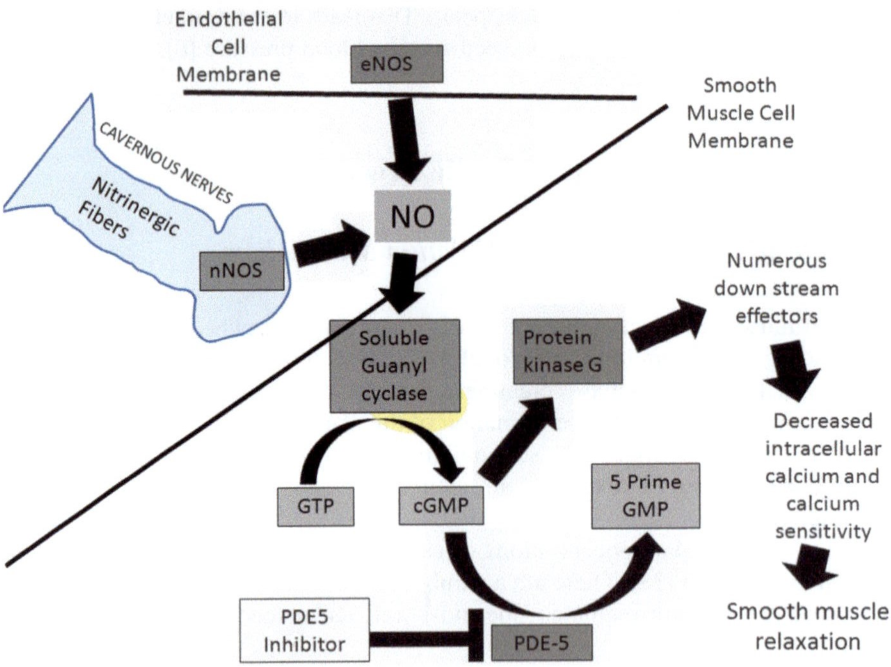

Fig. 1.2 The NO/cGMP pathway in erectile physiology. Molecules are presented in *light gray boxes*, enzymes in *dark gray boxes*, pathways in *black arrows*

which hyperpolarize the smooth muscle cells in turn causing closure of voltage-dependent calcium channels. This activity between adjacent cells is synchronized by the presence of gap junctions which allow for rapid communication of signaling [6]. The net effect of these various processes is at least the transient reduction in intracellular calcium [33].

NO release in smooth muscle also has effects on the activity of inositol triphosphate (IP3), phospholipase C, endothelin, and the Rho kinase pathways [33, 36]. These pathways (partially detailed below) are also important in erectile physiology.

PDE5

The phosphodiesterases are a class of enzymes that degrade cyclic nucleotides such as cGMP and cAMP. There are at least 11 known isoforms encoded on 21 different genes found in different tissues throughout the body [39]. Within the penile tissues, the most important isoform is PDE type 5 (PDE5), which acts exclusively on cGMP [40]. PDE5 is composed of two domains, a regulatory domain and a catalytic domain, the latter of which degrades cGMP by hydrolysis to 5 prime GMP

[39]. PDE5 breaks down cGMP continuously as the molecule is produced, providing constant negative regulation on the erectile process [39]. As PDE5 reduces the amount of available cGMP, intracellular calcium concentration tends to increase, which promotes smooth muscle contraction. Detumescence is thus driven in a large part by PDE5 activity.

PDE5 is the target molecule of the class of drugs known as PDE5 inhibitors (PDE5I) which includes sildenafil, vardenafil, tadalafil, udenafil, avanafil, mirodenafil, and lodenafil [41, 42]. These drugs are competitive inhibitors of PDE5 and thus tend to elevate cytosolic levels of cGMP [41]. The net result of increased cGMP activity is decreased intracellular calcium and subsequent smooth muscle relaxation, leading to prolongation of vasodilation. Because PDE5I act to maintain preexisting levels of cGMP, it is clear that these drugs cannot act without some form of sexual stimulation and/or an intact means to generate cGMP in penile tissues.

Other Mediators

A number of other molecular agents have been shown to have roles in the erection process. Many of these are areas of active research and will thus be mentioned briefly here.

The cyclic AMP, another cyclic nucleotide, is shown to have a similar action as cGMP on the smooth muscle cells of the penile vasculature. Like cGMP, cAMP is degraded by PDEs and promotes a decrease in intracellular calcium levels by its action on protein kinase A. Cyclic AMP is upregulated by a family of eicosanoides, the prostaglandins, specifically PGE1 [43]. The prostaglandins have widespread effects throughout the body; however, a few subtypes including PDE1 have been shown to act on various penile tissues. PGE1 has been utilized as therapeutic injection or intraurethral suppository in the treatment of ED [1].

Inositol triphosphate (IP3) levels are increased in response to the neurologic stimulation of protein phospholipase C. IP3 in turn stimulates the release of calcium from the sarcoplasmic reticulum, tending to promote smooth muscle contraction [44]. Carbon monoxide (CO) is a gaseous second messenger compound with activity somewhat similar to NO [45]. CO has an effect on vascular tone and may stimulate production of cAMP and cGMP [45, 46]. The natriuretic peptides (atrial, brain, and c-type natriuretic peptides) function in the regulation of the cardiovascular system and seem to have relaxing effects in the cavernous smooth muscle; their role in physiological erection in vivo is unclear [47].

The Rho A/Rho kinase calcium sensitization pathway has been a topic of some interest in recent years [48]. Rho A is a molecule that activates Rho kinase. Rho kinase in turn phosphorylates myosin light chain phosphorylase (MLCP); this has the net effect of decreasing MLCP activity [48, 49]. MLCP is responsible for removing phosphate groups from the myosin light chain. The increased phosphorylation of myosin light chain tends to increase the actin–myosin cross bridge formation in response to intracellular calcium and hence promotes smooth muscle contraction [49].

Endothelin, which is present within smooth muscle, is also felt to potentiate the effects of the catecholamines in promoting smooth muscle contraction [50]. Prostaglandin F2-alpha and angiotensin II have also been shown to play a role in the maintenance of smooth muscle tone in response to sympathetic input. These factors together are thought to maintain baseline penile flaccidity [51].

Conclusions

Erectile physiology is of great importance to the fertility specialist as ED is common in infertile men and may pose a substantial barrier to conception. Penile erection is fundamentally dependent on the actions of neural and vascular pathways both centrally and peripherally. An understanding of the complex physiology of penile erection enables to the infertility practitioner to address issues of sexual dysfunction in their patients.

References

1. Andersson KE. Mechanisms of penile erection and basis for pharmacological treatment of erectile dysfunction. Pharmacol Rev. 2011;63(4):811–59.
2. Lotti F, et al. Clinical correlates of erectile dysfunction and premature ejaculation in men with couple infertility. J Sex Med. 2012;9(10):2698–707.
3. O'Brien JH, et al. Erectile dysfunction and andropause symptoms in infertile men. J Urol. 2005;174(5):1932–4. discussion 1934.
4. Shindel AW, et al. Sexual function and quality of life in the male partner of infertile couples: prevalence and correlates of dysfunction. J Urol. 2008;179(3):1056–9.
5. Smith JF, et al. Sexual, marital, and social impact of a man's perceived infertility diagnosis. J Sex Med. 2009;6(9):2505–15.
6. Dean RC, Lue TF. Physiology of penile erection and pathophysiology of erectile dysfunction. Urol Clin North Am. 2005;32(4):379–95. v.
7. Brock G, et al. The anatomy of the tunica albuginea in the normal penis and Peyronie's disease. J Urol. 1997;157(1):276–81.
8. Lue TF, et al. Hemodynamics of erection in the monkey. J Urol. 1983;130(6):1237–41.
9. Fournier GR, et al. Mechanisms of venous occlusion during canine penile erection – an anatomic demonstration. J Urol. 1987;137(1):163–7.
10. Hoznek A, et al. The suspensory ligament of the penis: an anatomic and radiologic description. Surg Radiol Anat. 1998;20(6):413–7.
11. Gurbuz N, Mammadov E, Usta MF. Hypogonadism and erectile dysfunction: an overview. Asian J Androl. 2008;10(1):36–43.
12. Breza J, et al. Detailed anatomy of penile neurovascular structures: surgical significance. J Urol. 1989;141(2):437–43.
13. Mulhall JP, Secin FP, Guillonneau B. Artery sparing radical prostatectomy – myth or reality? J Urol. 2008;179(3):827–31.

14. Chen SC, et al. The progression of the penile vein: could it be recurrent? J Androl. 2005;26 (1):53–60.
15. Mallick HN, Manchanda SK, Kumar VM. Sensory modulation of the medial preoptic area neuronal activity by dorsal penile nerve stimulation in rats. J Urol. 1994;151(3):759–62.
16. Sanna F, et al. Dopamine D2-like receptor agonists induce penile erection in male rats: differential role of D2, D3 and D4 receptors in the paraventricular nucleus of the hypothalamus. Behav Brain Res. 2011;225(1):169–76.
17. Paick JS, et al. The role of prolactin levels in the sexual activity of married men with erectile dysfunction. BJU Int. 2006;98(6):1269–73.
18. Melis MR, et al. Prevention by morphine of apomorphine- and oxytocin-induced penile erection and yawning: involvement of nitric oxide. Naunyn Schmiedebergs Arch Pharmacol. 1997;355(5):595–600.
19. Diamond LE, et al. Co-administration of low doses of intranasal PT-141, a melanocortin receptor agonist, and sildenafil to men with erectile dysfunction results in an enhanced erectile response. Urology. 2005;65(4):755–9.
20. Melis MR, et al. The activation of gamma aminobutyric acid(A) receptors in the paraventricular nucleus of the hypothalamus reduces non-contact penile erections in male rats. Neurosci Lett. 2001;314(3):123–6.
21. Giuliano F, Rampin O. Neural control of erection. Physiol Behav. 2004;83(2):189–201.
22. Bialy M, et al. Blockade of androgen receptor in the medial amygdala inhibits noncontact erections in male rats. Physiol Behav. 2011;103(3–4):295–301.
23. Hull EM, et al. Hormone-neurotransmitter interactions in the control of sexual behavior. Behav Brain Res. 1999;105(1):105–16.
24. Park K, et al. A new potential of blood oxygenation level dependent (BOLD) functional MRI for evaluating cerebral centers of penile erection. Int J Impot Res. 2001;13(2):73–81.
25. Marson L, McKenna KE. A role for 5-hydroxytryptamine in descending inhibition of spinal sexual reflexes. Exp Brain Res. 1992;88(2):313–20.
26. Halata Z, Munger BL. The neuroanatomical basis for the protopathic sensibility of the human glans penis. Brain Res. 1986;371(2):205–30.
27. McKenna KE. Central control of penile erection. Int J Impot Res. 1998;10 Suppl 1:S25–34.
28. Pettus JA, et al. Preservation of ejaculation in patients undergoing nerve-sparing postchemotherapy retroperitoneal lymph node dissection for metastatic testicular cancer. Urology. 2009;73(2):328–31. discussion 331–2.
29. Nijman JM, et al. The treatment of ejaculation disorders after retroperitoneal lymph node dissection. Cancer. 1982;50(12):2967–71.
30. Walsh PC. The discovery of the cavernous nerves and development of nerve sparing radical retropubic prostatectomy. J Urol. 2007;177(5):1632–5.
31. Lue TF. Erectile dysfunction. N Engl J Med. 2000;342(24):1802–13.
32. Wier WG, Morgan KG. Alpha1-adrenergic signaling mechanisms in contraction of resistance arteries. Rev Physiol Biochem Pharmacol. 2003;150:91–139.
33. Chitaley K, Webb RC, Mills TM. The ups and downs of Rho-kinase and penile erection: upstream regulators and downstream substrates of rho-kinase and their potential role in the erectile response. Int J Impot Res. 2003;15(2):105–9.
34. Ignarro LJ, et al. Nitric oxide and cyclic GMP formation upon electrical field stimulation cause relaxation of corpus cavernosum smooth muscle. Biochem Biophys Res Commun. 1990;170 (2):843–50.
35. Burnett AL, et al. Nitric oxide: a physiologic mediator of penile erection. Science. 1992;257 (5068):401–3.
36. Burnett AL. Novel nitric oxide signaling mechanisms regulate the erectile response. Int J Impot Res. 2004;16 Suppl 1:S15–9.
37. Hurt KJ, et al. Akt-dependent phosphorylation of endothelial nitric-oxide synthase mediates penile erection. Proc Natl Acad Sci U S A. 2002;99(6):4061–6.

38. Arnal JF, et al. Endothelium-derived nitric oxide and vascular physiology and pathology. Cell Mol Life Sci. 1999;55(8–9):1078–87.
39. Sung BJ, et al. Structure of the catalytic domain of human phosphodiesterase 5 with bound drug molecules. Nature. 2003;425(6953):98–102.
40. Corbin JD, Francis SH, Webb DJ. Phosphodiesterase type 5 as a pharmacologic target in erectile dysfunction. Urology. 2002;60(2 Suppl 2):4–11.
41. Carson CC, Lue TF. Phosphodiesterase type 5 inhibitors for erectile dysfunction. BJU Int. 2005;96(3):257–80.
42. Shindel AW. 2009 update on phosphodiesterase type 5 inhibitor therapy part 2: updates on optimal utilization for sexual concerns and rare toxicities in this class. J Sex Med. 2009;6 (9):2352–64. quiz 2365–6.
43. Narumiya S, FitzGerald GA. Genetic and pharmacological analysis of prostanoid receptor function. J Clin Invest. 2001;108(1):25–30.
44. Carsten ME, Miller JD. Ca2+ release by inositol trisphosphate from Ca2+-transporting microsomes derived from uterine sarcoplasmic reticulum. Biochem Biophys Res Commun. 1985;130(3):1027–31.
45. Abdel Aziz MT, et al. Putative role of carbon monoxide signaling pathway in penile erectile function. J Sex Med. 2009;6(1):49–60.
46. Ryter SW, et al. Heme oxygenase/carbon monoxide signaling pathways: regulation and functional significance. Mol Cell Biochem. 2002;234–235(1–2):249–63.
47. Kuthe A, et al. Expression of guanylyl cyclase B in the human corpus cavernosum penis and the possible involvement of its ligand C-type natriuretic polypeptide in the induction of penile erection. J Urol. 2003;169(5):1918–22.
48. Wang H, et al. RhoA-mediated Ca2+ sensitization in erectile function. J Biol Chem. 2002;277 (34):30614–21.
49. Jin L, Burnett AL. RhoA/Rho-kinase in erectile tissue: mechanisms of disease and therapeutic insights. Clin Sci (Lond). 2006;110(2):153–65.
50. Ritchie R, Sullivan M. Endothelins & erectile dysfunction. Pharmacol Res. 2011;63(6):496–501.
51. Becker AJ, et al. Plasma levels of angiotensin II during different penile conditions in the cavernous and systemic blood of healthy men and patients with erectile dysfunction. Urology. 2001;58(5):805–10.

Chapter 2
Physiology of Ejaculation

Geraldine Sheu, Louis M. Revenig, and Wayland Hsiao

Abbreviations

BNST	Bed nucleus of the stria terminalis
CCK	Cholecystokinin
cGMP	Cyclic guanosine monophosphate
DCN	Dorsal central autonomic nucleus
fMRI	Functional magnetic resonance imaging
IML	Intermediolateral cell column
LCTF	Lateral central tegmental field
LSt cells	Lumbar spinothalamic cells
MEA	Medial amygdala
MPOA	Medial preoptic area
NO	Nitric oxide
nPGi	Nucleus paragigantocellularis
NPY	Neuropeptide Y
PDE5-I	Phosphodiesterase-5 inhibitor
PET	Positron emission tomography
PVN	Paraventricular nucleus of the hypothalamus
SPFp	Parvocellular subparafascicular thalamic nucleus
VIP	Vasoactive intestinal peptide
VTA	Ventral tegmental area

W. Hsiao (✉)
Department of Urology, Kaiser Permanente, Oakland Medical Center, 3600 Broadway, Oakland, CA 94611, USA
e-mail: wayland.hsiao@kp.org

J.P. Mulhall and W. Hsiao (eds.), *Men's Sexual Health and Fertility*,
DOI 10.1007/978-1-4939-0425-9_2, © Springer Science+Business Media New York 2014

Introduction

Despite being one of the most prevalent sexual dysfunctions [1–3], ejaculatory dysfunction is often misdiagnosed or disregarded. Additionally, no therapies currently exist as definitive "cures" for these disorders. This is likely due to the fact that despite its pervasiveness, surprisingly little is still understood regarding the physiology of ejaculation (for review see [4]). New research continues to provide findings that contribute to our insight and thus potential treatment approaches. This chapter aims to provide an overview of the anatomy as well as contemporary theories of peripheral and central neurophysiology of ejaculation.

Ejaculation is the forcible ejection of seminal fluid from the urethral meatus that commonly accompanies sexual climax and orgasm. *Ejaculation, however, should not be confused with orgasm.* Orgasm is a distinct entity from ejaculation characterized by a physical and emotional sensations experienced at the peak of sexual arousal usually after stimulation of a sexual organ. Orgasm is a purely cerebral and emotional cortical occurrence, though in normal male physiology, orgasm coincides with ejaculation. It should be noted that even in the published literature and among experts, there seems to oftentimes be confusion between these two terms.

To understand the complex process of ejaculation, it is important to understand the myriad of systems required for normal ejaculation. We will first review the gross anatomy of the pelvis as it pertains to the ejaculatory mechanism as well as the dynamic changes that occur with ejaculation. We then review the neuroanatomy of the spinal cord and the brain that are responsible for ejaculatory function. Finally, we will review the neurotransmitters implicated in ejaculatory function and dysfunction.

Gross Anatomy of Ejaculation

The process of ejaculation can be divided into two distinct phases: emission and expulsion. We will first review the anatomical structures and their actions, which contribute specifically to each phase.

Emission (Seminal Emission)

Emission is a physiologic process involving the distal epididymis, the vas deferens, the seminal vesicles, the prostate gland, the prostatic urethra, and the bladder neck (Fig. 2.1). The initial step in emission commences with closure of the bladder neck due to sympathetic innervation of the base of the bladder. This action prevents the retrograde flow of ejaculate into the bladder. After bladder neck closure, secretion of fluid from the prostate, laden with acid phosphatase, citric acid, and zinc mixes

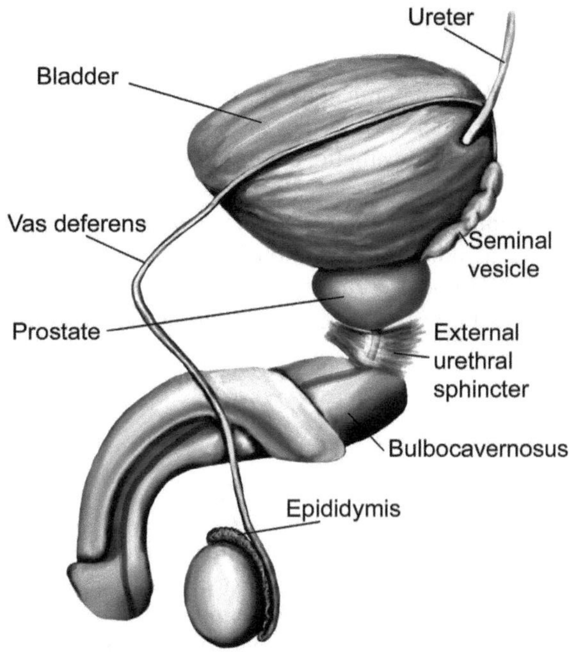

Fig. 2.1 Gross anatomy of the structures involved in ejaculation

with spermatozoa-rich fluid from the vas deferens in the prostatic urethra. Subsequent contribution of seminal vesicle fluid replete with fructose alkalinizes the final ejaculatory product. A minor component of the emission phase also includes excretion of fluid from both Cowper's glands and periurethral glands. In total, the composition of ejaculate consists of prostatic fluid (10 % of volume), vasal fluid (10 % of volume), seminal vesicle fluid (75–80 % of volume), and fluid from the Cowper's and periurethral glands (or glands of Littre) [5].

Expulsion (Propulsatile Expulsion)

Expulsion consists of discharge of the products of emission from the urethra through the coordinated actions of the bladder neck, urethra, and pelvic striated muscles. The expulsion phase follows the emission phase. Relaxation of the external urinary sphincter (with a closed bladder neck) is followed by clonic contractions of the prostate, bulbospongiosus muscle, ischiocavernosus, levator ani, and transverse perineal muscles [6–8]. Through rhythmic contractions lasting 0.6–1.0 s with latency time of 0.7 s between, and a total mean duration of contraction lasting 4.2 s, semen is expelled from the urethra [8].

Neuroanatomy of Ejaculation

Beyond the anatomical details of the ejaculatory response, an intact spinal cord and peripheral nervous system are essential to coordinate the numerous steps in the reflex. The sympathetic, parasympathetic, and somatic nervous systems all contribute to the ejaculatory response. Generally, the sympathetic nervous system regulates emission, while the somatic nervous system moderates expulsion. The role of parasympathetic innervation in ejaculation has still not been clearly elucidated, though it does certainly play a role in secretion of seminal fluids from epithelial cells and accessory sex glands during sexual arousal.

Emission

The pelvic plexus, also known as the inferior hypogastric plexus, is composed of dense sympathetic and parasympathetic nerve fibers, which innervates the organs involved in emission. This plexus consists of fibers that flank the rectum and can be found posterolateral to the seminal vesicles. Sympathetic innervation originates from the intermediolateral cell column (IML) and the dorsal central autonomic nucleus (DCN) of the thoracolumbar spine at T10–L2 coalesces in the lumbar sympathetic ganglia of the paravertebral sympathetic trunk and then passes posterior to the vena cava into the interaortocaval space on the right or lateral to the aorta on the left. The nerve fibers then combine anterior to the aortic bifurcation and course caudally on the anterior surface of L5 to form the superior hypogastric plexus (adrenergic nerves), which then terminate at postganglionic fibers that innervate the bladder neck, prostate, vas deferens, and seminal vesicles. These fibers are responsible for the emission events such as bladder neck closure and seminal vesicle emission [9]. The superior hypogastric plexus continues on inferiorly and splits into the bilateral inferior hypogastric plexuses. Familiarity with this functional anatomy is important in retroperitoneal surgeries, such as retroperitoneal lymphadenectomies for testis cancer or aortoiliac vascular operations, as disruption of the sympathetic fibers of either the superior or inferior hypogastric plexuses can result in disordered emission and retrograde ejaculation (see Fig. 2.2).

Expulsion

Expulsion is a spinal cord reflex that is mediated by somatic motor components of the perineal branch of the pudendal nerve that originate from nerve roots S2–S4 as well as by concurrent relaxation of external urethral sphincter and urogenital diaphragm. Specifically, the perineal nerve, which consists of afferent and efferent axons, innervates the bulbospongiosus muscle. Motor neurons in the pudendal

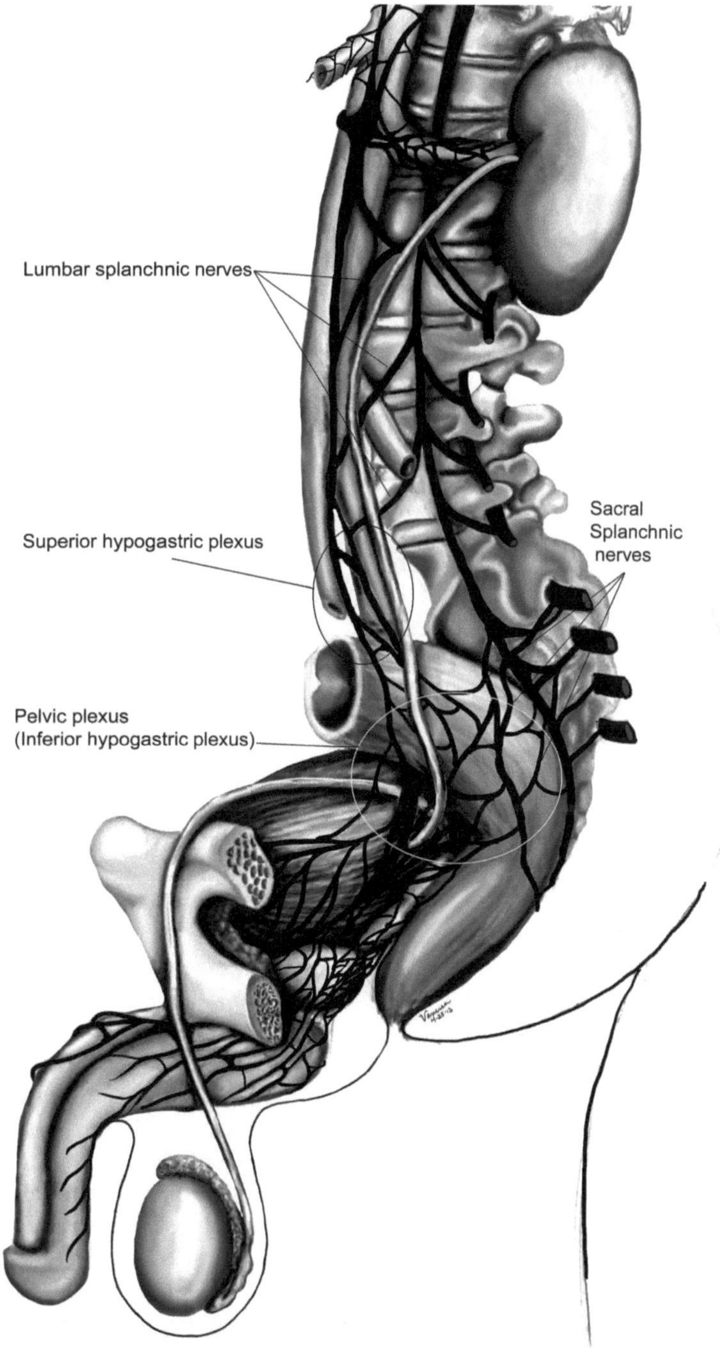

Fig. 2.2 Peripheral nerves and tracts involved in emission and ejaculation

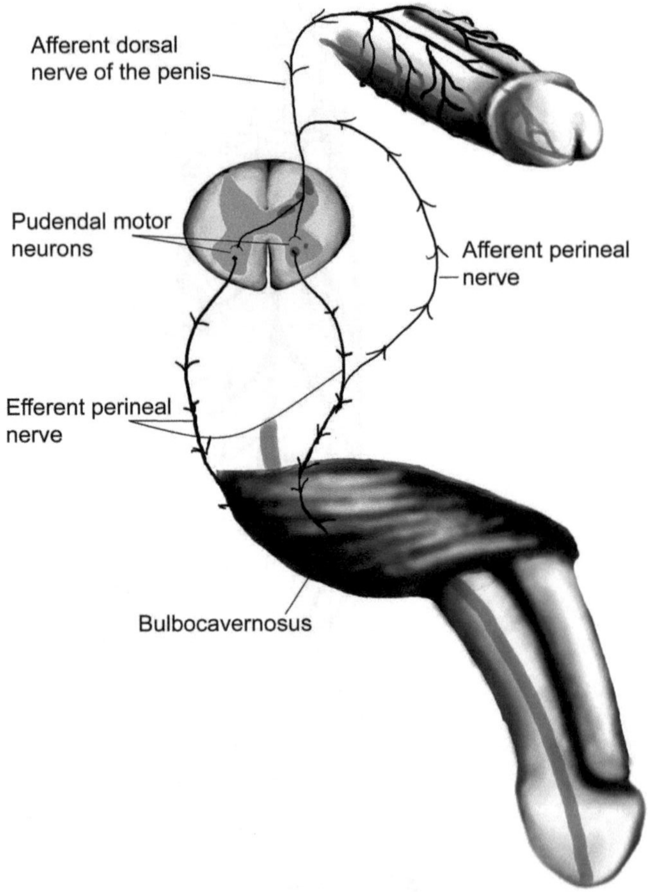

Fig. 2.3 Reflex circuit necessary to elicit ejaculation and bulbospongiosus contraction

nucleus that reside in sacral segments of the conus medullaris, specifically the nucleus of Onuf, supply these sensory axons of the perineal nerve as well as receive synaptic input from two sets of diverging axons of the dorsal nerve of the penis. One set of axons courses along the dorsolateral aspect of the penis and innervates the penile shaft and glans, while the other set of axons branches ventrolaterally and innervates the anterior urethra. These neural pathways are arranged in reflex circuits that are necessary to elicit ejaculation and bulbospongiosus contraction [10]. In essence, the sensory axons of the afferent perineal nerve and the dorsal and ventrolateral branches of the dorsal nerve of penis synapse on pudendal motor neurons in the conus medullaris. The efferent portion of the circuit exits the spinal cord via the perineal nerve to terminate on muscle fibers of the bulbospongiosus muscle for somatic reflex control of these muscles leading to ejaculation [11] (Fig. 2.3).

While both the bladder neck and proximal portion of the urethra are richly comprised of smooth muscle fibers with both sympathetic and parasympathetic innervation, the external urethral sphincter and pelvic floor striated muscles are controlled exclusively by the somatic nervous system. Although the somatic nervous system is typically under voluntary control, it is unclear whether the expulsion phase of ejaculation can be voluntarily controlled. Additionally, the evidence is undecided on which afferent signals are essential for the action of the spinal reflex controlling expulsion. While some data suggested that the viscerosensory deposition of semen in the bulbous urethra itself may trigger clonic contraction of the pelvic striated muscles fundamental to expulsion [12], other results suggest emission is not a required sensory stimulus as demonstrated by the occurrence of dry ejaculation as well as the presence of rhythmic pelvic striated muscle contractions despite a history of prostatectomy, vesiculectomy, or urethrectomy [8, 13]. Studies in rats have also shown maintenance of ejaculatory motor patterns despite urethral anesthetization or seminal emission reduction through medical [14] or surgical means [15]. Meanwhile, studies in humans have shown bulbospongiosus muscle contractions in response to electrical stimulation of the penile dorsal nerve, mechanical distension of the bulbar urethra, and magnetic stimulation of the sacral root [16–18].

Studies have also been performed evaluating the role of the unique somatosensory input from tactile penile stimulation. While the penis contains a high density of sensory nerve fibers, it has a lower tactile sensitivity than the skin of other body parts [19] but increases greatly during erection [20–22]. This plasticity may be explained by the presence of encapsulated nerve endings known as lamellated corpuscles that are distinctive to the glans penis [23–25]. While free nerve endings that sense deep pressure and pain comprise the main variety of nerve fibers in the glans, lamellated corpuscles (also known as Pacinian corpuscles) that sense vibration and pressure have also been found in a 10:1 ratio to free nerve fibers. This is in contrast to the Meissner's and Merkel cell corpuscles, the mechanoreceptor counterparts in the glabrous skin of the fingerpads, which direct tactile sensitivity and are rarely found, if at all, in the glans.

Additionally, the human penile afferent innervations are mainly composed of thinly, myelinated Aδ and unmyelinated C fibers that mediate fast and slow afferent conduction, respectively, and form the majority of the free nerve endings. This nerve variety may contribute to the adaptive response of the penis to low force vs. noxious high threshold stimulation. These high threshold sensory fibers may exert an inhibitory effect on reflex penile muscle contractions [26–29]. While the presence of these nerve receptors has been identified, their specific role in the complex interplay of sensory mechanisms responsible for initiating ejaculation remains ambiguous.

Central Neurophysiology of Ejaculation

Spinal Network

The presence of a spinal ejaculatory generator that coordinates peripheral afferents and somatic and sympathetic efferents has been proposed for at least the past decade and may provide a cohesive explanation of the physiology behind ejaculation. Control of ejaculation at the spinal cord level is indicated by the ability to induce ejaculation in patients with complete spinal cord transection above the tenth thoracic level (T10) through penile vibratory stimulation. This demonstrates the endurance of emission reflexes even after spinal cord trauma as well as coordinated control of pelvic floor and bulbospongiosus muscles despite the disconnection of neural pathways from supraspinal control [30–32].

Research in rats have identified a group of spinal neurons, known as lumbar spinothalamic (LSt) cells, which are integral to the generation of ejaculation. Anatomically, these interneurons are located in lumbar spinal cord (L3–4) and are clustered in laminae 10 and 7 located near the central canal of the spinal cord. They also have thalamic projections, hence their name. Functionally, LSt cells have also been found to be under both inhibitory and excitatory control by supraspinal areas, highlighting the facilitatory and inhibitory influence of supratentorial centers and the presence of an LSt-forebrain pathway.

Brain Network

It is important to note that much of the studies on ejaculation have been performed on animals, mostly rats. While these are mammalian models and offer a close representation of the human neural network, these studies have not been performed on primates or dogs that have prostates with more comparable anatomy. However, the results still provide a foundation for the elucidation of human supraspinal activity during ejaculation.

Neuronal mapping studies in rats have used Fos protein, a marker of neuronal activation, to determine expression patterns in brain structures during general sexual activity as well as ejaculation [33, 34]. Various subdivisions of the medial preoptic area (MPOA), the bed nucleus of the stria terminalis (BNST), the medial amygdala (MEA), and the posterior thalamus have been found to be activated during general sexual activity [35, 36]. Ejaculation-specific Fos activity has been localized to regions in the MEA, the BNST, and the medial portion of the parvocellular subparafascicular thalamic nucleus (SPFp) located in the posterior thalamus [36–38]. However, studies utilizing lesion techniques suggest that these brain structures may not be ejaculation-specific but rather associated with transmission of copulatory information or even inhibition of signals in the post-ejaculatory refractory period [39].

In humans, PET and fMRI studies showed strong activation in the ventral tegmental area (VTA) (a known reward center), the subparafascicular nucleus, ventromedial posterior thalamic nucleus, intralaminar nuclei, and lateral central tegmental field specifically during ejaculation. Activation of the lateral putamen, various aspects of the prefrontal, temporal, parietal, and insular cortex; as well as the cerebellum have been seen during ejaculation and orgasm. The parietal cortex, in particular, receives information from the pudendal sensory nerve fibers, bolstering the suggestion of its involvement in ejaculation [40, 41]. Interestingly, no activation was found in the hypothalamus or preoptic area as has been reported in rat studies. Only the lateral central tegmental field (LCTF) and the SPFp were found to be activated in both humans and rats. Deactivation of the medial aspect of the amygdala was also noted during all aspects of sexual activity including ejaculation [42]. This amygdalar finding correlates with our current knowledge of the amygdala's role in processing fear and the near-inability of humans to achieve ejaculation while sensing danger or fear, despite penile vibratory stimulation. In essence, animal and human imaging studies confirm a definite role of midbrain structures in regulating ejaculation in facilitatory and inhibitory manners, though the exact mechanisms are still unclear.

Retrograde tract-tracing studies suggest a connection between the medial aspect of the SPFp supraspinally and the spinal LSt cells. These neurons express the neuropeptides galanin and cholecystokinin (CCK) [43, 44]. These galanin-specific nerve fibers have also been found to correlate with ejaculation-associated neurons with strong Fos activity, providing further support for a spinothalamic pathway of ejaculation [38]. Galanin may be responsible for the inhibition of sexual activity after ejaculation as determined by brain infusion studies [45]. Additional evidence for a LSt-medial SPFp-forebrain pathway is bolstered by findings that (a) LSt cells have projections to pudendal motoneurons [26, 46], (b) Lst cells have been found to be post-ejaculation specific and are not present in female rats [47], (c) administration of a 5-HT1A receptor agonist known to specifically target ejaculation yielded positive LSt cell and associated supraspinal FOS [47–50], and (d) selective Lst inhibition and lesion testing solely produces decreases in ejaculation without changes in general sexual activity [51]. These findings support the central role of Lst neurons in the coordination of supratentorial and spinal control of ejaculation.

Other supraspinal centers have been implicated in inhibitory and excitatory control over the spinal ejaculatory center. Studies in rats have shown that the paraventricular nucleus (*PVN*) of the hypothalamus may yield excitatory influences over seminal emission, though it may not necessarily be compulsory in the erectile or ejaculatory process [52, 53]. The *MPOA* also appears to play an excitatory role in ejaculatory reflexes through dopaminergic actions on D2 receptors and resultant contraction of pelvic striated muscles along with erection [54–56]. The nucleus paragigantocellularis (nPGi) in the rat medulla, on the other hand, appears to affect an inhibitory control over ejaculatory reflexes through its serotonergic projections to the spinal ejaculation generator in the lumbosacral spinal cord [57, 58]. Therefore, other brain centers may influence the spinal ejaculatory center, either through a spinal pathway or by an even as yet undiscovered mechanism. It is important to note that these brain areas implicated in rat models have not, and may never be, confirmed in humans due to ethical research standards. However, they provide insight into possible human neural pathways taking into account for species differentiation.

Neurotransmitters

Neurochemical Regulation

Besides knowledge of cholinergic and noradrenergic pathways and other neurotransmitters (VIP, NO, NPY) known to be present at these nerve terminals [59–61], the exact function of these chemicals have been difficult to determine due to species variability, inconsistent study results, and receptor subtype polymorphism. The most studied in animal models (dopamine and serotonin) have highlighted the vital role of these neurotransmitters in the control of ejaculation. Furthermore, the association of SSRI antidepressants with delayed ejaculation and the excitatory sexual side effects of dopamine agonists in Parkinsonian patients have highlighted this clinically.

Dopamine

Dopamine appears to play an excitatory role in ejaculation. This was first suggested when stimulation of sexual behavior was incidentally observed in male Parkinson's patients receiving L-DOPA and then confirmed in rats [62–64]. Interestingly, not only did Parkinson's patients given L-DOPA find resolution of their motor symptoms, they also experienced hypersexuality in the form of increased libido, masturbation, sexual hallucinations, and spontaneous nocturnal erections. The specificity of the dopamine receptor involved was established with experiments using a 5-HT1a agonist known to stimulate ejaculation; however, with the administration of a D2 receptor antagonist, it lost this ability [65, 66].

Studies in rats show increased sexual activity and ejaculation with increased MPOA dopamine levels, though its temporal relationship remains unclear [67]. Correspondingly, injection of the dopamine agonist apomorphine into the MPOA increased ejaculation frequency [68, 69], while injection of the dopamine antagonist flupenthixol decreased ejaculatory occurrence [70]. Of the five dopamine g-protein-coupled receptor subtypes, D_1 and D_5 couple positively with adenylate cyclase (AC) activity while D_{2-4} couple negatively. The AC negatively coupled receptors appear to mediate the dopaminergic effects on ejaculation, demonstrated by experiments showing D_1 antagonists and D_2/D_3 agonists stimulate seminal emission and ejaculation [54, 71–75]. While the excitatory role of dopamine in sexual behavior has long been established, these studies implicate the generally stimulatory effect of dopamine on the ejaculatory process.

These biochemical findings further correlate with clinical findings of ejaculatory delay in patients treated with dopaminergic antagonists for schizophrenia or anxiety [71, 72]. Dopamine antagonists such as haloperidol, thioridazine, and sulpiride have been found to delay ejaculation. A double-blind crossover study in patients with premature ejaculation found significant improvement in ejaculation latency after administration of dopamine antagonists metoclopramide hydrochloride or sulpiride. Similar results were found with dose-dependent amounts of risperidone, a dopamine and serotonin receptor antagonist, and levosulpiride, a dopamine antagonist [73].

Serotonin

In contrast, serotonin generally exerts an inhibitory effect in the neuromodulation of ejaculation, though this varies depending on receptor subtype. Of the 15 known 5-HT receptors, 5-HT_{1A}, 5-HT_{1B}, and 5-HT_{2c} have consistently been shown to be involved in the regulation of ejaculation. Due to their heterogeneity, 5-HT receptors have been grouped into seven major families (5-HT_{1-7}) based on function and location. All are G-protein-coupled receptors except for the 5-HT_3 receptor. Similarly, all receptors are located postsynaptically, except for 5-HT_{1A}, 5-HT_{1B}, and 5-HT_{1D} receptors which are presynaptic and involved in negative feedback. Immunocytochemical studies have confirmed the ubiquitous presence of these 5-HT receptors throughout the central and peripheral nervous system, from the brainstem, hypothalamus (MPOA), and BDNT to the dorsal horns of the spinal cord and even structures involved in ejaculation such as the seminal vesicles, vas deferens, urethra, and prostate [74–76].

Somatodendritic 5-HT_{1A} receptor activation appears to abbreviate ejaculation latency times [77] while presynaptic 5-HT_{1B} and postsynaptic 5-HT_{2c} stimulation may increase ejaculatory latency times [78, 79]. However, 5-HT_{1A} at other neural sites, such as the brain, spinal cord, and autonomic ganglia, may exert either excitatory or inhibitory effects on ejaculation [80].

Nitric Oxide

The role of nitric oxide in *erection* (specifically the activation of guanylate cyclase resulting to an increase in cyclic GMP and subsequent smooth muscle relaxation of the corporal cavernosal blood vessels) is well established. However, the role of nitric oxide in the *ejaculatory* process has come to light in the recent debate over the use of phosphodiesterase-5 inhibitors (PDE5-I) for premature ejaculation. While PDE5-Is, which inhibit cGMP degradation and thus increase perfusion to the penis, are established in the treatment of erectile dysfunction, the suggestive effects of

PDE5-Is on ejaculatory dysfunction merits a look into the role of nitric oxide in ejaculation [81, 82].

The mechanism of action of nitric oxide in ejaculation is best approached centrally vs. peripherally. Studies on both humans and animals have found that nitric oxide (an inhibitory mediator) can act centrally by decreasing sympathetic drive as well as peripherally by inhibiting sympathetic vasoconstriction and inducing smooth muscle dilation of the vas deferens and seminal vesicles [83]. Specifically, central manipulation through intrathecal injection of sildenafil in rats has shown a resultant increase in NO and cGMP levels in the MPOA [84]. Increased NO activity in the MPOA in turn decreases sympathetic tone in the periphery which can inhibit ejaculation [85]. Alternatively, microinjection of *N*-nitro-L-arginine methyl-ester (NAME), an inhibitor of nitric oxide synthase, increased the number of seminal emissions and decreased the latency to first seminal emission in rats [86].

Peripherally, nitronergic innervation and nitric oxide synthase/cGMP and cAMP signaling pathways have been identified in human skeletal muscle as well as the smooth muscle of the vas deferens, seminal vesicles, prostate, and urethra [87–91]. As such, drugs such as PDE5-Is or NO donors that increase intracellular cGMP or cAMP diminish human seminal vesicle contraction and inhibit seminal emission in rats [86]. Conversely, NO inhibitors, such as L-nitro-arginine-methyl-ester, decrease the contractile response of human seminal vesicles [92] and guinea pig vas deferens [93], as well as reduce the latency to emission in rats [94]. Further, knockout mice with a homozygous deletion in the gene encoding endothelial NOS have decreased latency to emission with less stimulation than their wild-type counterparts [95].

While the action of nitric oxide in some central and peripheral pathways has been identified, the clinical application of NO modulators has yet to be elucidated. An understanding of these pathways as well as the physiology of ejaculation will build a foundation for future approaches to the treatment of ejaculatory disorders.

Summary

- Ejaculation consists of two phases: emission (deposition of seminal fluids and sperm in the posterior urethra) and ejaculation (propulsion of this ejaculate out of the urethra).
- Ejaculation culminates through the interaction of supraspinal, spinal, and peripheral neural pathways.
- A spinal ejaculation generator containing LSt cell has been discovered that appears to be a pivotal mediator in the ejaculatory process.
- Many neurotransmitters have been identified in the ejaculatory neuraxis; however, laboratory and clinical evidence support a general excitatory and inhibitory role of dopamine and serotonin, respectively, and an inhibitory role of nitric oxide.

– Little is still known regarding the physiology of ejaculation. Better understanding will assist with future clinical therapies for ejaculatory dysfunction, the most commonly reported sexual complaint.

References

1. Hendry WF. Disorders of ejaculation. Ann R Coll Surg Engl. 1999;81(5):352–8.
2. Althof SE. Prevalence, characteristics and implications of premature ejaculation/rapid ejaculation. J Urol. 2006;175(3 Pt 1):842–8.
3. Lewis RW, Fugl-Meyer KS, Bosch R, Fugl-Meyer AR, Laumann EO, Lissa E, Martin-Morales A. Definitions, classifications and epidemiology of sexual dysfunction in sexual medicine sexual dysfunctions in men and women. In: Lue TF, Basson R, Rosen R, Giuliano F, Khoury S, Montorsi F, editors. Sexual medicine sexual dysfunctions in men and women. Oxford: Health Publication Ltd; 2004. p. 37–72.
4. Mulhall J. Premature ejaculation. In: Wein AJ, Kavoussi L, Novick AC, Partin AW, Peters CA, editors. Campbell-Walsh urology. 10th ed. Philadelphia, PA: Elsevier Saunders; 2011. p. 770–9.
5. Master VA, Turek PJ. Ejaculatory physiology and dysfunction. Urol Clin North Am. 2001;28 (2):363–75. x.
6. Yang CC, Bradley WE. Somatic innervation of the human bulbocavernosus muscle. Clin Neurophysiol. 1999;110(3):412–8.
7. Gerstenberg TC, Levin RJ, Wagner G. Erection and ejaculation in man. Assessment of the electromyographic activity of the bulbocavernosus and ischiocavernosus muscles. Br J Urol. 1990;65(4):395–402.
8. Vaucher L, Bolyakov A, Paduch DA. Evolving techniques to evaluate ejaculatory function. Curr Opin Urol. 2009;19(6):606–14.
9. Lipshultz LI, Howards SS, Niederberger CS. Infertility in the male. 4th ed. Cambridge, UK: Cambridge University Press; 2009.
10. Yang CC, Bradley WE. Innervation of the human anterior urethra by the dorsal nerve of the penis. Muscle Nerve. 1998;21(4):514–8.
11. Wieder JA, Brackett NL, Lynne CM, Green JT, Aballa TC. Anesthetic block of the dorsal penile nerve inhibits vibratory-induced ejaculation in men with spinal cord injuries. Urology. 2000;55(6):915–7.
12. McKenna KE, Chung SK, McVary KT. A model for the study of sexual function in anesthetized male and female rats. Am J Physiol. 1991;261(5 Pt 2):R1276–85.
13. Bergman B, Nilsson S, Petersen I. The effect on erection and orgasm of cystectomy, prostatectomy and vesiculectomy for cancer of the bladder: a clinical and electromyographic study. Br J Urol. 1979;51(2):114–20.
14. Holmes GM, Sachs BD. The ejaculatory reflex in copulating rats: normal bulbospongiosus activity without apparent urethral stimulation. Neurosci Lett. 1991;125(2):195–7.
15. Larsson K, Swedin G. The sexual behavior of male rats after bilateral section of the hypogastric nerve and removal of the accessory genital glands. Physiol Behav. 1971;6(3):251–3.
16. Nordling J, Andersen JT, Walter S, Meyhoff HH, Hald T, Gammelgaard PA. Evoked response of the bulbocavernosus reflex. Eur Urol. 1979;5(1):36–8.
17. Opsomer RJ, Caramia MD, Zarola F, Pesce F, Rossini PM. Neurophysiological evaluation of central-peripheral sensory and motor pudendal fibres. Electroencephalogr Clin Neurophysiol. 1989;74(4):260–70.
18. Shafik A, El-Sibai O. Mechanism of ejection during ejaculation: identification of a urethrocavernosus reflex. Arch Androl. 2000;44(1):77–83.
19. Symonds C. Studies in neurology. London: Oxford University Press; 1970.

20. Johnson RD. Efferent modulation of penile mechanoreceptor activity. Prog Brain Res. 1988;74:319–24.
21. McKenna K. Ejaculation. In: Knobil E, Neill JD, editors. Encyclopedia of reproduction. New York: Academic; 1999. p. 1002–8.
22. Hull E, Meisel R, Sachs B. Male sexual behavior. In: Pfaff D, Arnold A, Etgen A, Fahrbach S, Rubin R, editors. Hormones, brain and behavior. New York: Academic; 2002. p. 3–137.
23. Johnson RD, Halata Z. Topography and ultrastructure of sensory nerve endings in the glans penis of the rat. J Comp Neurol. 1991;312(2):299–310.
24. Johnson R, Dugan V. Responses of spine associated penile mechanoreceptors to tangential mechanical stimulation. Soc Neurosci Abstr. 1988;14:726.
25. Gray BW, Beckett SD, Henry DF. Microscopic characteristics of genital end bulbs in the penis of bulls. Am J Vet Res. 1985;46(11):2393–8.
26. De Groat WC, Steers WD. Autonomic regulation of the urinary bladder and sexual organs. In: Loewy AD, Spyer K, editors. Central regulation of autonomic function. Oxford: Oxford University Press; 1990. p. 310–33.
27. Halata Z, Munger BL. The neuroanatomical basis for the protopathic sensibility of the human glans penis. Brain Res. 1986;371(2):205–30.
28. Calaresu FR, Mitchell R. Cutaneous mechanoreceptors in the glans penis of the rat. Brain Res. 1969;15(1):295–7.
29. Kitchell RL, Gilanpour H, Johnson RD. Electrophysiologic studies of penile mechanoreceptors in the rats. Exp Neurol. 1982;75(1):229–44.
30. Sonksen J, Biering-Sorensen F, Kristensen JK. Ejaculation induced by penile vibratory stimulation in men with spinal cord injuries. The importance of the vibratory amplitude. Paraplegia. 1994;32(10):651–60.
31. Brackett NL, Ferrell SM, Aballa TC, Amador MJ, Padron OF, Sonksen J, et al. An analysis of 653 trials of penile vibratory stimulation in men with spinal cord injury. J Urol. 1998;159 (6):1931–4.
32. Biering-Sorensen F, Laeessoe L, Sonksen J, Bagi P, Nielsen JB, Kristensen JK. The effect of penile vibratory stimulation on male fertility potential, spasticity and neurogenic detrusor overactivity in spinal cord lesioned individuals. Acta Neurochir Suppl. 2005;93:159–63.
33. Newman SW. The medial extended amygdala in male reproductive behavior. A node in the mammalian social behavior network. Ann N Y Acad Sci. 1999;877:242–57.
34. Pfaus JG, Heeb MM. Implications of immediate-early gene induction in the brain following sexual stimulation of female and male rodents. Brain Res Bull. 1997;44(4):397–407.
35. Coolen LM, Peters HJ, Veening JG. Fos immunoreactivity in the rat brain following consummatory elements of sexual behavior: a sex comparison. Brain Res. 1996;738(1):67–82.
36. Coolen LM, Peters HJ, Veening JG. Distribution of Fos immunoreactivity following mating versus anogenital investigation in the male rat brain. Neuroscience. 1997;77(4):1151–61.
37. Veening JG, Coolen LM. Neural activation following sexual behavior in the male and female rat brain. Behav Brain Res. 1998;92(2):181–93.
38. Coolen LM, Veening JG, Petersen DW, Shipley MT. Parvocellular subparafascicular thalamic nucleus in the rat: anatomical and functional compartmentalization. J Comp Neurol. 2003;463 (2):117–31.
39. Coolen LM. Neural control of ejaculation. J Comp Neurol. 2005;493(1):39–45.
40. Perretti A, Catalano A, Mirone V, Imbimbo C, Balbi P, Palmieri A, et al. Neurophysiologic evaluation of central-peripheral sensory and motor pudendal pathways in primary premature ejaculation. Urology. 2003;61(3):623–8.
41. Arnow BA, Desmond JE, Banner LL, Glover GH, Solomon A, Polan ML, et al. Brain activation and sexual arousal in healthy, heterosexual males. Brain. 2002;125(Pt 5):1014–23.
42. Holstege G, Georgiadis JR, Paans AMJ, Meiners LC, VanderGraaf FHCE, Reinders AATS. Neural correlates of human male ejaculation. J Neurosci. 2003;23:9185–93.
43. Nicholas AP, Zhang X, Hokfelt T. An immunohistochemical investigation of the opioid cell column in lamina X of the male rat lumbosacral spinal cord. Neurosci Lett. 1999;270(1):9–12.

44. Ju G, Melander T, Ceccatelli S, Hokfelt T, Frey P. Immunohistochemical evidence for a spinothalamic pathway co-containing cholecystokinin- and galanin-like immunoreactivities in the rat. Neuroscience. 1987;20(2):439–56.
45. Truitt WA, Dominguez JM, Adelman J, Coolen LM. Galanin infusions into the medial parvocellular parafascicular thalamic nucleus inhibit male sexual behavior. Horm Behav. 2003;44:81.
46. Allard J, Truitt WA, McKenna KE, Coolen LM. Spinal cord control of ejaculation. World J Urol. 2005;23(2):119–26.
47. Truitt WA, Shipley MT, Veening JG, Coolen LM. Activation of a subset of lumbar spinothalamic neurons after copulatory behavior in male but not female rats. J Neurosci. 2003;23(1):325–31.
48. Ahlenius S, Larsson K, Svensson L, Hjorth S, Carlsson A, Lindberg P, et al. Effects of a new type of 5-HT receptor agonist on male rat sexual behavior. Pharmacol Biochem Behav. 1981;15(5):785–92.
49. Lee RL, Smith ER, Mas M, Davidson JM. Effects of intrathecal administration of 8-OH-DPAT on genital reflexes and mating behavior in male rats. Physiol Behav. 1990;47(4):665–9.
50. Coolen LM, Olivier B, Peters HJ, Veening JG. Demonstration of ejaculation-induced neural activity in the male rat brain using 5-HT1A agonist 8-OH-DPAT. Physiol Behav. 1997;62 (4):881–91.
51. Truitt WA, Coolen LM. Identification of a potential ejaculation generator in the spinal cord. Science. 2002;297(5586):1566–9.
52. Wagner CK, Clemens LG. Projections of the paraventricular nucleus of the hypothalamus to the sexually dimorphic lumbosacral region of the spinal cord. Brain Res. 1991;539(2):254–62.
53. Wagner CK, Clemens LG. Neurophysin-containing pathway from the paraventricular nucleus of the hypothalamus to a sexually dimorphic motor nucleus in lumbar spinal cord. J Comp Neurol. 1993;336(1):106–16.
54. Hull EM, Warner RK, Bazzett TJ, Eaton RC, Thompson JT, Scaletta LL. D2/D1 ratio in the medial preoptic area affects copulation of male rats. J Pharmacol Exp Ther. 1989;251(2):422–7.
55. Hull EM, Eaton RC, Markowski VP, Moses J, Lumley LA, Loucks JA. Opposite influence of medial preoptic D1 and D2 receptors on genital reflexes: implications for copulation. Life Sci. 1992;51(22):1705–13.
56. Sato Y, Christ GJ. Differential ICP responses elicited by electrical stimulation of medial preoptic area. Am J Physiol Heart Circ Physiol. 2000;278(3):964–70.
57. Marson L, List MS, McKenna KE. Lesions of the nucleus paragigantocellularis alter ex copula penile reflexes. Brain Res. 1992;592(1–2):187–92.
58. Marson L, McKenna KE. A role for 5-hydroxytryptamine in descending inhibition of spinal sexual reflexes. Exp Brain Res. 1992;88(2):313–20.
59. Grundemar L, Hakanson R. Effects of various neuropeptide Y/peptide YY fragments on electrically-evoked contractions of the rat vas deferens. Br J Pharmacol. 1990;100(1):190–2.
60. Zoubek J, Somogyi GT, De Groat WC. A comparison of inhibitory effects of neuropeptide Y on rat urinary bladder, urethra, and vas deferens. Am J Physiol. 1993;265(3 Pt 2):R537–43.
61. Domoto T, Tsumori T. Co-localization of nitric oxide synthase and vasoactive intestinal peptide immunoreactivity in neurons of the major pelvic ganglion projecting to the rat rectum and penis. Cell Tissue Res. 1994;278(2):273–8.
62. Gessa GL, Tagliamonte A. Role of brain monoamines in male sexual behavior. Life Sci. 1974;14(3):425–36.
63. Tagliamonte A, DeMontis G, Olianas M, Vargiu L, Corsini GU, Gessa GL. Selective increase of brain dopamine synthesis by sulpiride. J Neurochem. 1975;24(4):707–10.
64. Giuliano F, Allard J. Dopamine and male sexual function. Eur Urol. 2001;40(6):601–8.
65. Clement P, Bernabe J, Kia HK, Alexandre L, Giuliano F. D2-like receptors mediate the expulsion phase of ejaculation elicited by 8-hydroxy-2-(di-N-propylamino)tetralin in rats. J Pharmacol Exp Ther. 2006;316(2):830–4.

66. Matuszewich L, Lorrain DS, Trujillo R, Dominguez J, Putnam SK, Hull EM. Partial antagonism of 8-OH-DPAT'S effects on male rat sexual behavior with a D2, but not a 5-HT1A, antagonist. Brain Res. 1999;820(1–2):55–62.
67. Hull EM, Du J, Lorrain DS, Matuszewich L. Extracellular dopamine in the medial preoptic area: implications for sexual motivation and hormonal control of copulation. J Neurosci. 1995;15(11):7465–71.
68. Hull EM, Bitran D, Pehek EA, Warner RK, Band LC, Holmes GM. Dopaminergic control of male sex behavior in rats: effects of an intracerebrally-infused agonist. Brain Res. 1986;370(1):73–81.
69. Scaletta LL, Hull EM. Systemic or intracranial apomorphine increases copulation in long-term castrated male rats. Pharmacol Biochem Behav. 1990;37(3):471–5.
70. Pehek EA, Warner RK, Bazzett TJ, Bitran D, Band LC, Eaton RC, et al. Microinjection of cis-flupenthixol, a dopamine antagonist, into the medial preoptic area impairs sexual behavior of male rats. Brain Res. 1988;443(1–2):70–6.
71. Compton MT, Miller AH. Sexual side effects associated with conventional and atypical antipsychotics. Psychopharmacol Bull. 2001;35(3):89–108.
72. Peeters M, Giuliano F. Central neurophysiology and dopaminergic control of ejaculation. Neurosci Biobehav Rev. 2008;32(3):438–53.
73. Sato Y, Horita H, Kurohata T, Adachi H, Tsukamoto T. Effect of the nitric oxide level in the medial preoptic area on male copulatory behavior in rats. Am J Physiol. 1998;274(1 Pt 2):R243–7.
74. Azmitia E, Gannon P. The ultrastructural localization of serotonin immunoreactivity in myelinated and unmyelinated axons within the medial forebrain bundle of rat and monkey. J Neurosci. 1983;3(10):2083–90.
75. Descarries L, Beaudet A, Watkins KC. Serotonin nerve terminals in adult rat neocortex. Brain Res. 1975;100(3):563–88.
76. Kim SW, Paick JS. Peripheral effects of serotonin on the contractile responses of rat seminal vesicles and vasa deferentia. J Androl. 2004;25(6):893–9.
77. Rowland DL, Houtsmuller EJ. 8-OH-DPAT interacts with sexual experience and testosterone to affect ejaculatory response in rats. Pharmacol Biochem Behav. 1998;60(1):143–9.
78. Hillegaart V, Ahlenius S. Facilitation and inhibition of male rat ejaculatory behaviour by the respective 5-HT1A and 5-HT1B receptor agonists 8-OH-DPAT and anpirtoline, as evidenced by use of the corresponding new and selective receptor antagonists NAD-299 and NAS-181. Br J Pharmacol. 1998;125(8):1733–43.
79. Foreman MM, Hall JL, Love RL. The role of the 5-HT2 receptor in the regulation of sexual performance of male rats. Life Sci. 1989;45(14):1263–70.
80. Giuliano F, Clement P. Physiology of ejaculation: emphasis on serotonergic control. Eur Urol. 2005;48(3):408–17.
81. Wang WF, Minhas S, Ralph DJ. Phosphodiesterase 5 inhibitors in the treatment of premature ejaculation. Int J Androl. 2006;29(5):503–9.
82. Chen J, Keren-Paz G, Bar-Yosef Y, Matzkin H. The role of phosphodiesterase type 5 inhibitors in the management of premature ejaculation: a critical analysis of basic science and clinical data. Eur Urol. 2007;52(5):1331–9.
83. Asimakopoulos AD, Miano R, Finazzi Agro E, Vespasiani G, Spera E. Does current scientific and clinical evidence support the use of phosphodiesterase type 5 inhibitors for the treatment of premature ejaculation? A systematic review and meta-analysis. J Sex Med. 2012;9(9):2404–16.
84. Sato Y, Zhao W, Christ GJ. Central modulation of the NO/cGMP pathway affects the MPOA-induced intracavernous pressure response. Am J Physiol Regul Integr Comp Physiol. 2001;281(1):R269–78.
85. Pfaus JG. Neurobiology of sexual behavior. Curr Opin Neurobiol. 1999;9(6):751–8.
86. Hull EM, Lumley LA, Matuszewich L, Dominguez J, Moses J, Lorrain DS. The roles of nitric oxide in sexual function of male rats. Neuropharmacology. 1994;33(11):1499–504.

87. Dixon JS, Jen PY. Development of nerves containing nitric oxide synthase in the human male urogenital organs. Br J Urol. 1995;76(6):719–25.
88. Hedlund P, Ekstrom P, Larsson B, Alm P, Andersson KE. Heme oxygenase and NO-synthase in the human prostate—relation to adrenergic, cholinergic and peptide-containing nerves. J Auton Nerv Syst. 1997;63(3):115–26.
89. Jen PY, Dixon JS, Gosling JA. Co-localization of nitric oxide synthase, neuropeptides and tyrosine hydroxylase in nerves supplying the human post-natal vas deferens and seminal vesicle. Br J Urol. 1997;80(2):291–9.
90. Kaminski HJ, Andrade FH. Nitric oxide: biologic effects on muscle and role in muscle diseases. Neuromuscul Disord. 2001;11(6–7):517–24.
91. Uckert S, Bazrafshan S, Scheller F, Mayer ME, Jonas U, Stief CG. Functional responses of isolated human seminal vesicle tissue to selective phosphodiesterase inhibitors. Urology. 2007;70(1):185–9.
92. Bultmann R, Klebroff W, Starke K. Nucleotide-evoked relaxation of rat vas deferens: possible mechanisms. Eur J Pharmacol. 2002;436(1–2):135–43.
93. Kato K, Furuya K, Tsutsui I, Ozaki T, Yamagishi S. Cyclic AMP-mediated inhibition of noradrenaline-induced contraction and Ca^{2+} influx in guinea-pig vas deferens. Exp Physiol. 2000;85(4):387–98.
94. Bialy M, Beck J, Abramczyk P, Trzebski A, Przybylski J. Sexual behavior in male rats after nitric oxide synthesis inhibition. Physiol Behav. 1996;60(1):139–43.
95. Kriegsfeld LJ, Demas GE, Huang PL, Burnett AL, Nelson RJ. Ejaculatory abnormalities in mice lacking the gene for endothelial nitric oxide synthase (eNOS−/−). Physiol Behav. 1999;67(4):561–6.

57. Dixon IS, [illegible] (19[illegible]) Development of nerves containing nitric oxide synthase in the human male urogenital organs. Br J Urol [illegible] 719–25.
58. [illegible]
59. [illegible] supplying [illegible]
60. [illegible]
61. [illegible] selective phosphodiesterase [illegible]
62. [illegible] Sildenafil [illegible]
63. [illegible]
64. [illegible]

Chapter 3
Physiology of Testosterone Production

Joseph W. McQuaid and Cigdem Tanrikut

In 1889, Charles Brown-Séquard reported before the Sociéte de Biologie in Paris the improved vitality, strength, and mental facility he had experienced after self-administering the testicular extracts of dogs and guinea pigs [1]. Although his work was not rigorously reproduced, it marked the start of a long effort to isolate this unknown male sex hormone, an accomplishment for which Ruzicka and Butenandt were awarded the Nobel Prize in Chemistry in 1939 [2]. Today, the effects of testosterone are better understood but no less impressive. Androgens play an essential role in the development of male reproductive organs, the maintenance of male fertility, and the preservation of secondary male sexual characteristics.

This chapter explores the physiology of testosterone production, beginning with its intracellular synthesis and steroidogenic conversion, and then following testosterone's transport across the cell membrane and into circulation. Regulation of this system via the hypothalamic–pituitary–gonadal (HPG) axis is reviewed. Finally, this discussion concludes with two increasingly prevalent clinical circumstances in which testosterone physiology is altered: the metabolic syndrome and the aging male.

Testosterone Production

Testosterone is the predominant circulating androgen in men, with roughly 6–7 mg produced per day. Over 95 % of testosterone originates from within the testes, where 400 million Leydig cells process cholesterol through the steroidogenic pathway [3]. The adrenal glands contribute the remainder of circulating testosterone. As a result of this synthetic effort from both sites, the relatively inert

C. Tanrikut (✉)
Department of Urology, MGH Fertility Center, Massachusetts General Hospital, Harvard Medical School, 55 Fruit Street, YAW-10A, Boston, MA 02114, USA
e-mail: ctanrikut@partners.org

J.P. Mulhall and W. Hsiao (eds.), *Men's Sexual Health and Fertility*,
DOI 10.1007/978-1-4939-0425-9_3, © Springer Science+Business Media New York 2014

cholesterol molecule is oxidized into a variety of biochemically active androgens, including testosterone.

Both functionally and anatomically the testis has two compartments: (1) the avascular seminiferous tubules that are home to Sertoli cells and spermatogenesis, and (2) the interstitium that is composed of blood vessels, lymphatics, immune cells, nerves, connective tissue, and Leydig cells. Three periods of Leydig cell development and function have been proposed after birth: neonatal, prepubertal, and pubertal [4]. During the neonatal period, Leydig cell numbers increase in response to gonadotropins secreted by the pituitary gland. The number of cells peaks at 2–3 months of age with a concomitant peak in testosterone levels. Immediately thereafter, however, Leydig regression ensues and, by 1 year of age, the prepubertal period starts, with a lifetime testosterone nadir that persists until the onset of puberty [4, 5]. At puberty, the Leydig cells are primed for steroid biosynthesis and conversion. Cytologically this is made apparent by the so-called organelle association of large, anastomosing tubules of smooth endoplasmic reticulum with many mitochondria and well-developed Golgi bodies [6]. Often, intracellular inclusions called Reinke's crystals may be visualized, but their nature and possible function is not well understood.

With pubertal maturation, Leydig cells increase their enzymatic oxidation of cholesterol to testosterone. Given the greatly limited storage potential of these cells, this process must occur on a continuous basis with rapid mobilization of this cholesterol [7]. For this reason, Leydig cells have developed great functional capacity for endogenous cholesterol synthesis from acetate. In addition, they are able to mobilize intracellular stores of cholesterol as needed from lipid droplets that contain cholesterol esters and to obtain extracellular sources of cholesterol via endocytosis of intravascular lipoproteins.

Testosterone Biosynthesis

From the most basic perspective, the biosynthesis of testosterone consists of several oxidative steps that result in the cleavage of a 27 carbon (C_{27}) substrate, cholesterol, down to the 19-carbon (C_{19}) product, testosterone (Fig. 3.1). Cytochrome $P450_{SCC}$ (CYP11A) catalyzes the first step in this process—two separate hydroxylations that result in the biochemically inactive, C_{21} steroid pregnenolone [8]. This is the only enzymatic reaction that occurs within the inner membrane of the mitochondria, and as such, it allows for a means of regulating testosterone biosynthesis. The aqueous intermembrane space of the mitochondria proves a major barrier for cholesterol transport to the CYP11A enzyme, which is located in the inner membrane. However, a lipophilic environment is created by a 30 kDa steroidogenic acute regulatory protein (StAR), which actively facilitates translocation of cholesterol [9]. While the precise mechanisms involved in its expression and function are not fully understood, it is now accepted that StAR regulates the rate-limiting step in steroid biosynthesis and represents the point of convergence for several hormonal and

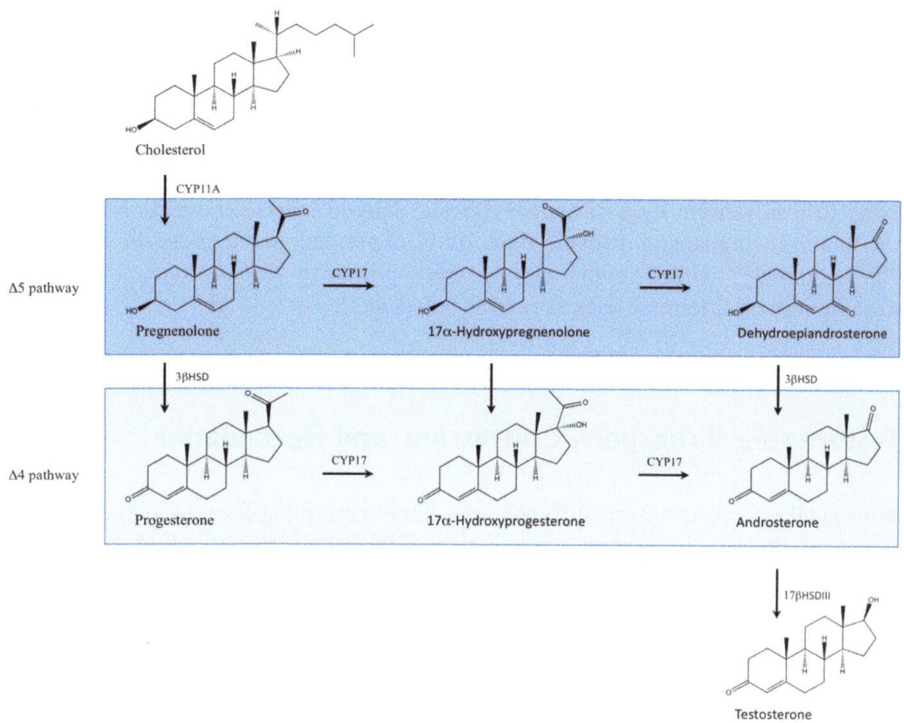

Fig. 3.1 The steroidogenic pathway

signaling pathways within the cell [10]. This is underscored by patients suffering from lipoid congenital adrenal hyperplasia, an autosomal recessive disorder that results in inactivation of the StAR gene and consequent severe impairment in steroid biosynthesis [11].

After this first side chain cleavage of cholesterol, pregnenolone is transported to the endoplasmic reticulum, where it is further metabolized by a variety of enzymes to make additional C_{19} and C_{21} steroids. Two of these pathways potentially lead to the ultimate production of testosterone: the Δ4 pathway and the Δ5 pathway; the notations Δ4 and Δ5 correspond to the location of the double bond on the steroid. Regardless of which pathway is utilized, two reactions must be completed including: (1) a 17α-hydroxylation of the C_{21} steroid, and (2) a cleavage of the C_{17-20} bond to produce a C_{19} steroid [8]. In the Δ5 pathway these steps are accomplished using pregnenolone as a direct substrate, which is transformed to 17 α-hydroxypregnenolone and then to dehydroepiandrosterone (DHEA). The Δ4 pathway requires an additional step, as pregnenolone is first converted to progesterone by 3β-hydroxysteroid dehydrogenase/isomerase. This steroid, in turn, undergoes similar hydroxylation and conversion by lyase to produce 17 α-hydroxyprogesterone and androstenedione, respectively. Contrary to what has previously been believed, both the Δ4 and Δ5 pathways are catalyzed by a single enzyme: cytochrome $P450_{C17}$ (CYP17) [12]. Furthermore, the human and bovine forms of this enzyme show a preference for the substrate 17 α-hydroxypregnenolone—the Δ5 pathway—and ultimately end up producing DHEA primarily [13]. In the end, DHEA is still converted to androstenedione, again by 3-β-hydroxysteroid dehydrogenase/isomerase.

The final step in the biosynthesis of testosterone is the reduction of androstenedione to testosterone by 17β-hydroxysteroid dehydrogenase. Several isoenzymes are found in humans; however, type III is expressed exclusively in the testes [8]. Ultimately, while Leydig cells secrete primarily testosterone, any of the aforementioned intermediaries may leak out as well.

Testosterone Transport, Conversion, and Degradation

After synthesis, testosterone diffuses from the interstitial space that bathes Leydig cells into the venous system via the pampiniform plexus, at which point it is available to affect target tissues. More precisely, the biologically available testosterone is available to affect target tissues. Of the total testosterone in circulation, 2 % remains free, or unbound, and 98 % is associated with plasma proteins. This includes the ~54 % bound to albumin and ~44 % bound to sex hormone binding globulin (SHBG). According to the free hormone hypothesis, it is only the unbound, free testosterone that is able to passively diffuse across cell membranes and cause downstream effects. Therefore in order for bound testosterone to contribute an appreciable effect, it must first dissociate from its binding protein [14]. In the case of testosterone bound to SHBG, this quantity is negligible as the binding affinity is too high to dissociate a significant amount of hormone. Conversely in the case of albumin, which has a dissociation constant many orders of magnitude lower, this does impact the total amount of testosterone available to cells. Thus, bioavailable testosterone is typically defined as unbound hormone *plus* albumin-bound hormone.

From a laboratory perspective, total testosterone can be easily assayed and is the initial step for the evaluation of androgen insufficiency. Assessment of free testosterone is more expensive and time consuming, generally requiring the use of equilibrium dialysis or precipitation assays [15]. Despite the well-established hypotheses regarding bioavailable testosterone, there is now some evidence suggesting the existence of endocytotic cellular uptake pathways for carrier-bound steroids; however, these are likely to play a role only in limited tissues under specific physiologic conditions [16].

The total level of testosterone is dependent upon the relative rates of its production and metabolism. In terms of metabolism, testosterone may follow one of three enzymatic pathways (Fig. 3.2). In the first, cytochrome $P450_{arom}$ (CYP19) aromatizes testosterone to create the C_{18} estrogen estradiol. While this conversion primarily takes place in adipose tissues, CYP19 is expressed in a number of tissues, including Leydig cells [8].

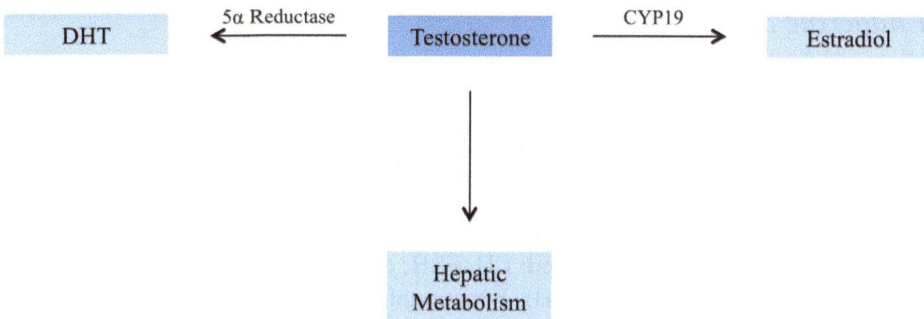

Fig. 3.2 Testosterone conversion and metabolism

Alternatively, testosterone may be reduced to 5α-dihydrotestosterone (DHT) by 5α reductase. Both testosterone and 5α-dihydrotestosterone bind to the same androgen receptor; however, DHT, as the most potent natural androgen, binds with much greater affinity [17]. Both molecules are essential to embryologic and pubertal development of the male genitourinary system, with testosterone responsible for maturation of the Wolffian ducts and DHT responsible for external virilization both in utero and during puberty. Thus far, two forms of 5α reductase have been identified: isoenzymes I and II. Type I 5α reductase is predominantly expressed in the liver and somatic tissue, whereas type II 5α reductase is predominantly found in the prostate, epididymis, seminal vesicles, and genital skin [18]. Pharmacologic inhibitors of 5α reductase have been used to relieve prostatic obstruction and consequently alleviate lower urinary tract symptoms in some patients. Two examples of such medications are finasteride, which is selective for the type II isoenzyme, and dutasteride, which is nonselective and inhibits both forms of 5α reductase.

Lastly, both testosterone and DHT can be degraded in the liver by a number of enzymes that will not be elaborated upon here. The end result of this process is to generate steroids conjugated with a glucuronide or sulfate group that are ultimately excreted by the skin or the kidneys.

Hormonal Regulation of Testosterone Production

The regulation of testosterone synthesis by the Leydig cells of the testis falls into two broad categories. The first includes endocrine signaling by the gonadotropins, primarily luteinizing hormone, which are secreted by the anterior pituitary gland and are the key mediators of the HPG axis. The second includes more discrete paracrine signaling by locally produced factors within the interstitial compartment of the testis.

Endocrine Signaling

The gonadotropins luteinizing hormone (LH) and follicle stimulating hormone (FSH) belong to a larger family of heterodimeric proteins known as glycoprotein hormones. As heterodimers, these molecules are composed of two different subunits. The α subunit is common to every member of the glycoprotein family; however, depending upon the β subunit that is chosen for dimerization, a variety of related hormones may be created: LH, FSH, chorionic gonadotropin (hCG), and thyroid stimulating hormone (TSH). Functionally, LH exerts its effects on testosterone production by binding to the G protein-coupled receptors on Leydig cells, and FSH exerts its effects on spermatogenesis by binding to the G protein-coupled receptors on Sertoli cells. This entire axis is tightly regulated by a negative feedback system in which testosterone plays a pivotal role (Fig. 3.3).

Gonadotropin-releasing hormone (GnRH), produced by the neurons of the hypothalamus, empties into the hypothalamic hypophyseal portal system to make its way to the anterior pituitary, where it acts to stimulate gonadotropin release. This process occurs in a pulsatile, coupled manner: GnRH pulses are followed by shorter-lived pulses of LH [19]. This episodic secretion is essential to the male reproductive axis, and continuous GnRH administration fails to achieve the same effect [20]. Yet the pulsatility of GnRH secretion is not constant throughout life. Recall that during the neonatal period, Leydig cell numbers increase and testosterone levels peak in response to GnRH and LH release at 2–3 months of life [4]. Thereafter, LH and GnRH levels drop and the neuronal GnRH generator goes dormant for the rest of prepuberty. With the onset of puberty, pulsatile GnRH secretions resume, and LH levels begin to rise as well—initially only at night but eventually throughout the day, as well [21].

After its pulsatile secretion, LH travels to the testes where it induces steroid synthesis in both an acute and a chronic manner. Binding of LH to the LH receptor, a G protein coupled receptor (GPCR), results in activation of adenylyl cyclase with a subsequent rise in cAMP and concomitant activation of the protein kinase A (PKA) pathway. There is evidence that multiple other pathways may be upregulated by this GPCR; however, in Leydig cells most investigators agree that these steroidogenic effects are primarily regulated by the GPCR/adenylyl cyclase/cAMP/PKA pathway [22]. Activated PKA in turn results in two major downstream effects. The first consists of increased translocation of cholesterol to the mitochondrial inner membrane secondary to upregulation of the acute regulatory protein (StAR) [11]. The second includes increased activation of the cholesterol side-chain cleavage system, mediated both by CYP11A and CYP17 [23].

While LH is accepted as being primarily responsible for the endocrine control of testosterone production by Leydig cells, there is some evidence FSH may play a role as well, albeit on a more limited scale. This likely occurs via the direct effect of Sertoli cells (triggered by FSH) on Leydig cells [4].

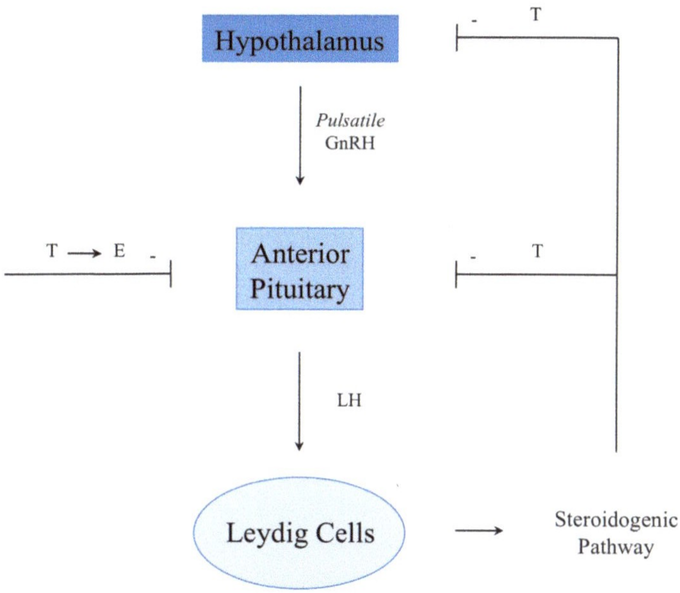

Fig. 3.3 The hypothalamic–pituitary–testis axis

Paracrine Signaling

Several non-pituitary, locally produced factors are identified as further regulators of Leydig cell function. Insulin-like growth factor 1 (IGF-1) and tumor growth factor beta (TGFβ) have well-established influences in this regard [4]. Both in vitro and in vivo studies demonstrate the important role IGF-1 plays in Leydig cell development and function [24, 25]. Furthermore, while the in vivo evidence is not as cogent, animal studies suggest that TGFβ modulates both steroidogenesis and Leydig cell proliferation [26]. A myriad of other potential local regulators are identified in vitro in rat models; however, studies on these molecules are often difficult to definitively translate to human Leydig cells [4].

More recently, additional regulators are generating increased attention including insulin-like factor 3 (INSL3), ghrelin, and leptin [27]. INSL3 is a peptide that belongs to the insulin-like growth factor (IGF) and relaxin family of hormones. It previously had an established role in testicular descent with uncertain biological significance in adults [28]; however, more recent human studies have shown a correlation between INSL3 levels and Leydig cell functional status [29, 30]. While the autocrine and paracrine effects of this peptide remain to be more fully elucidated, in data collected from adult men it appears that INSL3 operates outside of the HPG axis, reflecting both differentiation status and absolute number of Leydig cells [31].

Leptin and ghrelin have more firmly established roles in testosterone production and physiology than does INSL3. While the primary function of leptin and ghrelin is to operate as a coordinated system regulating energy homeostasis, there is increasing evidence that they play a combined role in modulating testosterone levels as well [32]. In one model, rats fed a restricted diet with repeated administration of ghrelin showed decreased LH and testosterone with reduced testis weight [32, 33]. Conversely, ablation of ghrelin in leptin-deficient *ob/ob* mice resulted in increased steroidogenesis and reduction of testicular apoptosis [34]. Thus, it appears that unopposed ghrelin may exert an inhibitory effect on testosterone production. This occurs centrally, as demonstrated by decreased LH levels in rats given daily doses of ghrelin, and peripherally at the level of the Leydig cell, as shown by in vitro models showing a ghrelin-mediated inhibition of testosterone secretion in a dose-dependent fashion [34–36]. Further substantiating this hypothesis are data collected from human testicular samples showing an inverse correlation between ghrelin expression by Leydig cells and peripheral testosterone levels [37].

Negative Feedback Control

LH levels are maintained within a narrow physiologic range. Therefore, the pulsatile, stimulatory effects of GnRH must be balanced by a refined set of negative feedback mechanisms. These mechanisms act at both the level of the anterior pituitary and the hypothalamus, and they primarily are the result of circulating testosterone and estrogen (Fig. 3.3). Note that this discussion regarding negative feedback control only pertains to LH physiology. Control of FSH and Sertoli cells occurs in an analogous manner and, however, involves additional factors—primarily activin and inhibin B—which do not primarily affect LH secretion and which will not be discussed here.

One well-designed human study illustrates the interplay between testosterone, estrogen, and the aromatization of testosterone to estrogen in the negative feedback of LH secretion [38]. Prior to completion of this study, the respective contributions of these sex steroids to negative feedback control of LH were unclear. Furthermore, the precise sites of inhibition via testosterone and estrogen were uncertain. Thirteen men with idiopathic hypogonadotropic hypogonadism (IHH), who do not produce GnRH at baseline but who may be normalized with exogenous pulsatile GnRH administration, allowed the study authors to better answer these remaining questions. By measuring the peripheral LH levels of these individuals in response to exogenous sex steroids and then comparing these values to healthy volunteers, a site of action as well as the relative contributions of testosterone and estrogen could be inferred.

From the work of Pitteloud et al. several conclusions can be made: (1) Testosterone and estrogen independently inhibit LH secretion, (2) Testosterone does require aromatization to estrogen to inhibit LH secretion at the pituitary but not the hypothalamus, and (3) While estrogen can act at either location it predominantly functions at the level of the hypothalamus [38]. While these discoveries do not hold immediate clinical applications, they do clarify a long-standing source of confusion and better elucidate the contributions of testosterone and estrogen to negative feedback control.

Altered Testosterone Physiology

Previous discussion has focused on the physiology of testosterone production in the normal male. There are two instances of altered physiology that warrant particular attention because of their increasing prevalence: the metabolic syndrome and the aging male.

Metabolic Syndrome

Changes in diet and reductions in physical activity have resulted in a rising wave of global obesity, not only within developed countries but now around the world [39]. Not only does one's total body fat predict important comorbidities such as coronary artery disease, stroke, and diabetes, but the distribution of body fat also makes a difference as individuals with a greater percentage of visceral fat appear to have an increased risk of metabolic consequences, as in the metabolic syndrome [40]. Hypogonadism is often seen in this picture, and it has been suggested that testosterone replacement may improve lipid profiles and insulin resistance in men with the metabolic syndrome [41]. The hypogonadal-obesity cycle attempts to explain this relationship: increased adipose tissues lead to greater testosterone deficiency through increased conversion of testosterone to estradiol by aromatase. This relative deficiency of testosterone and excess of estradiol, in turn, leads to even greater fat deposition and subsequent further declines in testosterone [42]. In addition, overall abdominal obesity may lead to increased glucocorticoid turnover and production with disruption of the HPG/adrenal axis, thereby leading to mild hypogonadism [43].

Of interest, two of the paracrine signals discussed earlier—leptin and ghrelin—have been studied in some detail with regard to the metabolic syndrome. Leptin has been demonstrated to increase in obese individuals with an attendant fall in serum testosterone [42, 44]. Administration of exogenous testosterone appears to suppress leptin levels, but this effect is short-lived and leptin levels return to the pre-therapy range after cessation of testosterone [45]. The data regarding ghrelin is more limited; however, there is evidence that suggests that testosterone replacement raises ghrelin levels back to their normal range [42].

The Aging Male

After the age of 40, serum testosterone declines at a rate 0.4–2.6 % per year with an associated decrease in muscle mass, strength, sexual function, and bone mass [46]. This decline in testosterone independently predicts disturbances in insulin and glucose metabolism, potentially leading to the metabolic syndrome as discussed previously [47]. However, not all men will exhibit clinically significant symptoms associated with this decline in testosterone levels [48]. Using data from the Boston Area Community Health Survey (BACH), Araujo et al. found 24 % of their 1,475 subjects aged 30–79 to have low total testosterone (<300 ng/mL) and 5.6 % of the 1,475 patients to be symptomatic [46]. Prevalence of low testosterone increases with age. This is reflected by estimates obtained from the Massachusetts Male Aging Study (MMAS), an observational cohort of 1,709 subjects aged 40–70 and enrolled between 1987 and 1989 with two separate follow-up phases. While the initial crude prevalence of androgen deficiency at baseline was 6.0 %, this increased to 12.3 % during the first follow-up phase of the study between 1995 and 1997 [48].

Why there is a range in testosterone decline and its associated symptomatology remains an area of interest. For instance, in contradiction to the typical aging male with a diminishing testosterone and minimally elevated LH, there is a population of men who mount a large enough rise in their LH to maintain a normal serum testosterone [49]. An increased amount of attention is being paid to these men and to the androgen receptor itself, with particular research being devoted to the number of CAG trinucleotide repeats present in the transactivation exon of this gene. There is a demonstrated inverse correlation between the number of CAG repeats and both the transcriptional activity of the androgen-dependent genes and their downstream effects [50–52]. Furthermore, men with normal total testosterone concentrations and longer CAG repeats run a greater risk of developing andropausal symptoms [52].

Summary

Testosterone production is a finely balanced process with many points of potential regulation starting with the translocation of cholesterol across the mitochondrial membrane and ending with the ultimate negative feedback of testosterone in the HPG axis. Two scenarios in which this physiology is altered are becoming increasingly, clinically relevant: metabolic syndrome and the aging male.

References

1. Brown-Sequard CE. The effects produced on man by subcutaneous injections of liquid obtained from the testicles of animals. Lancet. 1889;134(3438):3.
2. Freeman ER, Bloom DA, McGuire EJ. A brief history of testosterone. J Urol. 2001;165(2): 371–3.
3. Petersen PM, Pakkenberg B. Stereological quantification of Leydig and Sertoli cells in the testis of old and young men. Image Anal Stereol. 2000;19(3):215–8.
4. Lejeune H, Habert R, Saez JM. Origin, proliferation and differentiation of Leydig cells. J Mol Endocrinol. 1998;20(1):1–25.
5. Nistal M, Paniagua R, Regadera J, et al. A quantitative morphological study of human Leydig cells from birth to adulthood. Cell Tissue Res. 1986;246(2):229–36.
6. Prince FP. Ultrastructural evidence of mature Leydig cells and Leydig cell regression in the neonatal human testis. Anat Rec. 1990;228(4):405–17.
7. Weinbauer G, Gromoll J, Simoni M, et al. Physiology of Testicular Function. In: Nieschlag E, Behre HM, Ahlen HV, editors. Andrology: male reproductive health and dysfunction. 2nd ed. New York: Springer; 2001.
8. Payne AH, Hales DB. Overview of steroidogenic enzymes in the pathway from cholesterol to active steroid hormones. Endocr Rev. 2004;25(6):947–70.
9. Clark BJ, Stocco DM. Steroidogenic acute regulatory protein: the StAR still shines brightly. Mol Cell Endocrinol. 1997;134(1):1–8.
10. Manna PR, Dyson MT, Stocco DM. Regulation of the steroidogenic acute regulatory protein gene expression: present and future perspectives. Mol Hum Reprod. 2009;15(6):321–33.
11. Lin D, Sugawara T, Strauss III JF, et al. Role of steroidogenic acute regulatory protein in adrenal and gonadal steroidogenesis. Science. 1995;267(5205):1828–31.
12. Nakajin S, Shively JE, Yuan PM, et al. Microsomal cytochrome P-450 from neonatal pig testis: two enzymatic activities (17 alpha-hydroxylase and c17,20-lyase) associated with one protein. Biochemistry. 1981;20(14):4037–42.
13. Brock BJ, Waterman MR. Biochemical differences between rat and human cytochrome P450c17 support the different steroidogenic needs of these two species. Biochemistry. 1999;38(5):1598–606.
14. Mendel CM. The free hormone hypothesis. Distinction from the free hormone transport hypothesis. J Androl. 1992;13(2):107–16.
15. Vermeulen A, Verdonck L, Kaufman JM. A critical evaluation of simple methods for the estimation of free testosterone in serum. J Clin Endocrinol Metab. 1999;84(10):3666–72.
16. Willnow TE, Nykjaer A. Cellular uptake of steroid carrier proteins—mechanisms and implications. Mol Cell Endocrinol. 2010;316(1):93–102.
17. Jin Y, Penning TM. Steroid 5alpha-reductases and 3alpha-hydroxysteroid dehydrogenases: key enzymes in androgen metabolism. Best Pract Res Clin Endocrinol Metab. 2001;15(1):79–94.
18. El-Awady MK, El-Garf W, El-Houssieny L. Steroid 5alpha reductase mRNA type 1 is differentially regulated by androgens and glucocorticoids in the rat liver. Endocr J. 2004;51 (1):37–46.
19. Hayes FJ, Crowley Jr WF. Gonadotropin pulsations across development. Horm Res. 1998;49 (3–4):163–8.
20. Matsumoto AM, Gross KM, Bremner WJ. The physiological significance of pulsatile LHRH secretion in man: gonadotrophin responses to physiological doses of pulsatile versus continuous LHRH administration. Int J Androl. 1991;14(1):23–32.
21. Delemarre-van de Waal HA. Regulation of puberty. Best Pract Res Clin Endocrinol Metab. 2002;16(1):1–12.
22. Ascoli M, Fanelli F, Segaloff DL. The lutropin/choriogonadotropin receptor, a 2002 perspective. Endocr Rev. 2002;23(2):141–74.

23. Dufau ML. Endocrine regulation and communicating functions of the Leydig cell. Annu Rev Physiol. 1988;50:483–508.
24. Baker J, Hardy MP, Zhou J, et al. Effects of an Igf1 gene null mutation on mouse reproduction. Mol Endocrinol. 1996;10(7):903–18.
25. Hu GX, Lin H, Chen GR, et al. Deletion of the Igf1 gene: suppressive effects on adult Leydig cell development. J Androl. 2010;31(4):379–87.
26. Lui WY, Lee WM, Cheng CY. TGF-betas: their role in testicular function and Sertoli cell tight junction dynamics. Int J Androl. 2003;26(3):147–60.
27. Svechnikov K, Landreh L, Weisser J, et al. Origin, development and regulation of human Leydig cells. Horm Res Paediatr. 2010;73(2):93–101.
28. Wikstrom AM, Bay K, Hero M, et al. Serum insulin-like factor 3 levels during puberty in healthy boys and boys with Klinefelter syndrome. J Clin Endocrinol Metab. 2006;91(11): 4705–8.
29. Bay K, Hartung S, Ivell R, et al. Insulin-like factor 3 serum levels in 135 normal men and 85 men with testicular disorders: relationship to the luteinizing hormone-testosterone axis. J Clin Endocrinol Metab. 2005;90(6):3410–8.
30. Foresta C, Bettella A, Vinanzi C, et al. A novel circulating hormone of testis origin in humans. J Clin Endocrinol Metab. 2004;89(12):5952–8.
31. Ivell R, Wade JD, Anand-Ivell R. INSL3 as a biomarker of Leydig cell functionality. Biol Reprod. 2013;88(6):147.
32. Zhu CC, Zhang H, Zhang JS, et al. Inhibition of ghrelin signaling improves the reproductive phenotype of male ob/ob mouse. Fertil Steril. 2013;99(3):918–26.
33. Sirotkin AV, Chrenkova M, Nitrayova S, et al. Effects of chronic food restriction and treatments with leptin or ghrelin on different reproductive parameters of male rats. Peptides. 2008;29(8):1362–8.
34. Sun Y, Asnicar M, Saha PK, et al. Ablation of ghrelin improves the diabetic but not obese phenotype of ob/ob mice. Cell Metab. 2006;3(5):379–86.
35. Fernandez-Fernandez R, Tena-Sempere M, Navarro VM, et al. Effects of ghrelin upon gonadotropin-releasing hormone and gonadotropin secretion in adult female rats: in vivo and in vitro studies. Neuroendocrinology. 2005;82(5–6):245–55.
36. Tena-Sempere M. Ghrelin as a pleotrophic modulator of gonadal function and reproduction. Nat Clin Pract Endocrinol Metab. 2008;4(12):666–74.
37. Ishikawa T, Fujioka H, Ishimura T, et al. Ghrelin expression in human testis and serum testosterone level. J Androl. 2007;28(2):320–4.
38. Pitteloud N, Dwyer AA, DeCruz S, et al. Inhibition of luteinizing hormone secretion by testosterone in men requires aromatization for its pituitary but not its hypothalamic effects: evidence from the tandem study of normal and gonadotropin-releasing hormone-deficient men. J Clin Endocrinol Metab. 2008;93(3):784–91.
39. Popkin BM, Adair LS, Ng SW. Global nutrition transition and the pandemic of obesity in developing countries. Nutr Rev. 2012;70(1):3–21.
40. Montague CT, O'Rahilly S. The perils of portliness: causes and consequences of visceral adiposity. Diabetes. 2000;49(6):883–8.
41. Zitzmann M, Nieschlag E. Effects of androgen replacement on metabolism and physical performances in male hypogonadism. J Endocrinol Invest. 2003;26(9):886–92.
42. De Maddalena C, Vodo S, Petroni A, et al. Impact of testosterone on body fat composition. J Cell Physiol. 2012;227(12):3744–8.
43. Walker BR. Steroid metabolism in metabolic syndrome X. Best Pract Res Clin Endocrinol Metab. 2001;15(1):111–22.
44. Al-Harithy RN. Relationship of leptin concentration to gender, body mass index and age in Saudi adults. Saudi Med J. 2004;25(8):1086–90.
45. Luukkaa V, Pesonen U, Huhtaniemi I, et al. Inverse correlation between serum testosterone and leptin in men. J Clin Endocrinol Metab. 1998;83(9):3243–6.

46. Araujo AB, Esche GR, Kupelian V, et al. Prevalence of symptomatic androgen deficiency in men. J Clin Endocrinol Metab. 2007;92(11):4241–7.
47. Laaksonen DE, Niskanen L, Punnonen K, et al. Testosterone and sex hormone-binding globulin predict the metabolic syndrome and diabetes in middle-aged men. Diabetes Care. 2004;27(5):1036–41.
48. Araujo AB, O'Donnell AB, Brambilla DJ, et al. Prevalence and incidence of androgen deficiency in middle-aged and older men: estimates from the Massachusetts Male Aging Study. J Clin Endocrinol Metab. 2004;89(12):5920–6.
49. Harkonen K, Huhtaniemi I, Makinen J, et al. The polymorphic androgen receptor gene CAG repeat, pituitary-testicular function and andropausal symptoms in ageing men. Int J Androl. 2003;26(3):187–94.
50. Chamberlain NL, Driver ED, Miesfeld RL. The length and location of CAG trinucleotide repeats in the androgen receptor N-terminal domain affect transactivation function. Nucleic Acids Res. 1994;22(15):3181–6.
51. Beilin J, Ball EM, Favaloro JM, et al. Effect of the androgen receptor CAG repeat polymorphism on transcriptional activity: specificity in prostate and non-prostate cell lines. J Mol Endocrinol. 2000;25(1):85–96.
52. Liu CC, Lee YC, Wang CJ, et al. The impact of androgen receptor CAG repeat polymorphism on andropausal symptoms in different serum testosterone levels. J Sex Med. 2012;9(9): 2429–37.

Chapter 4
The Effects of Vaginal Lubricants on Sperm Function

Landon W. Trost, Daniel H. Williams IV, and John P. Mulhall

Abbreviations

CASA	Computer-assisted sperm analysis
LM	Light microscopy

Introduction

Personal lubricants encompass a large number of friction-reducing substances that are used in several settings relevant to male fertility including sexual intercourse, sperm extraction, and vaginal ultrasonography. The prevalence of lubricant use with sexual intercourse remains understudied. Results from a US survey of women reported that 62 % of women had previously used lubrication with intercourse, while 25.3 % noted use within the past month [1]. Among women trying to conceive, 25 % self-reported routine use of vaginal lubricants on baseline questionnaires, while subsequent prospective observation obtained from self-maintained diaries identified actual use in 43 % of women [2].

Classes of Lubricants

Lubricants may be broadly classified as water soluble, oil soluble, or silicone based. See Table 4.1 for a listing of lubricants with data evaluating their effects on sperm

J.P. Mulhall (✉)
Department of Urology, Memorial Sloan-Kettering Cancer Center, 353 E 68th St, Rm 531, New York, NY 10065, USA
e-mail: mulhalj1@mskcc.org

J.P. Mulhall and W. Hsiao (eds.), *Men's Sexual Health and Fertility*,
DOI 10.1007/978-1-4939-0425-9_4,

parameters. Although variations exist within classes, water-soluble compounds are generally condom-safe and frequently include additive substances to retain moisture, balance osmolarity and/or pH, provide thickening or viscosity, alter sensation (e.g., warming, cooling), and give fragrance. Water-soluble agents are prone to rapid drying and may require reapplication or addition of moisture/saliva, which may result in deposition of additional substances or further concentrate the product applied. Oil-based lubricants frequently incorporate fewer additional substances and are often not compatible with condom use. Silicone-based lubricants are less commonly utilized and are less prone to skin absorption or dehydration. They are often incompatible with condoms and may adversely affect other silicone-containing compounds upon contact. No data is currently available reporting the impact of silicone-based lubricants on semen parameters or fertility.

Mechanism for Fertility Impairment

Lubricants have demonstrated varied effects on sperm including reduced viability, altered morphology, DNA damage, and impaired motility/progression [3–8]. Several mechanisms for lubricant-induced impairments have been proposed including increased viscosity, creation of a barrier effect, direct cytotoxicity, or indirect cellular damage via altered pH and osmolarity [3–5, 8].

Despite these hypothesized mechanisms, there are currently limited data reporting the etiologic role of osmolarity and/or pH on impairing sperm motility/progression. Rossato and colleagues evaluated and compared seminal osmolarity among normospermic and oligospermic males and noted that seminal plasma is slightly hyperosmolar (336 mOsm/L) compared to serum plasma (291 mOsm/L) [9]. Men with normospermia were found to have significantly lower seminal osmolarity values (318 mOsm/L vs. 345 mOsm/L) compared to asthenospermic patients. The authors additionally noted dose-dependent impairments in motility with increasing levels of osmolarity, with 50 % reductions noted in solutions >400 mOsm/L.

To assess the impact of varied osmolarity lubricants on semen parameters, Kutteh and colleagues performed an in vitro comparison of four water-based lubricants (KY Jelly®, Astroglide®, Replens®, Touch®), canola oil, and olive oil on normospermic samples [5]. Results demonstrated significant reductions in sperm motility with higher osmolarity agents (Astroglide®, KY Jelly®, Replens®, Touch®) compared to relatively iso-osmolar agents. These findings are consistent with other studies which demonstrated a minimal impact on motility with Pre-Seed® (iso-osmolar), compared to various hyper-osmolar agents [3, 4].

However, other studies have reported contradictory results, suggesting a less significant role for osmolarity on sperm motility. In the previously cited study by Kutteh and colleagues, despite relatively equivalent osmolality and pH levels for canola and olive oils (canola 378 mOsm, 7.6 pH; olive 390 mOsm, 7.4 pH), greater impairments were noted with the olive oil (42 % vs. 70 % motility) [5]. Similarly, in

Table 4.1 Lubricants with published data evaluating impact on semen parameters or fertility

Water-based lubricants
Aquasonic Gel® (Parker Laboratories, Inc., Fairfield, NJ)
Astroglide® (Biofilm Management, Inc., Vista, CA)
Femglide® (Wallace O'Farrell, Inc., Puyallup, WA)
Glycerin
H-R Lubricating Jelly® (HR Pharmaceuticals, Inc., York, PA)
Keri Lotion® (Novartis Pharmaceuticals, Basel, Switzerland)
K-Y Jelly® (Johnson & Johnson, New Brunswick, NJ)
Lubifax® (E. Fougera & Co, Melville, NY)
Ortho-Gynol® (Personal Products Co, Skillman, NJ)
Pre-Seed® (INGfertility, Valleyford, WA)
Replens® (Vifor SA, Villars-sur-Glane, Switzerland)
Saliva
Surgilube® (E. Fougera & Co, Melville, NY)
Oil-based lubricants
Alpha-Keri® (Mentholatum Co Ltd, Melbourne, Australia)
Baby oil (Mineral oil; Johnson & Johnson, New Brunswick, NJ)
Canola oil
Olive oil
Peanut oil
Petroleum jelly
Safflower oil
Vegetable oil
Other/unknown
Egg white
pHisonex®
Searle Skin Lotion®

comparing baby oil (hyperosmolar), KY Jelly® (hyperosmolar), olive oil (iso-osmolar), and saliva (hypo-osmolar), baby oil had the least impact on sperm motility, while saliva had the greatest effect, opposite of what would be expected based on osmolarity alone [7]. These findings question the significance of osmolarity and suggest that alternative factors are likely responsible for a portion of sperm impairment observed with lubricants.

The role of lubricant pH on semen impairment is also currently understudied. The optimal pH for sperm transport through the female genital tract is reported at 7.0–8.5, with cervical pH increasing to similar ranges during ovulation [10, 11]. However, this is of unclear clinical significance given that the majority of lubricants are within the 7.0 pH range and that the native vaginal pH is <4.5–5.5.

Lubricants

Impact on Semen Parameters

Several studies have evaluated the impact of various lubricants on semen parameters in vitro. See Table 4.2 for the effect of common lubricants on semen parameters and/or fertility. Given the large number of lubricants currently available, the current review will only focus on agents with published data available, with additional information provided on more commonly utilized agents. Although the majority of lubricants discussed are used with sexual intercourse or for extraction of semen samples via masturbation, additional substances used during surgery, ultrasonography, and/or intrauterine insemination will also be discussed due to their relevance in routine fertility practice.

Water-Based/Soluble Lubricants

Aquasonic Gel®

Aquasonic Gel® is a high-viscosity coupling gel commonly utilized in ultrasonography applications, including transvaginal imaging. In the only in vitro study evaluating its effect on sperm, Vargas and colleagues combined 0.1, 1, 5, and 10 % Aquasonic Gel® with normospermic samples from three to five donors diluted to achieve a total sperm concentration of 10–20 million/mL [3]. Following an incubation period of 1 or 24 h, sperm motility and osmolality were assessed and compared to controls. Results demonstrated an increase in total osmolality to 408 mOsm/kg in the 10 % group only, with the lower concentrations remaining under a predefined threshold of 400 mOsm/kg. In the 1 % group, total motility was unchanged at 1 h, and significantly reduced by 46 % at 24 h compared to controls. The authors concluded that despite its labeling as nonspermicidal, Aquasonic Gel® could result in significant impairments to sperm motility at concentrations as low as 1 %.

Astroglide®

Astroglide® is a water-soluble lubricant which contains water, glycerin, propylene glycol, polyquaternium 15, methylparaben, and propylparaben. Alternative versions of Astroglide® are available, including silicone based and formulations without glycerine or paraben; however, all currently published reports have evaluated the water-soluble, glycerin-containing version only.

Several studies have compared Astroglide® to various agents including KY Jelly®, Replens®, Touch®, FemGlide®, Pre-Seed®, canola oil, and olive oil

Table 4.2 Summary of data on the effect of vaginal lubricants on semen parameters and fertility

Agent/date (Author)	Population (n=)	Study design	Outcome measure	Duration of exposure	Result	Notes
Aquasonic Gel®						
2011 (Vargas)	Norm	In vitro; comparison of 0.1 %, 1 %, 5 %, 10 % Aquasonic Gel®, Felis®, Pre-Seed®, Replens® to controls	SA via CASA	1, 24 h	1 h—mot unchanged 24 h—↓ mot 46 %	Used predominantly with U/S
Astroglide®						
2012 (Steiner)	15 Tx 221 Cont Women aged 30–44 No history of infertility	Prospective, observational; in vivo comparison of lubricant vs. non-lubricant users	Fec at 6 cycles of attempts	Natural intercourse	72.7 % Fec (lubricant users) 68 % Fec (non-lubricant users) $p = 0.87$	Lubricant users include multiple types of lubrication
2008 (Agarwal)	13 Norm	In vitro; comparison of 10 % Astroglide®, FemGlide®, Pre-Seed®, Replens®, KY Jelly®	SA via LM; DNA frag	30 min	↓ mot 99 %	Greatest impact on mot of four agents tested
1996 (Kutteh)	Norm	In vitro; compared 30 % Astroglide®, canola oil, KY Jelly®, olive oil, Replens®, and KY Touch® to pos and neg cont	SA via CASA; viability	1, 15, 30, 60 min	No mot, non-viable at 60 min	Astroglide® and Replens® with greatest impact on mot and viability

(continued)

Table 4.2 (continued)

Agent/date (Author)	Population (n=)	Study design	Outcome measure	Duration of exposure	Result	Notes
1992 (Frishman)	10 Norm	In vitro; comparison of Astroglide® and KY Jelly® at 100, 50, 25, and 12.5 %	SA via LM	1, 15, 30 min	Dose dependent decrease in progressive motility	No sig difference between Astroglide® and KY Jelly® except with KY Jelly® at 12.5 %
Baby oil						
1998 (Anderson)	16 Norm semen samples[a]	In vitro; compared baby oil, olive oil, KY Jelly®, saliva to control at 12.5 and 6.25 %	SA characteristics; LM	5, 15, 30 min	No sig effect on mot, vel, head mov at 12.5 or 6.25 % conc	Least impact of four agents tested
Canola oil						
1996 (Kutteh)	Norm	In vitro; compared 30 % Astroglide®, canola oil, KY Jelly®, olive oil, Replens®, and KY Touch® to pos and neg cont	SA via CASA; viability	1, 15, 30, 60 min	No sig effect on mot, viability	Least impact of agents tested
FemGlide®						
2008 (Agarwal)	13 Norm	In vitro; comparison of 10 % Astroglide®, FemGlide®, Pre-Seed®, Replens®, KY Jelly®	SA via LM; DNA frag	30 min	↓ mot 23 %, ↑ DNA frag 14 %	

Felis®						
2011 (Vargas)	Norm	In vitro; comparison of 0.1 %, 1 %, 5 %, 10 % Aquasonic Gel®, Felis®, Pre-Seed®, Replens® to controls	SA via CASA	1, 24 h	1 h—mot unchanged 24 h—↓ mot 48 %	
KY Jelly®/Touch®						
2012 (Steiner)	33 Tx 221 Cont	Prospective, observational; in vivo comparison of lubricant vs. non-lubricant users	Fec at 6 cycles of attempts	Natural intercourse	72.7 % Fec (lubricant users) 68 % Fec (non-lubricant users) $p = 0.87$	Lubricant users include multiple types of lubrication
2008 (Agarwal)	13 Norm	In vitro; comparison of 10 % Astroglide®, FemGlide®, Pre-Seed®, Replens®, KY Jelly®	SA via LM; DNA frag	30 min	↑ DNA frag 10 %	
1998 (Anderson)	16 Norm semen samples[a]	In vitro; compared baby oil, olive oil, KY Jelly®, saliva to control at 12.5 and 6.25 %	SA via LM	5, 15, 30 min	12.5 % Conc: ↓ mot 74 % at 30 min; ↓ vel 52 % at 30 min; ↓ head mov 37 % at 5 min 6.25 % Conc: no sig effect on mot, ↓ vel 27 % at 30 min, ↓ head mov 33 % at 5 min	More impact than baby oil; less impact than saliva

(continued)

Table 4.2 (continued)

Agent/date (Author)	Population (*n*=)	Study design	Outcome measure	Duration of exposure	Result	Notes
1996 (Kutteh)	Norm	In vitro; compared 30 % Astroglide®, canola oil, KY Jelly®, olive oil, Replens®, and Touch® to pos and neg cont	SA via CASA; viability	1, 15, 30, 60 min	KY Jelly® with no mot at 60 min KY Touch® with 10 % mot at 60 min KY Jelly® and Touch® with min impact on viability	
1992 (Frishman)	10 Norm	In vitro; comparison of Astroglide® and KY Jelly® at 100, 50, 25, and 12.5 %	SA via LM	1, 15, 30 min	Dose dependent decrease in progressive motility No sig impact on motility with KY Jelly® at 12.5 % No sig difference between 1, 15, and 30 min time points	No sig difference between Astroglide® and KY Jelly® except with KY Jelly® at 12.5 %
1975 (Goldenberg)	20	In vitro; compared Alpha-Keri®, glycerin, H-R Jelly®, Keri Lotion®, KY Jelly®, Lubifax®, olive oil, Ortho-Gynol®, peanut oil, petroleum jelly, pHisohex®, safflower oil, Searle Skin Lotion®, Surgilube®, vegetable oil	Motility using scale 0 to 4+ (0 = no mot; 4+ = cont mot)	15, 120 min	15 min: 0 mot 120 min: 0 mot	

1972 (Tagatz)	20 semen samples from 24 to 36 year old infertile couples	In vitro; compared 50 mg of KY Jelly® or Surgilube® to control	SA via LM	15, 30 min	No mot at 15 min with KY Jelly® or Surgilube® No viability at 15 min with KY Jelly® or Surgilube®	Compared norm to abnormal SA with similar impact on motility and viability
Olive oil						
1998 (Anderson)	16 Norm semen samples[a]	In vitro; compared baby oil, olive oil, KY Jelly®, saliva to control at 12.5 and 6.25 %	SA via LM	5, 15, 30 min	12.5 % Conc: ↓ mot 91 % at 30 min; ↓ vel 38 % at 30 min; ↓ head mov minimally 6.25 % Conc: mot, vel, head mov unchanged at 30 min	More impact than baby oil; less impact than saliva
1996 (Kutteh)	Norm	In vitro; compared 30 % Astroglide®, canola oil, KY Jelly®, olive oil, Replens®, and Touch® to pos and neg cont	SA via CASA; viability	1, 15, 30, 60 min	40 % mot at 60 min No impact on viability	Greater impact than canola oil. Lesser than KY Jelly® and Replens®
1975 (Goldenberg)	20	In vitro; compared Alpha-Keri®, glycerin, H-R Jelly®, Keri Lotion®, KY Jelly®, Lubifax®, olive oil, Ortho-Gynol®, peanut oil, petroleum jelly, pHisohex®, safflower oil, Searle Skin Lotion®, Surgilube®, vegetable oil	Motility using scale 0 to 4+ (0 = no mot; 4+ = cont mot)	15, 120 min	15 min: 2+ mot 120 min: 3+ mot	

(continued)

Table 4.2 (continued)

Agent/date (Author)	Population (n=)	Study design	Outcome measure	Duration of exposure	Result	Notes
Petroleum jelly						
1975 (Goldenberg)	20	In vitro; compared Alpha-Keri®, glycerin, H-R Jelly®, Keri Lotion®, KY Jelly®, Lubifax®, olive oil, Ortho-Gynol®, peanut oil, petroleum jelly, pHisohex®, safflower oil, Searle Skin Lotion®, Surgilube®, vegetable oil	Motility using scale 0 to 4+ (0 = no mot; 4+ = cont mot)	15, 120 min	15 min: 2 to 3+ mot 120 min: 3 to 4+ mot	Petroleum jelly and glycerin with least impact among agents tested
Pre-Seed®						
2013 (Agarwal)	22 Norm	Paired, randomized, crossover; obtained samples with or without use of Pre-Seed® lubricant	SA; viability, DNA frag	Used during masturbation	No sig effect on mot, viability, DNA frag	Unclear extent of SA contamination with Pre-Seed®
2012 (Steiner)	7 Tx 221 Cont	Prospective, observational; in vivo comparison of lubricant vs. non-lubricant users	Fec at 6 cycles of attempts	Natural intercourse	72.7 % Fec (lubricant users) 68 % Fec (non-lubricant users) $p = 0.87$	Lubricant users include multiple types of lubrication
2011 (Vargas)	Norm	In vitro; comparison of 0.1 %, 1 %, 5 %, 10 % Aquasonic Gel®, Felis®, Pre-Seed®, Replens® to controls	SA via CASA	1, 24 h	1, 24 h—mot unchanged	Least impact of agents tested

2008 (Agarwal)	13 Norm	In vitro; comparison of 10 % Astroglide®, FemGlide®, Pre-Seed®, Replens®, KY Jelly®	SA via LM; DNA frag	30 min	No sig effect on mot, DNA frag	Least impact of agents tested
Replens®						
2011 (Vargas)	Norm	In vitro; comparison of 0.1 %, 1 %, 5 %, 10 % Aquasonic Gel®, Felis®, Pre-Seed®, Replens® to controls	SA via CASA	1, 24 h	1 h—↓ mot 97 % 24 h—↓ mot 88 %	Greatest impact among agents tested
2008 (Agarwal)	13 Norm	In vitro; comparison of 10 % Astroglide®, FemGlide®, Pre-Seed®, Replens®, KY Jelly®	SA via LM; DNA frag	30 min	↓ mot 60 %	
1996 (Kutteh)	Norm	In vitro; compared 30 % Astroglide®, canola oil, KY Jelly®, olive oil, Replens®, and Touch® to pos and neg cont	SA via CASA; viability	1, 15, 30, 60 min	No mot, non-viable at 60 min	Astroglide® and Replens® with greatest impact on mot and viability
Saliva						
1998 (Anderson)	16 Norm semen samples[a]	In vitro; compared baby oil, olive oil, KY Jelly®, saliva to control at 12.5 and 6.25 %	SA via LM	5, 15, 30 min	12.5 % Conc: ↓ mot 95 % at 15 min; ↓ vel 100 % at 30 min; ↓ head mov 100 % at 15 min 6.25 % Conc: Sig ↓ mot, vel, head mov	Greater impact than baby oil, KY Jelly®, olive oil

(continued)

Table 4.2 (continued)

Agent/date (Author)	Population (n=)	Study design	Outcome measure	Duration of exposure	Result	Notes
1982 (Tulandi)	38 Norm	In vitro; 1, 2, 4, 10, 20 % saliva concentration	SA via LM	15, 30, 60, 120 min	Dose and time dependent ↓ mot and progression 20 % saliva at 30 min with 51 % mot vs. 69 % (control)	
Surgilube®						
1994 (Miller)	Norm semen samples, 7 females <40 year	RCT; 5-mL of Surgilube® per vagina at time of ovulation; tested at 5, 10, 20, 30 %	Post-coital test via LM at ovulation	0, 15, 30, 60, 120 min	Time and concentration dependent ↓ mot	
1972 (Tagatz)	20 Semen samples from 24 to 36 year old infertile couples	In vitro; compared 50 mg of KY Jelly® or Surgilube® to control	SA via LM	15, 30 min	No mot at 15 min with KY Jelly® or Surgilube® No viability at 15 min with KY Jelly® or Surgilube®	Compared norm to abnormal SA with similar impact on motility and viability

Others					
1984 (Tulandi)	15 Norm	In vitro; compared 16.7 % egg-white and 1, 2, 5, 10 % glycerin to control	SA via LM	15, 30, 60 min	Egg-white: at 60 min non-sig change in mot (62 % vs. 66 % control) and progression (51 % vs. 56 % control) Glycerin: at 30 min sig ↓ in mot and progression at 2 % and above (43 % mot vs. 72 % cont at 10 % conc)
1975 (Goldenberg)	20	In vitro; compared Alpha-Keri®, glycerin, H-R Jelly®, Keri Lotion®, KY Jelly®, Lubifax®, olive oil, Ortho-Gynol®, peanut oil, petroleum jelly, pHisohex®, safflower oil, Searle Skin Lotion®, Surgilube®, vegetable oil	Motility using scale 0 to 4+ (0 = no mot; 4+ = cont mot)	15, 120 min	H-R®: 1+, 0 Lubifax®: 0, 0 Surgilube®: 0, 0 Ortho-Gynol®: 0, 0 Alpha-Keri®: 0, 0 Keri Lotion®: 0 to 1+, 0 pHisonex®: 0, 0 Searle Skin Lotion®: 0 to 1+, 0 Vegetable oil: 3+, 2+ Safflower oil: 3+, 3+ Peanut oil: 3+, 3+ Glycerin: 3+, 3 to 4+

CASA computer-assisted semen analysis, *Conc* concentration, *Cont* controls, *Fec* fecundability, *Frag* fragmentation, *LM* light microscopy, *Mot* motility, *Mov* movement, *Neg* negative, *Norm* normospermic, *Pos* positive, *RCT* randomized controlled trial, *Retro* retrospective design, *SA* semen analysis, *Tx* treatment, *Vel* velocity

[a]Prepared by two-step discontinuous Percoll gradient centrifugation

[4–6]. All studies used an in vitro design with normospermic samples and lubricant concentrations ranging from 10 to 100 %. Samples were assessed following varied incubation periods (1, 15, 30, 60 min) using light microscopy (LM), computer-assisted sperm analyzer (CASA), and DNA fragmentation. Results demonstrated that among agents tested, Astroglide® had the greatest impact on fertility with dose-dependent decreases in motility achieving complete immotility at 30–60 min [4, 5]. Concentrations above 12.5 % resulted in similar impairments with KY Jelly®, Astroglide®, and Replens® [5, 6].

The mechanism for the significant impairment observed with Astroglide® has not been elucidated, with some suggesting that it may be due, in part, to the presence of glycerin [4]. Although an early report failed to identify decreases in motility with glycerin, several studies have subsequently noted significant reductions, with one author suggesting that the earlier findings were likely due to inadequate mixing of specimen [4, 5, 12, 13]. No studies to date have evaluated Astroglide® without glycerin to further isolate the individual impact of glycerin on observed findings.

In the only in vivo assessment of lubricants among couples attempting to conceive, Astroglide® accounted for 20 % of lubricants reported [2]. Although subset analyses were not performed on individual lubricants, overall results demonstrated no significant differences in fecundity among lubricant vs. non-lubricant users. Results from this study and its implications are discussed in greater detail in the "Overall Impact on Fertility" section.

FemGlide®

FemGlide® is a water-soluble lubricant containing water, polyethylene oxide, sodium carbomer, and methylparaben and is also manufactured under the trade name Slippery Stuff Gel®. One study using 13 normospermic samples compared the effect of 10 % FemGlide® on sperm motility and DNA fragmentation using 13 normospermic samples [4]. Following an incubation period of 30 min, motility was decreased by 23 %, and DNA fragmentation increased by 14 % compared to controls. In relation to other agents tested, FemGlide® had a lesser impact than Astroglide® and Replens® and greater impact than Pre-Seed® on overall motility (statistical assessments not performed between groups). DNA damage was similar between FemGlide® (14 %), KY Jelly® (10 %), and Pre-Seed® (7 %), although statistically significant increases in DNA damage were only noted with FemGlide® and KY Jelly® compared to controls.

Felis®

Felis® is a water-soluble lubricant with limited data available regarding its ingredients and properties. One in vitro, dose–response assessment of Felis® combined various concentrations (0.1, 1, 5, and 10 %) with normospermic samples

[3]. Concentrations of 5 % and 10 % resulted in significant increases in sample osmolality to 511 mOsm/kg and 734 mOsm/kg, respectively. At 10 %, no changes in motility were noted at 1 h, although a 48 % reduction occurred over the 24-h period of incubation. In comparing with other agents assessed, results were better than Replens® (88 % reduced), worse than Pre-Seed® (7 % reduced) and similar to Aquasonic Gel® (46 % reduced).

KY Jelly®/Touch®

KY brand lubricants are water-based products of various formulations, with published data evaluating the impact of KY Jelly® and Touch® on semen parameters. Ingredients vary based on formulation and product: KY Jelly® contains water, glycerin, hydroxyethylcellulose, chlorhexidine gluconate, gluconolactone, methylparaben, and sodium hydroxide; KY Touch® contains propylene glycol, PEG-8, hydroxypropylcellulose, and tocopherol. Alternative formulations are available without glycerin (KY Ultra®), although there are currently no data evaluating their impact on sperm or fertility parameters.

Several studies have assessed the effect of KY Jelly® and Touch® on sperm motility, morphology, viability, and DNA fragmentation [4–7, 13, 14]. Early studies by Tagatz and Goldenberg performed in vitro assessments of various compounds, including KY Jelly® and demonstrated no motility or viability of sperm on LM at 15 min [13, 14]. Frishman and colleagues subsequently evaluated varying concentrations of KY Jelly® and Astroglide® (12.5, 25, 50, 100 %) and reported a dose-dependent, time-independent reduction in motility [6]. At the 12.5 % concentration, a non-statistically significant decrease in motility was noted with KY Jelly® at 1 min, with no subsequent progressive decreases noted among agents over the remaining time points assessed (1, 15, 30 min). A further study by Anderson and colleagues compared KY Jelly® at 12.5 and 6.25 and reported no significant changes in motility with 6.25 %, while 12.5 % reduced motility by 74 % at 30 min [7]. Osmolarity at the 6.25 % concentration was noted to be 600 mOsm/L with the addition of sperm, reinforcing the idea that hyper-osmolarity alone does not result in reduced motility.

One study comparing 30 % KY Jelly® to KY Touch® demonstrated greater reductions in motility with KY Jelly® (100 % vs. 90 % at 60 min) [5]. Although these findings provide support for the possible detrimental effect of glycerin (present in KY Jelly® and absent in KY Touch®), given the varied ingredients between agents, direct comparisons are limited. KY Jelly® (10 % concentration) was also shown to increase DNA fragmentation by 10 % compared to controls, highlighting another potential mechanism for impaired sperm function [4].

In the previously discussed in vivo comparison of fecundity between lubricant users and nonusers, KY Jelly® accounted for 44 % of lubricants reported and represented the largest group [2]. Given the similar rates of conception identified between groups, this would suggest that despite contrasting in vitro data, use of KY Jelly® during attempted conception may not reduce successful fecundity.

Pre-Seed®

Pre-Seed® is a water-soluble, hydroxycellulose-based lubricant and currently represents the agent with the fewest detrimental effects on sperm parameters among tested, water-based substances. Ingredients include hydroxyethylcellulose, water, Pluronic (poloxamer), sodium chloride, arabinogalactan, sodium phosphate, potassium phosphate, carbomer, methylparaben, and sodium hydroxide.

Two recent studies compared Pre-Seed® to other compounds including Aquasonic Gel®, Astroglide®, Felis®, FemGlide®, Replens® and KY Jelly® at varied concentrations (0.1, 1, 5, 10 %) [3, 4]. Both studies demonstrated no significant reductions in sperm motility (incubation with 10 % Pre-Seed® for 30 min and 24 h) with a mild, non-statistically significant increase (7 %) in DNA fragmentation identified. Among the agents tested, Pre-Seed® was consistently noted to have the least impact on sperm parameters, with osmolality levels remaining below a pre-defined threshold of 400 mOsm/kg at all concentrations [3, 4].

Pre-Seed® was additionally evaluated for use during masturbation to produce sperm samples in a paired, randomized, crossover design study [8]. Samples were assessed for motility, viability, and DNA fragmentation, with results demonstrating no significant impairments compared to controls. Although the extent of semen contamination with any lubricant used during masturbation is unclear, these results provide support for the permissible use of Pre-Seed® during sample production.

In the in vivo trial comparing fecundity between lubricant users and nonusers, 9 % of the lubricant cohort endorsed using Pre-Seed®, representing the third most common lubricant reported [2]. As previously mentioned, no significant difference was noted in fecundity between groups, suggesting the acceptable use of lubricants among couples attempting to conceive.

Replens®

Replens® is a water-based lubricant which utilizes a polycarbophil polymer as an adhesive base to provide epithelial adherence. Ingredients include carbomer 934P, glycerin, hydrogenated palm oil glyceride, mineral oil, polycarbophil, water, methylparaben, sodium hydroxide, and sorbic acid. Compared to many of the previously discussed agents, Replens® has a significantly lower pH (2.8), although in vitro assessments with sperm at 5 % and 10 % concentrations resulted in increased pH levels of 6.6 and 5.5, respectively [3].

Three studies reported in vitro comparisons of Replens® to Aquasonic Gel®, Astroglide®, canola oil, Felis®, FemGlide®, KY Jelly®, KY Touch®, olive oil, and Pre-Seed® at concentrations of 0.1, 1, 5, 10, and 30 % [3–5]. Evaluation at varied time points (1, 15, 30, 60 min and 24 h) demonstrated consistent reductions in motility (60–100 %) and viability, with impairments identified at concentrations as low as 1 %. Among the agents tested, Replens® and Astroglide® were consistently noted to have the greatest impact on sperm function, with one author suggesting that this may be due, in part, to the shared ingredient glycerin [4]. However, the extent of the impairment attributable to glycerin alone is unknown.

Saliva

Two studies have assessed the impact of saliva on sperm parameters [7, 15]. Tulandi and colleagues compared various salivary concentrations (1, 2, 10, and 20 %) at 15, 30, 60, and 120 min and noted time- and concentration-dependent impairments in motility (51 % motility vs. 69 % control with 20 % concentration at 30 min) [15]. A subsequent study by Anderson and colleagues reported even greater reductions in sperm motility (95 % at 15 min), curvilinear velocity (100 % at 30 min), and lateral head movements (100 % at 15 min) at lower concentrations (12.5 % vs. 20 %) than the Tulandi study [7]. Compared to baby oil, KY Jelly®, and olive oil, saliva resulted in the greatest impairment in sperm parameters, despite favorable osmolality levels (274 mOsm/kg with sperm added). The etiology for the variable results between studies is unclear and may reflect differences in salivary compositions among individuals.

Surgilube®

Surgilube® is a common, water-based lubricant used in multiple applications in clinical medicine and surgery including with urinary catheter placements. Although a full list of ingredients is not readily available, it consists predominantly of water-soluble gums (viscous substances isolated from plant exudates) and chlorhexidine gluconate.

Two studies evaluated the effect of Surgilube® on sperm motility and viability [14, 16]. Tagatz and colleagues performed an in vitro assessment of Surgilube® and KY Jelly® compared to controls in 20 samples obtained from young infertile couples [14]. Sperm motility and viability assessed at 15 and 30 min demonstrated no motility or viability of sperm with either Surgilube® or KY Jelly® at the 15-min time point. Subset analysis of normal vs. abnormal semen samples showed similar impairments between groups. This study is significant in that it is the only one to assess samples from infertile couples and suggests that lubricant-induced impairments are independent of baseline fertility status.

Miller and colleagues subsequently performed an in vivo, randomized controlled evaluation of the impact of various concentrations of Surgilube® (5 mL of 5, 10, 20, 30 %) administered per vagina on sperm obtained from post-coital cervical mucus [16]. Results demonstrated time- and concentration-dependent decreases in sperm motility, with approximately 50, 60, 70, and 90 % reductions in motility at the 5, 10, 20, and 30 % concentrations, respectively. Similar reductions were noted within each concentration at each subsequent time point assessed (15, 30, 60, 120 min). As with the Aquasonic Gel®, these findings are relevant to clinical practice, given that Surgilube® is commonly used during clinical vaginal examinations and instrumentation.

Oil-Based/Soluble Lubricants

Baby Oil

Baby oil includes several varieties of lubricants which utilize mineral oil as a common ingredient. The only brand of baby oil with data evaluating its effect on sperm is produced by Johnson & Johnson (New Brunswick, NJ) and incorporates aloe vera, vitamin E, acetate, and additives for fragrance. In an in vitro comparison of baby oil, olive oil, KY Jelly®, and saliva at 6.25 and 12.5 % concentrations, baby oil had no significant effect on sperm motility, velocity, or head movement and was found to have the least impact among agents tested [7].

Plant Oils

Canola, olive, peanut, safflower, and vegetable oils are combination fatty acids obtained from various seeds and plants. In the earliest evaluation of the effect of various oils on sperm motility, Goldenberg and colleagues reported subjectively assessed sperm motilities (scale: 0 = no motility to 4+ = similar to controls) of olive, peanut, safflower, and vegetable oils [13]. At 15 and 120 min time points, reported motilities were similar among all oils tested: olive (15 min = 2+, 120 min = 3+); peanut (3+, 3+); safflower (3+, 3+); vegetable (3+, 2+). These results were superior to all water-based products assessed and slightly inferior to glycerin and petroleum jelly, although it is unclear if sufficient mixing was achieved with the non water-soluble agents.

Two additional in vitro trials were performed to evaluate the effect of olive and canola oils on sperm motility [5, 7]. Using a 30 % concentration of olive and canola oils, Kutteh and colleagues reported no significant impairments in sperm viability, with motility either unchanged (canola oil) or decreased by 40 % (olive oil) [5]. The authors concluded that canola oil had the least impact of the agents tested (Astroglide®, canola oil, KY Jelly®, olive oil, Replens®, Touch®). Anderson and colleagues similarly compared olive oil to baby oil, KY Jelly®, and saliva at 12.5 and 6.25 % concentrations [7]. Although motility, velocity, and head movements were all significantly reduced with olive oil at the 12.5 % concentration, no significant impairments were identified at 6.25 %. The authors noted that compared to the other agents, olive oil had a greater impact than baby oil and lesser impact than saliva at all concentrations.

Petroleum Jelly

Petroleum jelly is a semisolid mixture of hydrocarbons, with the most recognized brand being Vaseline® (Unilever N.V., Rotterdam, Netherlands). Very limited data is available on its effect on sperm parameters, with the only published study reported by Goldenberg and colleagues [13]. In their evaluation of multiple commercially available lubricants, the authors reported preserved motility of sperm at the 15 min (2 to 3+; scale 0 to 4+) and 120 min (3 to 4+) time points. Compared to all other agents, petroleum jelly and glycerin were noted to have the least impact on sperm motility. However, as glycerin has subsequently been shown to consistently impair sperm, some authors have questioned whether the Goldenberg study performed adequate mixing of samples, thus potentially underestimating the effect of glycerin (and by inference petroleum jelly) on sperm motility [4].

Other Lubricants

Egg white

Hen egg white has been reported as a potential lubricant for sexual intercourse with limited impact on fertility [17]. Although the origins for egg white as a lubricant are unclear, one of the earliest reports highlighted its use as a viable analog for cervical mucus in sperm penetration assays [18]. Subsequent introduction of hyaluronate resulted in the replacement of egg white due to improved passage of sperm, better linearity, and less lateral head displacement [19, 20].

In the only in vitro study evaluating the impact of egg white on sperm motility, Tulandi and colleagues noted no significant reductions in motility (62 % vs. 66 % controls) or progression (51 % vs. 56 % control) following 60 min of incubation [12].

Overall Impact on Fertility

Currently, there is very limited data on the in vivo impact of available lubricants on fertility. The only trial to assess fecundability as an end-point prospectively observed 296 females, aged 30–44 who were attempting to conceive for less than 3 months [2]. All participants completed a baseline questionnaire followed by a diary to record intercourse frequency and use of lubricants, among other factors. Prior to study initiation, 25 % of women reported use of vaginal lubricants while attempting to conceive, with 43 % subsequently utilizing lubrication during the 6-month study interval. Among users, the frequency of use varied, with 44, 31, and 24 % noting occasional, frequent, and every time use, respectively. Reported lubricants were Astroglide® (20 %), KY Jelly® (44 %), and Pre-Seed® (9 %), with the remainder not listed. After adjusting for age, partner race, and intercourse frequency during the fertile window, no differences were noted in fecundability in regards to women reporting use of lubricants overall (OR 1.23; CI 0.76–2.00) or during the fertile period (OR 1.05; CI 0.59–1.85).

As the only in vivo study evaluating the impact of lubricants on actual fecundability, this study highlights limitations inherent with in vitro assessments of the impact of lubricants on semen characteristics. Although several studies demonstrated the significant impacts of Astroglide® and KY Jelly® on reducing sperm motility and viability, these agents accounted for 64 % of lubricants reported during the 6-month in vivo study interval, suggesting that in actual use, their impact on fertility is negligible [2, 4–7, 13, 14].

Several possible factors may account for the discrepancy between in vitro and in vivo results. In vitro assessments consistently note concentration and time dependent effects of the various agents on sperm characteristics, with initial impairments evident as early as 5–15 min and significantly reduced motility at 60 min following exposure [5–7, 15]. As the majority of the lubricant is likely attenuated by vaginal secretions and remains in the entroitus/distal vagina, the actual concentration of lubricant reaching the cervical mucus and sperm is likely limited [2]. Similarly, given the rapid progression of sperm to the Fallopian tube (identified within 5 min of ejaculation), the duration of exposure to lubricant may be minimal [21]. In vitro assessments also poorly represent the in vivo vaginal milieu, in which factors such as pH and osmolarity would be rapidly reduced or negated. This likely overestimates the true impact of factors such as osmolarity and/or pH.

Study Limitations

Data on the effect of lubricants on fertility and sperm parameters is limited by the paucity of studies and significant heterogeneity of literature available. The far majority of studies are in vitro assessments using small numbers of normospermic samples, with unclear relevance of findings to couples with baseline impaired fertility. Comparisons between studies are also limited by varied study methodologies, including concentrations assessed, samples obtained, incubation periods, and methods of sperm evaluation. Similarly, as there is no consensus as to which sperm factors are most relevant to fertility, all in vitro evaluations are of unclear clinical utility. Given these limitations, further in vivo studies are required to determine the significance of in vitro observations.

Summary and Conclusions

Lubricants are commonly used by couples attempting to conceive and are important in clinical and operative settings. Available data on the effect of lubricants on sperm parameters and fertility are limited, with the majority of studies performing assessments on in vitro sperm samples. Results of in vitro studies consistently demonstrate effects on sperm motility and viability in a time- and concentration-dependent manner. Although data are unable to be compared between studies, individual results suggest that baby oil (mineral oil), canola oil, egg white, and Pre-Seed® do not result in significant reductions in sperm motility or other measured parameters. In contrast, Astroglide®, KY Jelly®/Touch®, Replens®, saliva, and Surgilube® all significantly impair sperm motility and/or other factors. In general, plant oils have minimal effects, with olive oil demonstrating slightly worse outcomes compared to canola oil. Limited data on Aquasonic Gel®, FemGlide®, and Felis® identify impaired motility at selected time points, while insufficient data is available to draw conclusions on the impact of petroleum jelly.

In vivo data is limited, with one study reporting no significant difference in the rate of fecundity between lubricant users and nonusers among couples attempting to conceive. The results are particularly relevant given that the majority of lubricants reported within the study have been shown in in vitro trials to significantly impair sperm. These data highlight the disparity between in vitro and in vivo assessments and underscore the need for additional in vivo studies to identify the true clinical impact of lubricant use in true-to-life settings.

References

1. Herbenick D, Reece M, Sanders SA, Dodge B, Ghassemi A, Fortenberry JD. Women's vibrator use in sexual partnerships: results from a nationally representative survey in the United States. J Sex Marital Ther. 2010;36(1):49–65. Epub 2010/01/12.
2. Steiner AZ, Long DL, Tanner C, Herring AH. Effect of vaginal lubricants on natural fertility. Obstet Gynecol. 2012;120(1):44–51. Epub 2012/08/24.
3. Vargas J, Crausaz M, Senn A, Germond M. Sperm toxicity of "nonspermicidal" lubricant and ultrasound gels used in reproductive medicine. Fertil Steril. 2011;95(2):835–6. Epub 2010/10/26.
4. Agarwal A, Deepinder F, Cocuzza M, Short RA, Evenson DP. Effect of vaginal lubricants on sperm motility and chromatin integrity: a prospective comparative study. Fertil Steril. 2008;89(2):375–9. Epub 2007/05/19.
5. Kutteh WH, Chao CH, Ritter JO, Byrd W. Vaginal lubricants for the infertile couple: effect on sperm activity. Int J Fertil Menopausal Stud. 1996;41(4):400–4. Epub 1996/07/01.
6. Frishman GN, Luciano AA, Maier DB. Evaluation of Astroglide, a new vaginal lubricant: effects of length of exposure and concentration on sperm motility. Fertil Steril. 1992;58(3):630–2. Epub 1992/09/01.
7. Anderson L, Lewis SE, McClure N. The effects of coital lubricants on sperm motility in vitro. Hum Reprod. 1998;13(12):3351–6. Epub 1999/01/14.

8. Agarwal A, Malvezzi H, Sharma R. Effect of an isotonic lubricant on sperm collection and sperm quality. Fertil Steril. 2013;99(6):1581–6. Epub 2013/03/16.
9. Rossato M, Balercia G, Lucarelli G, Foresta C, Mantero F. Role of seminal osmolarity in the reduction of human sperm motility. Int J Androl. 2002;25(4):230–5. Epub 2002/08/16.
10. World Health Organization. WHO laboratory manual for the examination of human semen and sperm-cervical mucus interaction. 4th ed. Cambridge: Cambridge University Press; 1999.
11. Guttmacher AF, Shettles LB. Cyclic changes in cervical mucus, and its practical importance. Hum Fertil. 1940;5(1):4–9. Epub 1940/02/01.
12. Tulandi T, McInnes RA. Vaginal lubricants: effect of glycerin and egg white on sperm motility and progression in vitro. Fertil Steril. 1984;41(1):151–3. Epub 1984/01/01.
13. Goldenberg RL, White R. The effect of vaginal lubricants on sperm motility in vitro. Fertil Steril. 1975;26(9):872–3. Epub 1975/09/01.
14. Tagatz GE, Okagaki T, Sciarra JJ. The effect of vaginal lubricants on sperm motility and viability in vitro. Am J Obstet Gynecol. 1972;113(1):88–90. Epub 1972/05/01.
15. Tulandi T, Plouffe Jr L, McInnes RA. Effect of saliva on sperm motility and activity. Fertil Steril. 1982;38(6):721–3. Epub 1982/12/01.
16. Miller B, Klein TA, Opsahl MS. The effect of a surgical lubricant on in vivo sperm penetration of cervical mucus. Fertil Steril. 1994;61(6):1171–3. Epub 1994/06/01.
17. Eggert-Kruse W, Gerhard I, Tilgen W, Runnebaum B. The use of hens' egg white as a substitute for human cervical mucus in assessing human infertility. Int J Androl. 1990;13 (4):258–66. Epub 1990/08/01.
18. Hansen KB, Hjort T. The penetration of antibody-covered spermatozoa into cervical mucus and egg white. Arch Androl. 1979;3(3):245–9. Epub 1979/11/01.
19. Tang S, Garrett C, Baker HW. Comparison of human cervical mucus and artificial sperm penetration media. Hum Reprod. 1999;14(11):2812–7. Epub 1999/11/05.
20. Engel S, Petzoldt R. Human sperm penetration in different media. Andrologia. 1999;31 (4):233–9. Epub 1999/09/02.
21. Settlage DS, Motoshima M, Tredway DR. Sperm transport from the external cervical os to the fallopian tubes in women: a time and quantitation study. Fertil Steril. 1973;24(9):655–61. Epub 1973/09/01.

Chapter 5
Sexually Transmitted Infections

Claire Brookings, David Goldmeier, and Hossein Sadeghi-Nejad

Introduction

Sexually transmitted infections (STIs) have a high prevalence worldwide. STIs and their complications are one of the top five reasons to attend healthcare in the developing world [1]. In 2008, the US incidence rate of new STI infections was 20 million with a prevalence of 110 million. In 2010, the medical costs in the USA were $16 billion [2]. The effect of untreated STIs on pregnancy is well documented, as is the association with pelvic inflammatory and female tubal infertility. The effect of STIs and male accessory gland infection on male fertility is less clear. The evidence to date is conflicting as to the extent of impact. Most STIs are easily treated, and those that are at present incurable such as HIV can be treated and controlled to allow couples to conceive without harm to each other or the child. Another consideration when assessing a couple for fertility issues is male sexual function. Erectile dysfunction can prohibit penetrative sex. The psychological impact of a diagnosis of a STI, whether current or in the past, may well cause psychological issues that if addressed may improve sexual function, and thus the ability to conceive. For quick reference for testing and US recommended treatment of specific STIs, please refer to Table 5.1 and 5.2, respectively.

HIV

In 2010, an estimated 34 million people were living with HIV infection [3]. The global epidemic seems to have stabilized with a drop in incidence. In 2010, there were an estimated 2.7 million new infections compared to the peak of 3.2 million in

H. Sadeghi-Nejad (✉)
Rutgers New Jersey Medical School, Hackensack University Medical Center, 20 Prospect Avenue, #711, Hackensack, NJ 07021, USA
e-mail: hossein@ix.netcom.com; http://www.hsadeghi.com

J.P. Mulhall and W. Hsiao (eds.), *Men's Sexual Health and Fertility*,
DOI 10.1007/978-1-4939-0425-9_5, © Springer Science+Business Media New York 2014

Table 5.1 Tests available for sexually transmitted infections, site specific

Chlamydial infection	
Endocervical swab	NAATs
Urethral swab	Cell culture
	Direct immunofluorescence
	EIA
	Nucleic acid hybridization tests
Urine	NAATs
Vaginal Swab	NAATs
Rectal swab	NAATs
Oropharyngeal swab	Nucleic acid hybridization tests
Gonococcal infections	
Male urethral swab	Gram stain
	Culture
	Nucleic acid hybridization tests
	NAATs
Endocervical swab	Culture
	NAATs
Vaginal swab	NAATs
Urine	NAATs
Oropharyngeal swab	NAATs (not FDA approved)
Rectal swab	
Conjunctival swab	
Herpes Simplex Virus	
Direct swab	Viral culture
	Viral PCR
Serology	HSV-specific glycoprotein 1 and 2 Abs
HIV	
Serology First Line	HIV 1 and 2 EIA
Serology Confirmation	Western Blot
	Indirect Immunofluorescence
	HIV RNA assay
	p24 antigen
HPV	
Cervical swab	NAATs
Syphilis	
Direct test	Dark-field microscopy
	T. pallidum PCR
Serology	Syphilis EIA
	fluorescent treponemal antibody absorbed tests [FTA-ABS] tests, *T. pallidum* passive particle agglutination [TP-PA] assay, with either
	Venereal Disease Research Laboratory (VDRL)
	RPR
Trichomoniasis	
Vaginal swab	Wet prep microscopy

(continued)

Table 5.1 (continued)

	Culture
	NAATs
	Point-of-care tests (nucleic acid probe test immunochromatographic capillary flow)
Urethral swab	Culture
Semen	NAATs
Urine	NAATs

Table 5.2 US recommended treatment for specific STIs

Chlamydial infections	
1st Line	Azithromycin 1 g orally in a single dose
	Doxycycline 100 mg orally twice a day for 7 days
Alternative	Erythromycin base 500 mg orally four times a day for 7 days
	Erythromycin ethylsuccinate 800 mg orally four times a day for 7 days
	Levofloxacin 500 mg orally daily for 7 days
	Ofloxacin 300 mg orally twice a day for 7 days
Gonococcal infections	
1st Line	Ceftriaxone 250 mg IM
	with
	Azithromycin 1 g stat or doxycycline 100 mg twice daily for 7 days
Herpes Simplex Virus	
Primary infection	Acyclovir 400 mg 3 times a day for 7–10 days
	Acyclovir 200 mg 5 times a day for 7–10 days
	Famciclovir 250 mg 3 times a day for 7–10 days
	Valacyclovir 1 g twice a day for 7–10 days
Recurrent infection	Acyclovir 400 mg orally 3 times a day for 5 days
	Acyclovir 800 mg orally twice a day for 5 days
	Famciclovir 125 mg orally twice a day for 5 days
	Famciclovir 1000 mg orally twice a day for 1 day
	Famciclovir 500 mg orally once then 250 mg twice daily for 2 days
	Valacyclovir 500 mg orally twice a day for 3 days
	Valacyclovir 1 g orally once a day for 5 days
Suppression	Acyclovir 400 mg orally twice a day
	Famciclovir 250 mg orally twice a day
	Valacyclovir 500 mg orally once a day
	Valacyclovir 1 g orally once a day
HIV-1[a]	
Treatment naive	Efavirenz/tenofovir disoproxil/emtricitabine
	Ritonavir-boosted atazanavir + tenofovir disoproxil/emtricitabine
	Ritonavir boosted darunavir + tenofovir disoproxil/emtricitabine
	Raltegravir + tenofovir disoproxil/emtricitabine
Virological resistance	Regimen tailored to resistance tests and previous treatment history
HPV	
Genital warts	Imiquimod 5 % cream
	Podophyllotoxin 0.15 %
	Cryotherapy

(continued)

Table 5.2 (continued)

	Excision
	Electrosurgery
	Laser surgery
Precancerous cells	Stage dependent
Syphilis	
Early syphilis	Benzathine penicillin G 2.4 million units IM in single dose
Early latent syphilis	Benzathine penicillin G 2.4 million units IM in single dose
Late latent syphilis	Benzathine penicillin G 7.2 million units total, administered as three doses of 2.4 million units each at 1-week intervals
Syphilis of unknown duration	Benzathine penicillin G 7.2 million units total, administered as 3 doses of 2.4 million units each at 1-week intervals
Tertiary syphilis	Benzathine penicillin G 7.2 million units total, administered as 3 doses of 2.4 million units each at 1-week intervals
Neurological syphilis	Aqueous crystalline penicillin G 18–24 million units per day, administered as three to four million units IV every 4 h or continuous infusion, for 10–14 days
	or
	Procaine penicillin 2.4 million units IM once daily for 10–14 days with Probenecid 500 mg orally four times a day for 10–14 days
Trichomoniasis	
1st Line	Metronidazole 2 g orally in a single dose
	or
	Tinidazole 2 g orally in a single dose
Alternative regimen	Metronidazole 500 mg twice daily for 7 days

CDC. Sexually Transmitted Diseases Guidelines, 2010. Morbidity and mortality weekly report December 2010. Vol 59. No. RR-12. http://www.cdc.gov/std/treatment/2010/STD-Treatment-2010-RR5912.pdf. Accessed 18 August 2013

[a]National Institutes of Health. Guidelines for the use of antiretroviral agents in HIV-1-infected adults and adolescents. http://aidsinfo.nih.gov/contentfiles/lvguidelines/aa_recommendations.pdf. Accessed 18 August 2013

1997. The prevalence of HIV infection in people aged 15–49 years has remained constant at 0.8 % worldwide, though worryingly in some areas such as central Asia and Eastern Europe the prevalence has doubled in 8 years [4]. With the increased availability of Highly Active Anti Retroviral Therapy (HAART), there are now more people living with HIV infection despite the reduction in incidence. There are two types of HIV virus, HIV-1 and HIV-2. HIV-2 is a much rarer virus, mainly confined to Western Africa. HIV-2 is less aggressive, with a lower rate of progression to AIDS and a lower transmission risk compared to HIV-1. Some Antiretrovirals (ARVs) are not effective against HIV-2. All subsequent discussion will be about HIV-1 unless specified.

HIV is a retrovirus, an RNA virus that infects and replicates in human CD4 T cells. It is a blood borne virus and is transmitted through blood, blood products, sexual fluids, and exposure to other bodily fluids such as amniotic fluid, spinal fluid, and breast milk. The common routes of transmission are via sexual intercourse, mother-to-child transmission and by sharing injecting equipment. Initial infection with HIV is most commonly asymptomatic. Symptomatic seroconversion illness consists of flu-like symptoms, myalgia, rash, headaches, and fevers. Later in the disease process, with the subsequent fall in CD4 count, other symptoms develop including loss of weight and then more specific opportunistic diseases associated with HIV infection. AIDS (Acquired Immunodeficiency Syndrome) is a diagnosis made using the CDC classification (Centers for Disease Control and Prevention). The individual has to have detectable HIV antibody and either an abnormal CD4 cell count (<200 cells/mm^3 or <14 % of all functioning lymphocytes) or an AIDS defining illness.

HIV infection can be diagnosed via a blood or saliva test. A confirmatory test (Western blot) is used after a positive HIV screening test. The fourth generation ELISA (enzyme-linked immunosorbent assay) is recommended for use in the UK by BHIVA (British HIV Association). This test detects not only antibodies to HIV 1 and 2 but also the p24 antigen, and thus, it can detect HIV infection before the patient becomes antibody positive. Rapid point-of-care tests for HIV infection are available. These are highly sensitive though not specific for HIV infection. Confirmatory testing is required for all reactive results.

The treatment for HIV-1 infection is HAART, normally a combination of three drugs that belong to at least two different classes. Recommendations for starting HAART and the choice of combinations are provided by BHIVA, EACS (European Aids Clinical Society), and the CDC.

HIV Infection and Conception

HAART has dramatically improved the life expectancy of those living with HIV. This and other advances in HIV care have reduced morbidity and increased survival. HAART has also had a dramatic affect on mother to child transmission (MTCT). A study in the UK of over 2,000 women virologically suppressed on HAART found the MCTC rate was 0.1 % [5]. With this in mind, fertility and conceiving with HIV infection has now become an important issue. In serodiscordant couples, where condom use is used to prevent transmission, options for safe conception are vital.

If the female is HIV positive in the serodiscordant couple, self-insemination is an option. To obtain the semen the HIV negative male can either ejaculate into a container or have sex using a non-spermicidal condom. Self-insemination with semen, using a sterile 10 ml syringe, can then be performed by the couple after about 30 min once the ejaculate has liquefied. In serodiscordant couples where the male is HIV positive sperm washing is the safest way to conceive. It protects the female partner and child from HIV infection. The technique separates the sperm from the seminal fluid and non-germinal cells that potentially carry HIV. The process uses centrifugation and a swim-up method that has been proven to provide spermatozoa that are HIV-1 RNA and proviral DNA negative [6]. This sperm is then used to fertilize the woman during ovulation via intrauterine insemination

(IUI) or, if needed, in vitro fertilization (IVF) or intracytoplasmic sperm injection (ICSI). A multicentered retrospective study of over 3,390 cycles of sperm washing has not shown seroconversion in either the female partner or the child [7].

In 2008 "The Swiss statement" published by the Swiss Federal Commission on AIDS Related Issues stated clearly that after reviewing the literature, an HIV-infected individual is sexually noninfectious provided the individual complies with antiretroviral therapy (ART), the viral load has been non-detectable for at least six months and there are no additional sexually transmitted diseases present [8]. An interim report from the HPTN 052 study of heterosexual couples was subsequently released and showed that earlier initiation of ART led to a 96 % reduction in HIV transmission to the HIV uninfected partner [9]. With this information, in situations where sperm washing is not an option, some couples may wish to try to conceive naturally. To limit the exposure of the HIV negative partner, BHIVA guidelines recommend discussion on the fertility cycle and timed conception. Additional screening for fertility should be offered before unprotected sex commences to ensure conception via natural methods is likely [10].

Pre-exposure chemoprophylaxis (PrEP) is the use of daily antiretroviral medication in HIV seronegative people to reduce the risk of becoming HIV seropositive through sexual exposure. The FDA has recently approved the combination of tenovofir and emtricitabine for use in PrEP. This would be an alternative option in serodiscordant couples. The "Partners in PrEP Study" led by the University of Washington's International Clinical Research Center showed a reduction in risk of HIV transmission by 75 % (95 % CI 55–87 % $p < 0.001$) using once daily tenofovir–emtricitabine (Truvada) [11].

HIV Infection and Fertility

HIV can affect fertility in a number of ways. There have been several studies showing abnormal semen parameters in HIV positive males. A relatively large study showed that ejaculate volume, sperm concentration, total count, progressive motility, and normal morphology were all significantly lower in HIV positive men. There was a significant positive correlation observed between CD4 count and sperm concentration, total count, motility, progressive motility, and post-preparation concentration and also a significant negative correlation with normal sperm morphology [12]. Interestingly, this same study showed that an HIV viral load of <1,000 copies/ml and receiving HAART significantly improved IUI outcome, indicating a secondary benefit from being on treatment. Other studies suggest HIV positive men have more viscous semen containing fewer motile sperm and more round cells [13]. It has been shown that with prolongation of survival in AIDS patients there was more pronounced loss of germ cells within the testes [14]. HIV infection is known to cause secondary hypogonadism and a thus a low testosterone level [15]. Low testosterone is associated with a reduction in sperm count. HIV positive men are more likely to suffer from erectile dysfunction and low sexual desire [16]. Patients on HAART were found to have raised estradiol levels that were associated with low sexual desire [16, 17]. Low sexual desire and erectile dysfunction may impact further on the ability to conceive. With regard to HIV positive females, prior to antenatal screening and HAART there was a 67 % increased risk of spontaneous abortion. In the HAART era, HIV positive women are still less likely to conceive, but when they do they have miscarriage rates similar to HIV negative women. Despite some ARVs being associated with preterm labor there has been an overall reduction in stillbirths and prematurity. Though IVF is available for HIV positive women the pregnancy rates are lower than the normal population. There is ovarian resistance to hyperstimulation which is independently associated with CD4 count [18]. There is also a theoretical risk to the embryo of HIV transmission with invasive techniques used but more evidence is required.

Herpes Simplex Virus Type I and II

Genital herpes is caused by Herpes Simplex Virus (HSV) type 1 and 2, members of the Herpesviridae family. The virus has an active and latent phase. After the primary infection the virus is transported along the sensory nerves to the nerve bodies where it multiplies. The virus travels back along the nerve axon to the skin continuously, though reoccurrence occurs only when the virus is no longer controlled by the CD8 dermal cells [19]. The episodes of active disease tend to reduce in frequency and severity over time. Up to 90 % of people who are HSV type 2 antibody positive have never knowingly had an outbreak of genital herpes [20]. Transmission is most likely during periods of active disease but asymptomatic shedding of the virus does occur without evidence of lesions [21].

HSV infection presents initially as erythema, progressing to blisters on the skin. These break down to form painful ulcers, most commonly on the genitals or around the mouth. There may be a preceding prodromal phase of flu like illness, aching in the groin or tingling over the skin prior to lesions appearing. The primary infection is often the most severe. This can be associated with fever, headache, malaise, and myalgia, and can lead to complications such as urinary retention or aseptic meningitis. It is also associated with miscarriage in pregnancy.

Diagnosis was previously made by viral isolation and culture. With the development of PCR techniques the diagnosis of HSV has improved. Serum antibody tests can be performed but this only confirms previous exposure to HSV 1 or 2 and does not predict whether the patient has symptomatic disease. Treatment of a primary episode is with antiviral medication such as acyclovir. Supportive treatment such as analgesia and topical lidocaine may also be needed. With recurrent episodes treatment needs to be implemented early to have maximal impact on the duration of symptoms. In frequent or severe recurrence, suppression therapy may be indicated with daily antivirals.

HSV and Fertility

Conclusive evidence for the association of HSV 1 and 2 on fertility is lacking. HSV DNA has been found more frequently in infertile men [22]. Studies have shown HSV is associated with significantly lower sperm count and motility [23–25]. In HSV positive men reduced citrate and alpha glucosidase levels, associated with impaired prostate and epididymal function, have also been observed [24]. Treatment of both couples for HSV with acyclovir has lead to pregnancy in some small studies [26, 27]. Other studies have shown no effect of HSV on sperm parameters [22, 27, 28]. Genital HSV transmission is via skin to skin contact. Though condoms offer a degree of protection depending on the site of viral shedding HSV transmission may still occur. HSV is a very stigmatizing disease, in part due to the incurable nature of the virus. In August 2011, a man was jailed in the UK for transmitting HSV-2 to his partner as he did not disclose his status. The psychological distress and psychosexual problems associated with a diagnosis of HSV infection and recurrent HSV infections have been well described in the literature, though there is some debate as to whether these are due to long term effects of HSV infection or whether some patients are predisposed to anxiety [29–31]. In recurrent genital herpes suppressive treatment with daily antiviral therapy has been shown to improve quality of life, reduce anxiety [32] and reduce transmission rates [33]. The reduction in transmission rate is important for serodiscordant couples who wish to conceive but normally rely on condoms to prevent transmission.

Human Papillomavirus

Many types of Human Papillomavirus (HPV) have been isolated that affect the genital region and are transmitted via sexual contact. The most common types are HPV 16 and 18, high-grade oncogenic viruses, and HPV 6 and 11, low-grade viruses responsible for genital warts. The prevalence of HPV infection in the USA has recently been estimated to be 26.8 % among females aged 14–59 years [34]. Genital warts are typically flesh colored raised or flat lesions, often with a typical roughened keratinized head. Genital warts are diagnosed by examination and infection with the high grade oncogenic HPV is diagnosed by DNA PCR. HPV infection in many cases is self-limiting and the virus is cleared without the need for medical attention. In the case of genital warts, patients may request treatment with cryotherapy or topical treatments. Condoms provide some, but not total protection from HPV.

HPV Infection and Fertility

Studies of HPV and male fertility have tended to isolate types 16 and 18, the high-grade oncogenic viruses, as the viruses associated with male infertility. Studies have shown a significant association with asthenospermia [35], a reduced total sperm count [24] and an effect on some aspects of sperm motility. Though not significant, a trend towards impaired sperm function was seen in several studies [34–36]. In contrast other studies have seen no effect on semen volume, sperm concentration or motility, or any associated oligospermia or asthenospermia [36, 37]. It is unclear if there is a direct effect on the sperm or whether the presence of HPV alters the pH of the semen, thus impairing sperm motility [36]. There is conflicting data as to whether HPV causes psychological problems including sexual enjoyment and frequency of intercourse [38–41]. In practice we often see young men complaining of sexual dysfunction after a diagnosis of HPV infection has been made.

Trichomonas vaginalis

Trichomonas vaginalis, a member of the Trichomonadidae family, is an anaerobic, flagellated protozoan that lives in the human urogenital tract. It is the most common sexually transmitted infection worldwide with an estimated 173 million cases in 1999 [42]. The estimated prevalence in the USA is 3.1 % [43]. Infection tends to be asymptomatic, only causing symptoms in about 30 % of cases. The symptoms in men include dysuria, irritation in the urethra, or urethral discharge. Diagnosis can be made by culture, wet mount, NAATs (nucleic acid amplification tests), and point-of-care tests. Wet mount examination is less reliable in men compared to women. Staining methods should have confirmatory testing. In most cases treatment consists of immediate administration of 2 g of metronidazole.

Trichomonas and Fertility

The association is controversial. Some research has shown that the presence of Trichomonas was associated with reduced sperm motility and viability with a reduction in the percentage of normal morphology when compared to men without Trichomonas. Treatment significantly improved these parameters in 50 % of men after one dose of metronidazole [44]. In vitro mixing of sperm with Trichomonas showed reduced sperm activity [45]; it has also been shown that a proteinaceous substance produced by Trichomonas kills sperm rapidly [46]. Conversely a study by Daly showed no effect on sperm number or motility with the presence of Trichomonas in vitro [47].

Syphilis

Syphilis is a relatively common STD, with approximately 12 million new infections each year worldwide [48]. There is wide geographic variation in the rates of syphilis. In the newly independent states of the former Soviet Union, rates have risen dramatically since 1990 from an estimated 5–15 per 100,000 to 120–170 per 100,000 in 1999. More recent data from surveillance of syphilis in the USA showed that there were 45,834 reported cases of syphilis in 2010, at a rate of 14.9 per 100,000 [49]. The majority of these cases were in urban areas or the Southern states. In the UK, the rates of infectious syphilis (primary, secondary or early latent) peaked in 2005 and were 5.6 per 100,000 in 2011 [50].

Syphilis is caused by infection with *Treponema pallidum*. Transmission occurs through direct inoculation from an infectious lesion (through sexual contact including vaginal and anal sex, oral sex, and mutual masturbation), mother to child in utero and also rarely through blood and blood products.

For classification, stages and clinical presentation of syphilis *see* Table 5.3.

Diagnosis can be made in early syphilis by direct visualization of spirochetes from a syphilitic lesion via dark-ground microscopy. There is also specific *T. pallidum* PCR that can be performed from a swab taken from a chancre. Most commonly syphilis is diagnosed by serological tests. Screening consists of using an automated treponemal test, usually the EIA (enzyme immunoassay) for IgG, with or without IgM, and confirmation with TPPA (*T. pallidum* particle agglutination assay) or TPHA (*T. pallidum* hemagglutination assay). Nonspecific tests include VDRL and RPR. These are indicators of infectivity and are normally raised in early syphilis. The subsequent fall in RPR is an important marker of successful treatment.

Treatment is with antibiotics, most evidence supporting a penicillin-based regime. The length, dose, and delivery of treatment with repository penicillin are dependent on the stage of disease and clinical scenario. There are alternative regimes such as doxycycline. The CDC, British Association for Sexual Health and HIV (BASHH), and International Union against Sexually Transmitted infections (IUSTI) provide up-to-date treatment guidelines available online [51–53].

Syphilis and Fertility

Testing both partners for syphilis and treating as required is imperative before proceeding with any form of fertility treatment. The effects of infectious syphilis on the unborn child are devastating and include spontaneous abortion and still birth in 50 %, with mortality of infected infants being over 10 % [54].

Though a direct effect of syphilis on male fertility is not described in the literature, complications of syphilis can affect fertility. Tabes dorsalis is a known cause of erectile dysfunction. Gummatous lesions within the testis can lead to destruction of the testicular tissue. Chronic obliterative endarteritis and interstitial

Table 5.3 Classification, stages, and clinical presentation of syphilis

Classification	Stages		Time	Clinical signs and symptoms
Acquired	Early	Primary syphilis	3–90 days after inoculation (normally 14–21 days)	Chancre (single painless ulcer) regional lymphadenopathy
		Secondary syphilis	4–10 weeks after primary infection	Generalized rash (macular, papular, or maculo-papular) Generalized lymphadenopathy Mucocutaneous lesions Condylomata lata Headaches Cranial nerve palsies Optic neuritis Anterior uveitis Hepatitis Glomerulonephritis Periosteitis
		Early latent	Acquired less than 1 year previously (CDC) <2 years (WHO)	Serological evidence without clinical features
	Late	Late latent	Acquired more than 1 year previously (CDC) >2 years (WHO)	Serological evidence without clinical features
		Meningovascular	2–7 years	Focal arteritis leading to infarction and presenting as a cerebral vascular accident
		Cardiovascular	10–30 years	Aortitis (commonly ascending aorta) Aneurysm formation Dilation of the aortic root Coronary ostial stenosis causing angina
		Neurological	10–25 years	General paresis (decline in memory and cognitive function, emotional liability and personality changes, psychosis, dementia, seizures, and hemiparesis) Tabes doralis (pain, paraesthesia, loss of reflexes, and sensory ataxia) Argyll Robertson pupils Optic atrophy
		Gummatous	1–46 years (average 15 years)	Destructive inflammatory granulomas occurring in any organ

(continued)

Table 5.3 (continued)

Classification	Stages	Time	Clinical signs and symptoms
Congenital	Early –	Presentation before 2 years of age	Hepatosplenomegaly Rash Generalized lymphadenopathy Hemorrhagic rhinitis Perioral fissures Osteochondritis Neurological involvement Non-immune hydrops
	Late –	Presentation >2 years after birth	Interstitial keratitis Hutchinson's incisors Mulberry molars Saddle nose deformity High palatal arch Saber shin Clutton's joints Neurological involvement Gummatous involvement

CDC Centers for Disease Control and Prevention, *WHO* World Health Organisation

inflammation can occur in congenital or tertiary syphilis, and lead to small, fibrotic testes [55]. Syphilitic epididymitis has also been described and classified into three forms: acute diffuse interstitial, chronic diffuse interstitial, and gummatous [56]. With a chronic inflammatory process there is fibrosis and scarring with the potential to cause obstruction of the epididymis. We postulate that, though rare, these complications and the psychological effect of having an STI may also have an adverse impact on male fertility.

Neisseria gonorrhea

Gonorrhea is caused by *Neisseria gonorrhea*, a gram-negative diplococcus. Worldwide there are an estimated 62 million people infected annually [57]. It accounted for 820,000 cases of STIs in the USA in 2008 [2]. Symptoms of genital infection include purulent discharge and dysuria. Infection can be asymptomatic, especially in the pharynx or rectum. Gonorrhea can cause conjunctivitis, epididymo-orchitis, prostatitis, or pelvic inflammatory disease through local spread or direct inoculation. Disseminated Gonococcal Infection (DGI) occurs in about 1 % of cases [57]. DGI commonly presents with a petechial or pustular rash, asymmetrical arthralgia, tenosynovitis, or septic arthritis. Rarely it can cause a perihepatitis, endocarditis, and meningitis.

Diagnosis is made by direct visualization on gram stain of a urethral, cervical, or rectal smear. It is then confirmed by culture. NAATs for gonorrhea are now widely used and are thought to have increased the diagnosis rate, especially in asymptomatic cases and extra-urethral sites.

A wide variety of antibiotics have been used to treat gonorrhea over the years. There have been issues with drug resistance. In view of this, it is always worth sending cultures for sensitivities whenever possible and following local guidelines on the use of antibiotics. Currently in the UK, ceftriaxone 500 mg IM injection is recommended for the treatment of gonorrhea. It is given with antibiotic cover for Chlamydia as 10 % of cases have both infections.

Gonorrhea and Fertility

Gonorrhea tends to cause an acute infective episode. The relationship between infection and infertility is due to the resultant PID in women. In men the subsequent scarring and obliteration of the epididymal canal following an acute infection is usually persistent even after cure. If bilateral, the infection can result in obstructive azoospermia [58].

Chlamydia trachomatis

Chlamydia trachomatis is a gram-negative, aerobic, intracellular bacterium. It is one of the most common sexually transmitted infections worldwide and the most commonly reported bacterial STI in England and the USA. Chlamydia is transmitted by sexual contact including the use of sex toys and also from mother to child. It can infect the cervix, urethra, rectum, pharynx, and conjunctiva. The majority of cases are asymptomatic. Male symptoms include urethral discomfort, pain on urination, urethral discharge, and testicular pain. The infection is normally confined to the urethra causing urethritis, but can ascend and cause prostatitis and epididymo-orchitis. NAATs are used widely to diagnose Chlamydia via a swab taken from the site of infection or first void urine sample (urethral infection). Other tests include culture, EIA, DFA (direct fluorescent antibody), and nucleic acid hybridization tests. Treatment is with a stat dose of azithromycin 1 g in most cases. Alternatives include doxycycline 100 mg bid for 1 week. If there is evidence of pelvic inflammatory disease or of ascending infection in the male (epididymitis, orchitis, or prostatitis), a longer course of antibiotics such as ofloxacin is recommended.

Chlamydia and Fertility

A common anxiety with a diagnosis of Chlamydia is the effect on a woman's fertility. Chlamydia is associated with pelvic inflammatory disease (PID) and female tubal infertility, though a recent study suggests the risk of developing PID with untreated Chlamydia is low with a relative risk of 0.17 (0.03–1.01) $p = 0.07$ after 1 year follow-up. PID was, in fact, seen more frequently in Chlamydia negative women [59]. With regard to male infertility, the connection is even less clear. There are several theories as to how Chlamydia may affect male fertility. These include a direct effect of the Chlamydia, the presence of associated inflammation, or the development of anti-sperm antibodies triggered by Chlamydia. The research has been contradictory and is inconclusive. It has been shown that the presence of elementary bodies of *C. trachomatis* serovar E within the lab setting caused a significant decrease in motile sperm with an increase of dead spermatozoa [60]. The detection of Chlamydia in either semen or urine has been associated with a reduction in sperm numbers [61], reduction of the percentage of progressively motile sperm [62–65], and abnormal morphology and viability [65].

Chlamydia has also been shown to cause sperm DNA fragmentation that improves with treatment [64]. Chlamydia has not been shown to affect the percentage of immotile or viable sperm [62], and there are other contrasting studies that show no association with DNA fragmentation [63] or effect on sperm concentration, motility, and/or morphology [66]. The presence of *C. trachomatis* antibodies, therefore, has not been shown to be conclusively linked to infertility, although there are studies suggesting an association [67], and others showing that despite an associated inflammatory response, there was no effect on sperm parameters [68].

Male Accessory Gland Infections

Male accessory gland infections (MAGIs) include urethritis, epididymitis, orchitis, and prostatitis. These infections are potentially curable causes of male infertility, though studies so far have not been conclusive in showing an effect on sperm quality and male fertility. A study has shown that MAGI with abnormal semen quality as the only abnormality was seen in 1.6 % of infertile couples. Sperm motility and morphology showed improvement over time whether treated or not, and this improvement did not seem to enhance the probability of conception [69].

Urethritis

Urethritis is most commonly caused by infections such as *C. trachomatis*, *N. gonorrhea*, *Ureaplasma urealyticum* and *Mycoplasma genitalium*. Other less common causes are *T. vaginalis* and *Herpes simplex* virus. Urethritis can also be caused by allergic reactions and trauma. The main symptoms include pain on voiding and urethral discharge. Diagnosis is made on the clinical presence of mucopurulent or purulent discharge, ≥ 5 granulocytes per microscopic high power field (1,000×) on a urethral smear, a positive leukocyte esterase test on first-void urine, or microscopic examination of first-void urine sediment demonstrating ≥ 10

WBC per high-power [70]. Both CDC and BASHH guidelines recommend the use of a single dose of Azithromycin 1 g if gonorrhea is excluded on urethral gram stain.

A recent study found that there were more abnormalities of semen parameters in attendees of genitourinary medicine clinics, especially those patients with asymptomatic, Chlamydia negative, nonspecific urethritis as compared with men attending a General Practitioner (Family Physician) for the first check for possible infertility [71]. There have also been several studies looking at the effect of the bacterial pathogens that are associated with urethritis on sperm quality and fertility. A recent study showed that semen contaminations with *Mycoplasma* spp. and Chlamydia were associated with decreased sperm concentrations, with Mycoplasma having the highest adverse effect on sperm quality (concentration, motility, morphology, and DNA condensation). Unfortunately, despite successful antibiotic therapy, semen quality parameters did not improve at least up to 3 months after the therapy. Sperm chromatin integrity assessed by the presence of DNA breaks was not seen with these infections [72]. Also, when looking at the prevalence of these infections, there was no difference comparing fertile to infertile couples [73].

Epididymitis

Acute inflammation of the epididymis is most commonly caused by bacterial infection. A sexually transmitted infection such as Chlamydia or Gonorrhea is the most common cause in men less than 35 years of age. In older men, especially those with a history of bladder outlet obstruction, *Escherichia coli* is more common. Rarer causes of epididymitis include *Mycobacterium tuberculosis*. Noninfectious causes include Behcet's disease, urethral manipulation, following vasectomy and as an adverse effect of amiodarone. With any inflammatory process there is the risk of scarring and fibrosis. Though uncommon, bilateral occlusion of the epididymis is a cause of azoospermia and, therefore, male infertility.

Orchitis

Orchitis is defined as inflammation of one or both testes. It may be caused by a variety of viral and bacterial infections. Symptoms include tenderness or swelling in the groin or testes, as well as pain on intercourse or urination. Treatment is supportive, with treatment of any specific underlying cause if identified. Complications of orchitis include testicular atrophy and testicular infarction. Both conditions can impair testicular function and may have an adverse impact on fertility. Mumps occurring after puberty is commonly associated with unilateral or bilateral orchitis. This can cause reduced fertility in men.

Prostatitis

Prostatitis is classified into four distinct conditions by the National Institute of Diabetes and Digestive and Kidney Diseases (NIDDK) of the National Institutes of Health (NIH). Acute bacterial prostatitis, chronic bacterial prostatitis, chronic prostatitis/chronic pelvic pain (this may be inflammatory or non-inflammatory), and, finally, asymptomatic inflammatory prostatitis are often found when investigating other urological conditions or fertility issues.

The impact of chronic prostatitis on male fertility has not been conclusively proven. Chronic prostatitis caused by *C. trachomatis* was shown in one study to result in significant differences in sperm concentration, motility, and morphology compared to the effect of prostatitis due to other uropathogens [74].

A study of 30 men, all with leucocytosis, who had undergone long-term treatment for chronic prostatitis with antimicrobials showed improvement or normalization of the sperm count in 70 % [75]. A study published in 1991 compared patients with a diagnosis of chronic abacterial prostatovesiculitis (current NIDDK classification of chronic prostatitis/chronic pelvic pain) to age-matched asymptomatic controls. All the patients in the prostatitis group had ultrasound evidence of chronic inflammatory changes. The study showed that patients in the prostatitis group had an increased incidence of disturbed sperm quality and azoospermia, though some were normospermic. Not all patients in the prostatitis group had leukospermia and the degree of the leukospermia could not predict the extent of the disturbance in semen quality [76]. Psychological stress is common in patients with prostatitis, with 43 % of men with symptomatic prostatitis complaining of erectile dysfunction and 24 % reporting low libido [77], thus impacting further the ability to conceive.

Conclusion

The role that STIs play in male infertility is not fully understood. Many studies to date have shown conflicting results and the differing techniques used to analyze sperm makes comparison of the various studies difficult. The lack of markers for previous infection in some STIs adds to these research difficulties. For example, we cannot test for previous Gonorrhea infections. As for Chlamydia, serum IgG for Chlamydia is not specific for genital infection. IgA in the semen may be a more specific test for previous genital infection. Finding IgG antibodies to HSV 1 and 2 does not imply active disease.

Now that the WHO has produced an internationally agreed definition of sperm abnormalities and with the improvement in diagnostic tests, hopefully, we can expect some of the questions posed by research to date to be answered in the near future. It will remain difficult to determine which of the various factors may be relevant to the possible development of male infertility for each specific STI. Is it an effect related to the specific pathophysiology of the organism, or to the inflammatory response provoked, or to the nonspecific damage to the male genital tract? Is it mediated by changes to the sperm or the seminal fluid? What part does the psychological impact of the concept of infection play in the function of the man or his partner? We must not forget that various multiple and complex factors play a part in the normal process of conception, which evidentially differ even at an individual level, providing ample opportunity for disturbance by the pathophysiology of disease.

In the meantime it is always prudent to screen and treat those at risk of STIs. In infertile couples the screening and treatment of any underlying pathology is a sensible approach in order to avoid where possible both any impact on fertility and also the known complications of pregnancy.

References

1. World Health Organisation. 10 facts on sexually transmitted diseases. WHO. October 2008. http://www.who.int/features/factfiles/sexually_transmitted_diseases/en/index.html. Accessed 14 Aug 2013.
2. CDC fact sheet. Incidence, prevalence, and cost of sexually transmitted infections in the United States. CDC. 2013. http://www.cdc.gov/std/stats/STI-Estimates-Fact-Sheet-Feb-2013.pdf. Accessed 14 Aug 2013.
3. UNAIDS. World AIDS day report. 2011. UNAIDS. ISBN: 978-92-9173-904-2 | UNAIDS/JC2216E 2011. http://www.unaids.org/en/media/unaids/contentassets/documents/unaidspublication/2011/JC2216_WorldAIDSday_report_2011_en.pdf. Accessed 3 Sept 2012.
4. UNAIDS. Global report: UNAIDS report on the global AIDS epidemic. 2010. UNAIDS UNAIDS/10.11E | JC1958E. http://www.unaids.org/documents/20101123_globalreport_em.pdf. Accessed 3 Sept 2012.
5. Townsend CL, Cortina-Borja M, Peckham CS, de Ruiter A, Lyall H, Tookey PA. Low rates of mother-to-child transmission of HIV following effective pregnancy interventions in the United Kingdom and Ireland, 2000–2006. AIDS. 2008;22:973–81.
6. Kato S, Hanabusa H, Kaneko S, Takakuwa K, Suzuki M, Kuji N, et al. Complete removal of HIV-1 RNA and proviral DNA from semen by the swim-up method: assisted reproduction technique using spermatozoa free from HIV-1. AIDS. 2006;20(7):967–73.
7. Bujan L, Hollander L, Coudert M, Gilling-Smith C, Vucetich A, Guibert J, et al. Safety and efficacy of sperm washing in HIV-1-serodiscordant couples where the male is infected: results from the European CREAThE network. AIDS. 2007;21(14):1909–14.
8. Vernazza P, Hirschel B, Bernasconi E, Flepp M. Les personnes séropositives ne souffrant d'aucune autre MST et suivant un traitment antirétroviral efficace ne transmettent pas le VIH par voie sexuelle. *Bulletin des médecins suisses Schweizerische Ärztezeitung Bollettino dei medici svizzeri* 2008;89: 5. English translation. http://www.edwinjbernard.com/pdfs/Swiss%20Commission%20statement_May%202008_translation%20EN.pdf. Accessed 3 Sept 2012.
9. National Institutes of Health. Treating HIV-infected people with antiretrovirals protects partners from infection. Findings result from NIH-funded International Study. http://www.niaid.nih.gov/news/newsreleases/2011/Pages/HPTN052.aspx. Accessed 3 Sept 2012.
10. Fakoya A, Lamba H, Mackie N, Nandwani R, Brown A, Bernard EJ, et al. British HIV Association, BASHH and FSRH guidelines for the management of the sexual and reproductive health of people living with HIV infection 2008. HIV Med. 2008;9:681–720.

11. Baeten J, Donnell D, Ndase P, Mugo N, Campbell J, Wangisi J, et al. Antiretroviral prophylaxis for HIV prevention in heterosexual men and women. N Engl J Med. 2012;367:399–410.
12. Nicopoullos JD, Almeida PA, Ramsay JW, Gilling-Smith C. The effect of human immunodeficiency virus on sperm parameters and the outcome of intrauterine insemination following sperm washing. Hum Reprod. 2004;19(10):2289–97.
13. Crittenden JA, Handelsman DJ, Stewart GJ. Semen analysis in human immunodeficiency virus infection. Fertil Steril. 1992;57(6):1294–9.
14. Shevchuk M, Pigato JB, Khalife G, Armenakas N, Fracchia J. Changing testicular histology in AIDS: it's implication for sexual transmission of HIV. Urology. 1999;53910:203–8.
15. Crum-Crianflone NF, Bavaro M, Hale B, Amling C, Truett A, Brandt C, et al. Erectile dysfunction and hypogonadism among men with HIV. AIDS Patient Care STDS. 2007;21:9–19.
16. Lamba H, Goldmeier D, Mackie NE, Scullard G. Antiretroviral therapy is associated with sexual dysfunction and with increased serum oestradiol levels in men. Int J STD AIDS. 2004;15:234–7.
17. Goldmeier D, Scuallard G, Kapembwa M, Lamba H, Frize G. Does increased aromatase activity in adipose fibroblasts cause low sexual desire in patients with HIV lipodystrophy? Sex Transm Infect. 2002;78:64–6.
18. Coll O, Suy A, Figueras F, Vernaeve V, Martinez E, Mataro D, et al. Decreased pregnancy rate after in-vitro fertilization in HIV-infected women receiving HAART. AIDS. 2006;20(1):121–33.
19. Schiffer J, Abu-Raddad L, Mark K, Zhu J, Selke S, Koelle D, et al. Mucosal host immune response predicts the severity and duration of herpes simplex virus-2 genital tract shedding episodes. Proc Natl Acad Sci U S A. 2010;107(44):18973–8.
20. Fleming D, McQuillan G, Johnson R, Nahmias A, Aral S, Lee F, et al. Herpes Simplex Virus Type 2 in the United States, 1976 to 1994. N Engl J Med. 1997;337:1105–11.
21. Wald A, Zeh J, Selke S, Warren T, Ryncarz A, Ashley R, et al. Reactivation of genital Herpes Simplex Virus Type 2 infection in asymptomatic seropositive persons. N Engl J Med. 2000;342:844–50.
22. Borai N, Masato I, Lefevre C, Naumova E, Sato B, Yamamura M. Detection of Herpes Simplex DNA in semen and menstrual blood of individuals attending an infertility clinic. J Obstet Gynaecol Res. 1997;1:17–24.
23. Kapranos N, Petrakou E, Anastasiadou C, Kotronias D. Detection of Herpes simplex virus I and II, Cytomeglovirus and Epstein-Barr virus in the semen of men attending an infertility clinic. Fertil Steril. 2003;79(3):1566–70.
24. Bezold G, Politch JA, Kiviat NB, Kuypers JM, Wolff H, Anderson DJ. Prevalence of sexually transmissible pathogens in semen from asymptomatic male infertility patients with and without leukocytospermia. Fertil Steril. 2007;87(5):1087–97.
25. Kotronias D, Kapranos N. Detection of herpes simplex virus DNA in human spermatozoa by in situ hybridization technique. In Vivo. 1998;12:391–4.
26. Kundsin RB, Falk L, Hertig AT, Horne HW. Acyclovir treatment of twelve unexplained infertility couples. Int J Fertil. 1987;32:200–4.
27. Borai N, Lefevre C, Inove M, Naumova EN, Sato K, Suzuki S, et al. Presences of HSV-1 DNA in semen and menstrual blood. J Reprod Immunol. 1998;41:137–48.
28. Bezold G, Schuster-Grusser A, Lange M, Gall H, Wolff H, Uwe Peter R. Prevalence of human herpesvirus type 1-8 in the semen of infertility patients and correlation with semen parameters. Fertil Steril. 2001;76(2):416–8.
29. Brookes JL, Hayward S, Green J. Adjustment to the psychological and social sequelae of recurrent genital herpes simplex infection. Genitourin Med. 1993;69:384–7.
30. Catotti DN, Clarke P, Catoe KE. Herpes revisited: still a cause for concern. Sex Transm Dis. 1993;20:77–80.

31. Rosenthal S, Zimet G, Leichliter J, Stanberry L, Fife K, Tu W, et al. The psychosocial impact of serological diagnosis of asymptomatic herpes simplex virus type 2 infection. Sex Transm Infect. 2006;82:154–7.
32. Carney O, Ross E, Ikkos G, Mindel A. The effect of suppressive oral acyclovir on the psychological morbidity associated with recurrent genital herpes. Genitourin Med. 1993;69:457–9.
33. Corey L, Wald A, Patel R, et al. Once-daily valacyclovir to reduce the risk of transmission of genital herpes. N Engl J Med. 2004;350:11–20.
34. Dunne EF, Unger ER, Sternberg M, McQuillan G, Swan DC, Patel SS, et al. Prevalence of HPV infection among females in the United States. JAMA. 2007;297(80):813–9.
35. Lai YM, Lee JF, Huang HY, Soong YK, Yang FP, Pao CC. The effect of human papillomavirus infection on sperm motility. Fertil Steril. 1997;67:1152–5.
36. Rintala MAM, Grenman SE, Pollanen PP, Suominen JJO, Syrjanen SM. Detection of high risk HPV DNA in semen and its association with the quality of semen. Int J STD AIDS. 2004;15:740–3.
37. Tanaka H, Karube A, Kodama H, Fukuda J, Tanaka T. Mass screening for human papilloma virus type 16 infection in infertile couples. J Reprod Med. 2000;45:907–11.
38. Conaglen HM, Hughes R, Conaglen JV, Morgan J. A prospective study of the psychological impact on patients of first diagnosis of human papillomavirus. Int J STD AIDS. 2001;12:651–8.
39. Maw RD, Reitano M, Roy M. An international survey of patients with genital warts: perceptions regarding treatment and impact on lifestyle. Int J STD AIDS. 1998;9:571–8.
40. Reed BD, Ruffin MT, Gorenflo DW, Zazove P. The psychosexual impact of human papillomavirus cervical infections. J Fam Pract. 1999;48:110–6.
41. Clarke P, Ebel C, Catotti DN, Stewart S. The psychosocial impact of human papillomavirus infection: implications for health care providers. Int J STD AIDS. 1996;7(3):197–200.
42. World Health Organisation. Global prevalence and incidence of selected curable sexually transmitted infections overview and estimates. http://www.who.int/hiv/pub/sti/who_hiv_aids_2001.02.pdf. Accessed 24 Sept 2012.
43. Sutton M, Sternberg M, Koumans EH, McQuillan G, Berman S, Markowitz LE. The prevalence of Trichomonas vaginalis infection among reproductive-age women in the United States, 2001–2004. Clin Infect Dis. 2007;45(10):1319–26.
44. Gopalkrishnan K, Hinduja IN, Anand Kumar TC. Semen characteristics of asymptomatic males affected by Trichomonas vaginalis. J In Vitro Fert Embryo Transf. 1990;7(3):165–7.
45. Tuttle J, Holbrook T, Derrick F. Interference of human spermatozoal motility by Trichomonas vaginalis. J Urol. 1977;118:1024–5.
46. Jarecki-Black J, Lushbaugh W, Golosov L, Glassman AB. Trichomonas vaginalis: preliminary characterization of sperm motility inhibiting factor. Ann Clin Lab Sci. 1988;18:484–9.
47. Daly JJ, Sherman JK, Green L, Hostetler TL. Survival of Trichomonas vaginalis in human semen. Genitourin Med. 1989;65:106.
48. World Health Organisation. Global prevalence and incidence of selected curable sexually transmitted infections overview and estimates. http://www.who.int/hiv/pub/sti/who_hiv_aids_2001.02.pdf. Accessed 24 July 2012.
49. Center for Disease Control and Protection. 2010. STD surveillance. http://www.cdc.gov/std/stats10/syphilis.htm. Accessed 24 July 2012.
50. Health Protection Agency. Sexually transmitted infections annual data. http://www.hpa.org.uk/stiannualdatatables/. Accessed 25 July 2012.
51. Center for Disease Control and Protection. Sexually transmitted diseases treatment guidelines. 2010. http://www.cdc.gov/std/treatment/2010/STD-Treatment-2010-RR5912.pdf. Accessed 25 July 2012.
52. British Association for Sexual Health and HIV. Guidelines. http://www.bashh.org/guidelines/. Accessed 25 July 2012.

53. International Union against Sexually Transmitted Infections. Guidelines/resources. http://www.iusti.org/regions/Europe/euroguidelines.htm. Accessed 25 July 2012.
54. World Health Organisation. Standards for maternal and neonatal care. Prevention of mother-to-child transmission of syphilis. Integrated management of pregnancy and childbirth (IMPAC). http://www.who.int/reproductivehealth/publications/maternal_perinatal_health/prevention_mtct_syphilis.pdf. Accessed 30 July 2012.
55. Cheng L, Bostwick DG (eds) Essentials of anatomic pathology. Totowa, NJ, Humana Press; 2002.
56. Micelson H.E. Syphilis of the epididymis. JAMA. 1919; 73(19): 1431–33. http://jama.jamanetwork.com/Issue.aspx?journalid=67&issueID=5672&direction=P.html. Accessed 25 July 2012.
57. World Health Organisation. http://www.who.int/vaccine_research/diseases/soa_std/en/index2.html. Accessed 8 Oct 2012.
58. Harkness AH. The pathology of gonorrhea. Br J Vener Dis. 1948;24940:137–47.
59. Oakeshott P, Kerry S, Aghaizu A, Atherton H, Hay S, Taylor-Robinson D, et al. Randomised controlled trial of screening for Chlamydia trachomatis to prevent pelvic inflammatory disease: the POPI (prevention of pelvic infection) trial. Br Med J. 2010;340:c1642. http://www.ncbi.nlm.nih.gov/pmc/articles/PMC2851939/. Accessed 12 Nov 2012.
60. Hosseinzadeh S, Brewis IA, Eley A, Pacey A. Co-incubation of human spermatozoa with Chlamydia trachomatis serovar E causes premature sperm death. Hum Reprod. 2001;2:293–9.
61. Rybar R, Prinosilova P, Kopecka V, Hlavicova J, Veznik Z, Zajicova A, et al. The effect of bacterial contamination of semen on sperm chromatin integrity and standard semen parameters in men from infertile couples. Andrologia. 2012;44 Suppl 1:410–8.
62. Kokab A, Akhondi MM, Sadeghi MR, Modarresi MH, Aarabi M, Jennings R, Pacey AA, Eley A. Raised inflammatory markers in semen from men with asymptomatic chlamydial infection. J Androl. 2010;31(2):114–20.
63. Gdoura R, Keskes-Ammar L, Bouzid F, Eb F, Hammami A, Orfila J. Chlamydia trachomatis and male infertility in Tunisia. Eur J Contracept Reprod Health Care. 2001;6(2):102–7.
64. Gallegos G, Ramos B, Santiso R, Goyanes V, Gosalvez J, Fernandez JL. Sperm DNA fragmentation in infertile men with genitourinary infection by Chlamydia trachomatis and Myoplasma. Fertil Steril. 2008;90(2):328–34.
65. Cengiz T, Aydoganli L, Baykam M, Mungan NA, Tuncbilek E, Dincer M, et al. Chlamydial infections and male infertility. Int Urol Nephrol. 1997;29(6):687–93.
66. Vigi P, Morales P. Chlamydia trachomatis infection in male partners of infertile couples: incidence and sperm function. Andrologia. 2002;34(3):155–61.
67. Joki-Korpela P, Sahrakorpi N, Halttunen M, Surcel HM, Paavonen J, Tiitinen A. The role of Chlamydia trachomatis infection in male infertility. Fertil Steril. 2009;91(4):1448–50.
68. Ochsendorf FR, Özdemir K, Rabenau H, Fenner T, Oremek R, Milbradt R, Doerr HW. Chlamydia trachomatis and male infertility: chlamydia-IgA antibodies in seminal plasma are C. trachomatis specific and associated with an inflammatory response. J Eur Acad Dermatol Venereol. 1999;12(2):143–52.
69. Comhaire F, Rowe P, Farley T. The effect of doxycycline in infertile couples with male accessory gland infection: a double blind prospective study. Int J Androl. 1986;9(2):91–8.
70. Centers for Disease Control and Protection. Sexually transmitted diseases treatment guidelines. 2010. http://www.cdc.gov/std/treatment/2010/urethritis-and-cervicitis.htm. Accessed 17 Sept 2012.
71. Carne CA, Chilcott S, Palmer C, Green O, Bridge S, Walsh R, et al. Low sperm counts in genitourinary medicine clinic attendees: results from a case–control study. Sex Transm Infect. 2012;88(6):422–6.
72. Rybar R, Prinosilova P, Kopecka V, Hlavicova J, Veznik Z, Zajicova A, Rubes J. The effect of bacterial contamination of semen on sperm chromatin integrity and standard semen parameters in men from infertile couples. Andrologia. 2012;44 Suppl 1:410–8.

73. Gunyeli I, Abike F, Dunder I, Aslan C, Tapisiz OL, Temizkan O, et al. Chlamydia, Mycoplasma and Ureaplasma infections in infertile couples and effects of these infections on fertility. Arch Gynecol Obstet. 2011;283(2):379–85.
74. Mazzoli S, Cai T, Addonisio P, Bechi A, Mondaini N, Bartoletti R. Chlamydia trachomatis infection is related to poor semen quality in young prostatitis patients. Eur Urol. 2010;57 (4):708–14.
75. Giamarellou H, Tympanidis K, Bitos N, Leonidas E, Daiko GH. Infertility and chronic prostatitis. Andrologia. 1984;16(5):417–22.
76. Christiansen E, Tollefsrud A, Purvis K. Sperm quality in men with chronic abacterial prostatovesiculitis verified by rectal ultrasonography. Urology. 1991;38(6):545–9.
77. Mehik A, Hellström P, Sarpola A, Lukkarinen O, Jarvelin MR. Fears, sexual disturbances and personality features in men with prostatitis: a population-based cross-sectional study in Finland. BJU Int. 2001;88(1):35–8.

Chapter 6
Erectile Dysfunction and Infertility

Vikram Soni, Alexander W. Pastuszak, and Mohit Khera

Introduction

Infertility and sexual dysfunction in men, specifically erectile dysfunction (ED), are distinct entities that share a complex and interdependent relationship with one another. This chapter discusses the similarities and differences between the etiologies and treatments for each condition and highlights the potential impact infertility may have on male sexual function. It is important to consider these as linked entities during evaluation of affected men and to structure treatment approaches while considering the numerous and varied causes of both ED and male infertility, given the close relationship between the two conditions.

Approximately 60–75 % of couples conceive within 6 months of initiating unprotected sexual intercourse, with 90 % conceiving within 1 year [1, 2]. Based on these data, infertility is defined as an inability to conceive after at least 12 months of regular, unprotected intercourse. Approximately 15 % of couples have fertility difficulties, with a male factor implicated in up to 50 % of these cases [3]. Extrapolated further, these data suggest that close to 8 % of all men of reproductive age will seek medical treatment for infertility at some point in their lives [4]. Clearly, these numbers are not insignificant. Fortunately the treatment of both male and female infertility has dramatically improved over the past three decades with the advent of assisted reproductive technologies (ART), including in vitro fertilization (IVF) and intracytoplasmic sperm injection (ICSI). These treatment methods have offered the ability to bypass many of the most vexing causes of male infertility but also come at a substantial cost: an estimated $1.8 billion dollars was spent on ART in the United States in the year 2000 alone [5]. According to a recent industry analysis, ART now results in more than 50,000 babies per year in the United States via more than 140,000 IVF procedures, a number that has nearly tripled since 1999.

M. Khera (✉)
Scott Department of Urology, Baylor College of Medicine, 6620 Main St, Suite 1325, Houston, TX, USA
e-mail: mkhera@bcm.edu

J.P. Mulhall and W. Hsiao (eds.), *Men's Sexual Health and Fertility*,
DOI 10.1007/978-1-4939-0425-9_6, © Springer Science+Business Media New York 2014

There are more than 450 infertility clinics, 100+ sperm banks, an unknown number of egg donors, and more than 1,700 reproductive specialists competing for a slice of a very lucrative business—the infertility services sector has swelled to an estimated $4 billion dollar industry [6].

However, these approaches often do not take into consideration the fundamental causes of male infertility, which are increasingly known to be genetic in nature, leading to an increased risk of genetic disease in the offspring as well as an increased risk of masking significant medical pathology in the male partner [7, 8]. The causes of male infertility are numerous and include a variety of congenital and acquired disorders (Table 6.1). Inherent to an inability to father a child naturally is the inability to have an erection sufficient for penetration and duration of sexual intercourse, and men with ED may have difficulties with fertility as a result not only due to the inability of vaginal penetration but also potentially due to dysregulation of the hypothalamic-pituitary-gonadal (HPG) axis which may result from hormonal imbalance, leading to both infertility and ED.

ED is defined as an inability to achieve or maintain an erection sufficient for satisfactory sexual intercourse [9]. ED is estimated to affect 30 million men in the United States and carries a 10–20 % worldwide prevalence rate [10, 11]. Despite a growing understanding of the pathophysiology of ED and persistent improvements in treatment modalities, ED prevalence rates continue to rise, and approximately 322 million men are expected to have ED by 2025, a large increase from 152 million men in 1995 [12]. Furthermore, the prevalence of ED increases with age and coincides with numerous chronic health conditions, including type II diabetes, cardiovascular disease, depression, dyslipidemia, hypertension, benign prostatic hypertrophy, lower urinary tract symptoms, and hypogonadism. Given the world's aging population and the increasing prevalence of the aforementioned comorbidities it is likely that the prevalence of ED will continue to increase [13–18]. As with infertility, ED also places a substantial economic burden on both patients and society. Between 1994 and 2000, expenditures for the management of ED, excluding the cost of pharmaceuticals, almost doubled from $185 million to $330 million [19, 20]. This increase in spending on ED treatment may represent an increased societal acceptance of ED as a treatable condition and a corresponding increase in self-reporting and acceptance of treatment on behalf of the male population [20]. With regard to incidence, a recent study found that during the period from 1995 to 2000 the incidence of ED increased from 5 to 6.5 % but has since stabilized at approximately 5 % per year [21]. However, as the prevalence of the above comorbidities continues to rise, we can expect the economic burden of ED to correspondingly increase.

Taken separately, infertility and ED have been well studied and treatment strategies for these two conditions have dramatically improved over the past two decades, coinciding with the development of ICSI in 1992 and the approval of phosphodiesterase-5 (PDE5) inhibitors in 1998. As the relationship between male infertility and ED becomes clearer, it is apparent that these conditions are inextricably linked. Evaluation and treatment of the infertile male may influence erectile function, and conversely, ED can impact a man's fertility. Given this relationship,

Table 6.1 Causes and distribution of male infertility

Hypothalamic-pituitary disorders (1–2 %)	
Congenital disorders	• Congenital GnRH deficiency (Kallmann syndrome) • Hemochromatosis • Multi-organ genetic disorders (Prader–Willi syndrome, Laurence–Moon–Biedl syndrome, familial cerebellar ataxia)
Acquired disorders	• Pituitary and hypothalamic tumors (macroadenoma, craniopharyngioma) • Infiltrative disorders (sarcoidosis, histiocytosis, tuberculosis, fungal infections) • Trauma, post-surgery, postirradiation • Vascular (infarction, aneurysm) • Hormonal (hyperprolactinemia, androgen excess, estrogen excess, cortisol excess) • Drugs (opioids and psychotropic medications, GnRH agonists or antagonists)
Systemic disorders	• Chronic illnesses • Nutritional deficiencies • Obesity
Primary gonadal disorders (30–40 %)	
Congenital disorders	• Klinefelter's syndrome (XXY) and its variants (XXY/XY; XXXY) • Cryptorchidism • Myotonic dystrophy • Functional prepubertal castrate syndrome (congenital anorchia) • Varicocele • Androgen-insensitivity syndromes • 5α-reductase deficiency • Y chromosome deletions
Acquired disorders	• Varicocele • Viral orchitis (mumps, echovirus, arbovirus) • Granulomatous orchitis (leprosy, tuberculosis) • Epididymo-orchitis (gonorrhea, chlamydia) • Drugs (e.g., alkylating agents, alcohol, marijuana, antiandrogens, ketoconazole, spironolactone, histamine2 receptor antagonists) • Ionizing radiation • Environmental toxins (e.g., dibromochloropropane, carbon disulfide, cadmium, lead, mercury, environmental estrogens, and phytoestrogens) • Hyperthermia • Immunologic disorders, including polyglandular autoimmune disease • Trauma • Torsion • Castration • Systemic illness (e.g., renal failure, hepatic cirrhosis, cancer, sickle cell disease, amyloidosis, vasculitis, celiac disease)
Disorders of sperm transport (10–20 %)	
	• Epididymal dysfunction (drugs, infection) • Abnormalities of the vas deferens (congenital absence, Young's syndrome, infection, vasectomy) • Ejaculatory dysfunction (spinal cord disease, autonomic dysfunction, premature ejaculation)
Idiopathic male infertility (40–50 %)	

the clinician should consider both conditions when developing a management plan for affected men.

In this chapter we provide a discussion of the similarities and differences between ED and male infertility—in terms of etiology and treatment—as well as the potential impact a diagnosis of infertility may have on male erectile function. Our goal is to provide clinicians and healthcare providers with a clearer understanding of the emerging links between ED and male factor infertility.

Differences and Common Links Between Male Infertility and Erectile Dysfunction

Numerous causes of ED and male infertility have been identified to date, though it is clear that not all etiologies are known for either condition. The causes of ED are frequently multifactorial, comprising a mix of organic and psychogenic factors [22] (Table 6.2). Many of the disorders in Table 6.2 are chronic and systemic in nature, leading to damage of multiple tissue types, including vascular and nervous, and often leading to effects on endocrine signaling. Together, the effects of these system-wide insults may result in ED [23–25]. Fortunately, the disease processes contributing to ED can often be identified and in some cases risk modification by way of smoking cessation, increased exercise, weight control, diet optimization, and modification of activities leading to penile and perineal trauma has been shown to significantly improve erectile function [26–33]. In cases where ED may be attributed to the effects of medications, drug substitution, dosage adjustment, drug holidays, or drug cessation may restore sexual function in some men [22, 34, 35]. If further treatment of ED symptoms is required, a multimodal therapeutic plan incorporating medications, lifestyle modification, and surgery may be implemented. Many treatment modalities for ED, including oral therapy via PDE5i's, intracavernous injections and intraurethral suppositories containing vasoactive medications, vacuum erection devices, and penile prostheses or revascularization surgery, have been extensively studied and efficacy rates clearly established [36–42]. This is helpful in giving both patients and clinicians a clear understanding of the benefits and risks of each therapeutic option.

Although many causes of male infertility are known (Table 6.1), 40–50 % of causes remain unidentified, despite significant improvements in our diagnostic armamentarium and the use of new technologies in diagnosis [43–45]. Without establishing a cause for a man's fertility difficulties, it is not possible to develop a targeted treatment plan. As a result, empiric pharmacotherapy is frequently utilized in affected men after limited laboratory evaluation of the HPG axis. Empiric therapies include GnRH-, FSH-, and LH-modulating drugs, antiestrogens (clomiphene citrate, tamoxifen citrate), aromatase inhibitors (testolactone, anastrozole), and antioxidants such as L-carnitine, α-tocopherol, ascorbic acid, and retinoids. Unfortunately, large-scale randomized, placebo-controlled studies in infertile men

Table 6.2 Classification of causes of erectile dysfunction

Organic	
Vasculogenic	• Atherosclerosis
	• Hypertension
	• Hypercholesterolemia
	• Diabetes mellitus
	• Pelvic/perineal trauma or irradiation
	• Smoking
	• Peyronie's disease
	• Venous shunts (may be acquired after penile surgery)
Neurogenic	• Stroke
	• Parkinson's disease
	• Alzheimer's disease
	• Encephalitis
	• Temporal lobe epilepsy
	• Spinal cord injury or associated CNS disorder (disc herniation, tumor, spina bifida, multiple sclerosis)
	• Pelvic trauma or surgery
	• Diabetic neuropathy
Endocrinologic	• Hypogonadism
	• Hyperprolactinemia
	• Hyper- and hypothyroidism
Drug induced	• Antihypertensives (diuretics, nonselective β-adrenergic blockers, spironolactone)
	• Antipsychotics (clozapine, risperidone, haloperidol)
	• Antidepressants (tricyclic antidepressants, monoamine oxidase inhibitors, selective serotonin reuptake inhibitors)
	• Lithium
	• Anxiolytics (benzodiazepines); newer anxiolytics (bupropion, buspirone) not associated with sexual side effects
	• Antiandrogens (LHRH agonists, finasteride, dutasteride)
	• Alcohol abuse
Psychogenic	
Generalized	• Primary lack of sexual arousability
	• Age-related decline in sexual arousability
Situational	• Performance anxiety
	• Depression
	• Partner related (lack of arousability, partner conflict)

of most of the above agents are lacking, and smaller studies have produced conflicting results as to the efficacy of these treatments [46–59]. Assisted reproduction has become an increasingly popular treatment option for couples in which a cause of infertility is not established or other therapies have failed. Intrauterine insemination (IUI) may be used to achieve conception in the setting of male subfertility, with a recent meta-analysis finding that couples were three times more likely to achieve a pregnancy through IUI when compared with timed intercourse [60]. Successful fertilization rates using ICSI have been reported to be 70–80 %, with corresponding pregnancy rates of up to 45 % [61]. What is frequently overlooked in both men and women with fertility difficulties is the possibility of a transmissible genetic lesion that may affect the couple's offspring. Recent data indicate that 10–30 % of male infertility is genetic in origin [62], yet testing for genetic lesions is rarely performed, in part due to a lack of clinically available assays to test for a broad range of genetic defects.

Despite the differences between many of the etiologies and treatments of ED and male factor infertility, numerous common links exist between the two conditions, and having an awareness of these is crucial to a thorough work-up of patients presenting with these conditions.

Any condition that interferes with signaling through the HPG axis can potentially result in both male infertility as well as ED [63, 64]. Disorders resulting in testosterone (T) deficiency are common causes of both conditions, as androgens influence the development of the male reproductive tract and affect libido and sexual behavior [65]. A study conducted in the Boston area reported a 5.6 % prevalence of symptomatic androgen deficiency (hypogonadism) in men between 30 and 79 years old. Of symptomatic men, ED was reported as the primary symptom in 16 % of cases [66]. Hypogonadism is generally diagnosed via serum total T levels $\leq$300 ng/dL on two consecutive blood samples, as well as the presence of hypogonadal symptoms, including fatigue, decreased energy and libido, ED, insomnia, and increased fat mass, and may contribute to both ED and infertility [64, 66–71]. Of the various forms of T deficiency, hypogonadotropic hypogonadism (HH) is the most common and best described [64]. HH may be subdivided into congenital, acquired, or idiopathic etiologies. Congenital causes of HH include Kallmann syndrome (KS), Prader–Willi and Laurence–Moon–Biedl syndromes, and hereditary hemochromatosis, with KS being the most common of these [64, 72, 73]. In cases of HH, T secretion from Leydig cells is diminished, which may result in both ED and infertility [74]. Furthermore, in cases of HH, a decline in FSH production leads to impaired spermatogenesis.

Hypogonadotropic hypogonadism may also be acquired secondary to hyperprolactinemia, defined as a serum prolactin of $\geq$20 ng/mL [64]. Excessive prolactin suppresses GnRH release, impairs binding of LH to receptors on Leydig cells, and may decrease ejaculate volumes, culminating in both infertility and ED [75, 76]. Hyperprolactinemia is most commonly caused by a prolactin-secreting pituitary adenoma but may also be secondary to conditions that interfere with the secretion of dopamine, which inhibits prolactin release. Lesions that inhibit dopamine secretion include tumors of the hypothalamus, infiltrative diseases such as sarcoidosis that damage dopamine-secreting cells in the central nervous system, or damage to the hypothalamic-pituitary stalk following trauma or surgery. Numerous drugs, including the antipsychotics risperidone and haloperidol, gastric motility agents such as metoclopramide and domperidone, and antihypertensive medications including methyldopa and verapamil, can also cause hyperprolactinemia and consequently HH [77].

Thyroid disease has also been implicated in ED and male factor infertility. Both hyper- and hypothyroidism are known to affect steroid hormone metabolism and sperm quality and have been associated with subfertility [78–80]. Hyperthyroidism in particular has been shown to be associated with ED, whereas hypothyroidism has been postulated to primarily affect sexual desire and ejaculatory function [81, 82].

Iatrogenic causes of both male infertility and ED have also been reported. Surgical procedures that violate the retroperitoneum may result in obstruction of the vas deferens or ejaculatory ducts or cause damage to the nerves involved in penile erection, seminal emission, and ejaculation [83]. Bilateral retroperitoneal lymphadenectomy can result in sympathetic nerve injury leading to anejaculation or retrograde ejaculation, having a clear impact on male fertility, and may also lead to ED [84, 85]. Radical prostatectomy and radical cystoprostatectomy also carry with them a risk of ED from neurovascular injury and infertility due to transection of the vas deferens, removal of the seminal vesicles, and injury to nerves involved in ejaculation and erection, as above [83]. Hormonal therapies for metastatic prostate carcinoma impact both male fertility and erectile function, given that these medications reduce serum testosterone levels [86]. An improved understanding of the neuroanatomy of the pelvis has resulted in modification of surgical techniques to lower the incidence of iatrogenically induced sexual dysfunction [87]. Indeed, nerve-sparing techniques during radical prostatectomy have decreased the incidence of ED from 43–100 % to 30–50 % following radical prostatectomy and to <10 % (from 15 to 100 %) after radical rectal surgery [87–92]. Similarly, use of nerve-sparing techniques during radical cystectomy has been shown to improve postoperative quality of life and sexual function, with preservation of erectile function in 62, 47, 43, and 20 % of men between the ages of 40 and 49, 50 and 59, 60 and 69, and 70 and 79 years old, respectively [93].

Other medications are also known to negatively impact both male fertility and sexual function. Spironolactone, a nonselective mineralocorticoid receptor antagonist, blocks both the epithelial and nonepithelial actions of aldosterone. With its moderate affinity for both progesterone and androgen receptors, spironolactone use carries with it a risk of sexual side effects, including ED, and, through inhibition of testosterone production, infertility [94, 95]. A variety of psychotherapeutic medications have also been shown to affect erectile function and fertility. Antidepressant medications including selective serotonin reuptake inhibitors (SSRIs), monoamine oxidase inhibitors (MAOIs), and tricyclic antidepressants (TCAs) may lead to both ED and ejaculatory dysfunction [96–98]. Antipsychotics such as phenothiazines and the mood-stabilizer lithium, owing to their anti-β-adrenergic, anticholinergic, and/or antidopaminergic effects within the CNS, may also disrupt the HPG axis, lead to ejaculatory and erectile dysfunction, and reduce libido [99, 100]. 5α-reductase inhibitors (5ARIs) often used in the treatment of benign prostatic hypertrophy, including finasteride and dutasteride, have also been associated with a reduction in semen volume, ejaculatory disturbances, and ED [101]. In addition, 5ARI usage has been associated with reduced libido, and several studies have reported this effect in up to 5 % of subjects. In some cases, persistent loss of libido even after discontinuation of the drug has been reported [102–106].

Although many of the above medications reduce serum androgen levels, the use of exogenous androgens may also affect male fertility. Exogenous androgen supplementation can impair spermatogenesis by suppressing GnRH secretion, and exogenous androgens can induce azoospermia, which may last for 6 months or longer and in some cases be irreversible following cessation of androgen administration [59]. While T therapy may be part of an appropriate treatment approach to the hypogonadal patient, its use should be limited in men desiring fertility, and alternative treatments, including antiestrogens and GnRH receptor blockers, should be considered instead. Alternatively, recent studies indicate that judicious use of exogenous androgen concomitantly with medications that stimulate testicular testosterone production, including human chorionic gonadotropin (hCG) and FSH, may preserve semen parameters in hypogonadal men [107, 108].

It should be noted that the links between male factor infertility and ED discussed above, and summarized in Table 6.3, do not represent the most common causes of infertility and/or ED. Though pathologies common to both male infertility and ED exist, most causes of both male infertility and ED are independent of one another (Tables 6.1 and 6.2). However, there is also a psychological relationship between an infertility diagnosis and ED that may pose interesting challenges to patients, their partners, and the clinicians treating them. This relationship is explored in the following section.

The Impact of Infertility on Erectile Dysfunction

Achieving a sense of sexual compatibility is integral to most intimate relationships, and in many of these relationships, one or both partners report a strong desire for a child [109]. While society's expectations of procreation may influence sexual behavior, at least to some degree, a feeling of sexual togetherness is important to overall sexual health and relationship stability. Thus, sexual satisfaction and the desire to have children are interrelated, and it seems intuitive, then, that a diagnosis of infertility, which can heighten anxiety and increase stress levels, may be associated with an increased incidence of male sexual dysfunction.

A diagnosis of male factor infertility is associated with a loss of self-esteem, increased anxiety, and overall diminished feelings of self-worth in the male partner [110]. Shindel et al., in a study of 121 infertile couples, found that male subjects reported significantly lower scores on the Mental Health subscale of the Short Form 36 (SF-36) questionnaire, a validated instrument for assessing one's perception of physical health, than the general population, indicating a poorer perception of their mental health. Furthermore, 11 and 12 % of men in this study reported moderate and severe depressive symptoms, respectively, as assessed by the Center for Epidemiologic Studies Depression Scale (CES-D) questionnaire, a validated tool for assessment of depressive symptoms. The same study found that while mean erectile function domain (EFD) scores of the International Index of Erectile Function (IIEF) questionnaire were above the cutoff value for a diagnosis of ED, 22 % of men had EFD scores <26, and of these, 18 and 4 % had mild and moderate ED, respectively [111]. Monga et al. similarly found that infertile men had significantly lower total and intercourse satisfaction scores on the IIEF compared with controls,

Table 6.3 Etiologies common to male infertility and ED

Category	Disorders	Mechanism of dysfunction
Endocrinologic	*Congenital hypogonadotropic hypogonadism (HH)*	In all cases gonadotropin deficiency results in T deficiency, impaired spermatogenesis, and sexual dysfunction (loss of libido, ED in some cases)
	Kallmann syndrome	
	Prader–Willi	
	Gonadotropin subunit mutation	
	DAX 1 mutation	
	GPR54 mutation	
	Leptin or leptin receptor mutation	
	Hyperprolactinemia	Excess prolactin inhibits GnRH secretion, leading to HH
	Pituitary adenoma	
	Hypothalamic tumors (i.e., craniopharyngiomas)	
	Section of hypothalamic-pituitary stalk	
	Antipsychotics (phenothiazines, haloperidol, pimozide, risperidone, molindone, olanzapine)	
	Antidepressants (clomipramine, desipramine)	
	Gastrointestinal drugs (cimetidine, metoclopramide)	
	Antihypertensives (methyldopa, reserpine, verapamil)	
	Hyper/hypothyroidism	Both impair steroid metabolism and lower sperm quality are associated with ED
Infiltrative disease	Sarcoidosis Langerhans cell histiocytosis Hemochromatosis	Deposition and accumulation of compounds in hypothalamus or pituitary damages GnRH-, LH-, or FSH-secreting cells leading to HH
Drug induced	*Suppression of gonadotropins*	Suppression of gonadotropins leads to HH
	Exogenous gonadal steroids	
	Glucocorticoids	
	Opiates	
	GnRH analogs	
	Psychotropic medication (SSRIs, MAOIs, TCAs)	ED, ejaculatory dysfunction, or orgasmic dysfunction plus infertility via CNS activity
	Antiandrogens (spironolactone, 5-α-reductase inhibitors)	Suppress production of T/DHT
Iatrogenic	Radical prostatectomy Radical cystectomy Bilateral pelvic lymphadenectomy	All pose risk of neurovascular injury and obstruction of sperm transport. Newer techniques have reduced incidence of such injuries, however

and Jain et al. found, in a survey of 175 infertile couples in India, that premature ejaculation, erectile dysfunction, decreased libido, and orgasmic failure were reported by 66, 15, 11, and 8 % of male partners, respectively [112, 113].

The stress induced by both the diagnosis and treatment of infertility may result in increased male sexual dysfunction and reduced sexual activity among infertile men [114]. When the male factor is identified as the sole cause of infertility in a couple, men experience greater distress and sexual dysfunction than when a female or a mixed etiology is responsible [115]. Furthermore, the prevalence of ED, determined by a score of <22 on the Sexual Health Inventory in Men (SHIM) questionnaire, and the frequency of hypogonadal symptoms, determined by a positive finding on the Androgen Deficiency in the Aging Male (ADAM) questionnaire, were both significantly higher among infertile men compared with men with proven fertility. The investigators further postulated that, due to the relatively young age and overall good health of the subjects in this study, as well as the lack of correlation between ED, hypogonadal symptoms, and serum T levels, both ED and hypogonadal symptoms were "likely multifactorial and probably largely due to psychogenic factors" related to infertility [116]. Given these associations, it is not surprising to find that a link exists between depression, anxiety, and stress and reduced sexual frequency, desire, and overall sexuality, particularly in men who already have diminished fertility [117–120]. Given that corporal smooth muscle contraction, and therefore detumescence, is mediated in part by noradrenaline, ED in this setting may be due to increased noradrenaline production in response to the stress associated with an infertility diagnosis.

Diagnostic tests performed as a result of a standard infertility work-up may also exacerbate difficulties with sexual function in men. Semen analysis, generally the first diagnostic test of an infertility work-up, frequently requires the patient to provide a semen sample in the clinic and under time constraints. Under these circumstances, transient ED and ejaculatory difficulties may be experienced by the male patient [121]. In addition, the identification of abnormal semen parameters on the first semen analysis can also lead to erectile and orgasmic difficulties. Saleh et al. observed that 11 % of men undergoing infertility evaluation experienced problems with erection or orgasm after detection of an abnormality in their first semen analysis [122].

Some clinics may try to ameliorate difficulties in obtaining a semen sample by offering patients the option to collect samples at home and bring them to the clinic within an hour. However, even in this scenario the potential for transient ED arises owing to the "forced" nature of sexual activity. Many couples are also advised to schedule sexual intercourse around the period of female ovulation, which may diminish the spontaneity of the sexual act and result in performance anxiety, ED, and ejaculatory dysfunction [123]. Owing to the "calculated" nature of the resulting sexual intercourse, many men have reported avoiding sex outside of this time frame, and a decline in libido has been reported in almost 10 % of men after fertility evaluation [120, 124].

It is important to note that the results of these studies do not necessarily establish a causal relationship between infertility and ED, and our aim here is not to make such a claim. Rather, the data show that an association between the two very well might exist and that the initial diagnosis and work-up of infertility can have a substantial impact on male sexuality. In addition, outside influences and social pressures related to successful reproduction may also have marked effects upon male psychosexual function and may ultimately lead to sexual dysfunction [125]. As such, it is important for the clinician to be aware of these associations and take proactive measures to counsel and treat these patients accordingly.

An Overview of the Evaluation of Erectile Dysfunction

The modern management of ED has been marked by a drive to establish evidence-based best practices that are both standardized and proceed in a stepwise, goal-orientated fashion. The current philosophy behind the management and treatment of ED revolves around a "patient-centered, goal-directed" approach, originally described by Lu [126, 127]. The foundations of this paradigm stress the importance of pursuing ED management and treatment in a methodical, evidence-based manner, beginning with a thorough medical, sexual, and psychosocial history followed by a focused physical examination and pertinent laboratory testing (Fig. 6.1) [128]. The clinician is then encouraged to present treatment options to the patient or the couple in a manner that is sensitive to the cultural, ethnic, and religious factors that may influence the patients' preferred treatment path [129]. The goal of this approach is to allow the patient or the couple to make an informed decision regarding treatment that is consistent with their view of sexual fulfillment [130, 131]. Since its initial description, this model has been further buoyed by a series of internationally accepted consensus meetings, chief among these being a series of reports generated from the International Consultations on Sexual Medicine (ICSM) [132–134].

A stepwise approach to the management and treatment of ED begins with the understanding that, unlike a variety of disease processes, a diagnosis of ED commonly hinges upon the subjective complaint(s) of the patient. Extensive diagnostic testing and objective data gathering are not necessarily required to initiate ED treatment, although such data may be helpful in guiding treatment in particular cases [135]. Regardless, an essential first step in ED management is a comprehensive sexual, medical, and psychosocial history [136–138].

Given the association between ED and several chronic medical conditions and adverse lifestyle habits (e.g., diabetes, cardiovascular disease (CVD), hypertension, prostate disease, obesity, sedentary lifestyle, cigarette smoking), the medical history of the ED patient should focus on elucidating the existence and extent of these underlying conditions [13–18, 139]. The third Princeton Consensus Guidelines Panel, acknowledging the frequent coexistence of ED and CVD, recommended that all men presenting with ED should undergo an initial cardiac assessment with stratification of their cardiac risk, regardless of the presence or the absence of overt cardiac symptoms [140]. This algorithm places ED patients into three

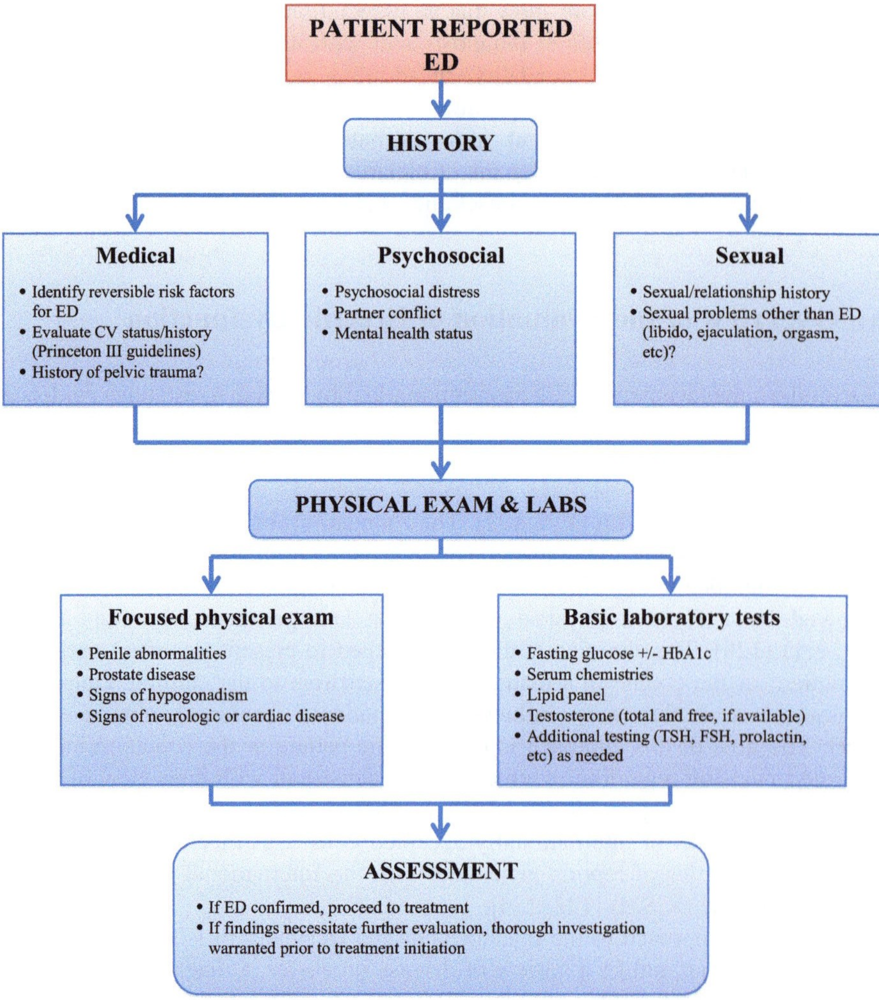

Fig. 6.1 Algorithm for the diagnostic evaluation of ED

categories—low, medium, or high cardiac risk—and guides management based upon this stratification (Fig. 6.2). A complete medical history would also include an assessment of the known organic causes of ED, such as neurologic disease, hypogonadism, thyroid disorders, pelvic trauma, and medication usage. These known organic causes of ED have been described previously and are presented in Table 6.2.

The sexual and psychosocial history of the ED patient is also of vital importance in framing the patient's overall sexual well-being and confirming the diagnosis [141]. This includes establishing the duration and severity of erectile dysfunction as well as assessing the entirety of the male sexual response cycle (i.e., libido, ejaculation, and orgasm). Partner sexual function and the patient's relationship

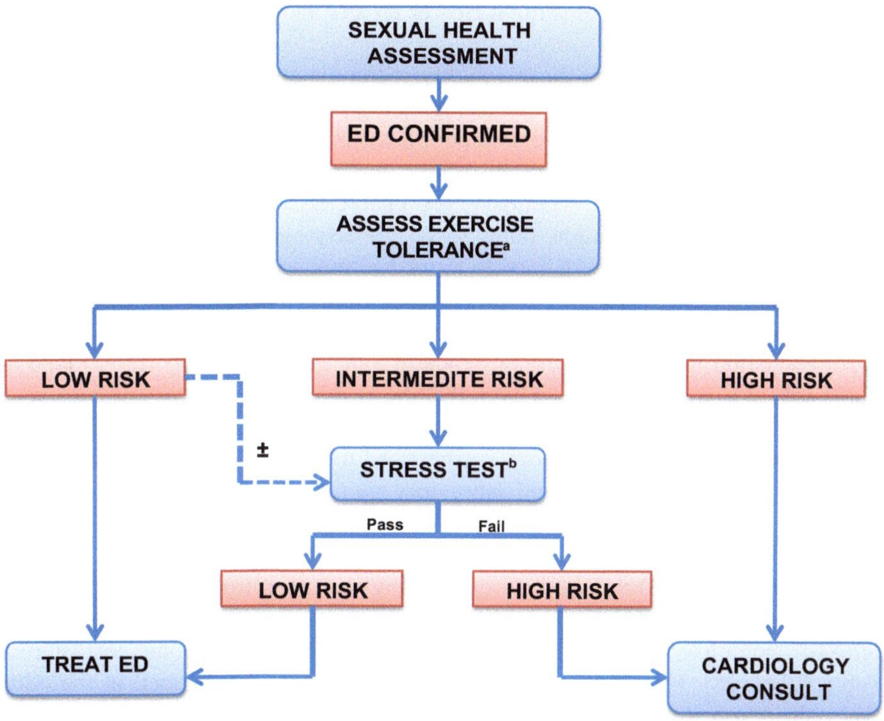

Fig. 6.2 Princeton III Consensus Panel recommendations for ED management in CVD. (*Superscript a*) Sexual activity is equivalent to walking one mile on flat surface in 20 min or briskly climbing two flights of stairs in 10 s. (*Superscript b*) Sexual activity is equivalent to 4 min of the Bruce treadmill protocol. Low-risk patients are those able to perform exercise of moderate intensity without symptoms. This group also includes patients with a history of successful revascularization, asymptomatic controlled hypertension, mild valvular dysfunction, and left ventricular dysfunction (NYHA class I and II). High-risk patients are those with moderate-to-severe cardiac symptoms, including unstable angina pectoris, uncontrolled hypertension, congestive heart failure (NYHA class IV), recent MI (<2 weeks), high-risk arrhythmia, severe cardiomyopathy, and moderate-to-severe valve disease [140]

satisfaction (both past and present relationships) are also important in establishing the broader picture of the patient's overall sexual health. Inquiring about potential sources of anxiety, depression, or relationship distress may serve to reveal emotional or environmental stressors that might contribute to, or exacerbate, ED [142]. Several validated, self-administered ED questionnaires, such as the IIEF and SHIM, exist and may provide useful information to supplement the history. The IIEF, mentioned previously, consists of 15 questions addressing five domains of sexual function—erectile function, orgasmic function, sexual desire, intercourse satisfaction, and overall satisfaction. The SHIM, a five-item questionnaire adapted from the IIEF, focuses specifically on erectile function and serves as a useful, brief, and easily administered ED screening tool. Information gleaned from patient responses to questionnaires may help stratify patients based on ED severity and can aid the clinician in establishing a clearer understanding of the patients' sexual health status [10, 143].

A focused physical exam is also highly recommended and should include an assessment of the cardiovascular, neurologic, and genital systems [129]. A finding of elevated blood pressure or reduced peripheral pulses, for example, may reveal undiagnosed cardiovascular disease concomitant with the patient's ED [23, 144]. The absence of secondary sex characteristics or the presence of a distinctive body habitus might point to an underlying endocrine disorder or a congenital abnormality (e.g., Klinefelter's or Kallmann syndrome). An evaluation of the genital system may uncover the evidence of pelvic trauma, penile deformity (Peyronie's disease), or testicular abnormality, while findings of an abnormal neurologic exam may suggest the presence of a peripheral neuropathy portending a diagnosis of diabetes mellitus. Given that the etiology of ED is often multifactorial, physical exam findings alone might not pinpoint a specific cause. Rather, the physical exam may help corroborate aspects of the history, provide direction to subsequent diagnostic testing and laboratory work, and in some cases uncover undiagnosed comorbidities [134, 138].

The choice of laboratory testing should be equally focused and flow from the information obtained from the history and physical examination. Recommended laboratory tests for the evaluation of ED include serum chemistries, fasting glucose, HgbA1c, complete blood count, lipid profile, and serum total testosterone (Table 6.3) [128]. In select cases, additional testing may be ordered at the clinician's discretion if particular etiologies, such as hypogonadism, thyroid disease, hyperprolactinemia, or others, are suspected [66, 71, 128, 134, 145–147].

Treatment Considerations for Erectile Dysfunction

Once a diagnosis of ED has been established appropriate treatment may commence (Fig. 6.3). Given the association between ED and comorbid health conditions such as diabetes, hypertension, and cardiovascular disease it is logical to presume that lifestyle modification might play a role in optimization of overall sexual health. Several reports have suggested such a beneficial effect. For example, smoking cessation, weight reduction, increased exercise, and adoption of a healthy diet have all been shown to provide a beneficial effect on erectile function [26, 28, 32, 148–150]. However, few data exist evaluating the effects of lifestyle modification on ED, and reports often differ on the efficacy of lifestyle changes and reversal of ED symptoms [30, 31]. However, it is advisable to counsel patients on the importance of adopting healthy lifestyle habits to improve sexual health, notwithstanding the need for pharmacotherapy or medical interventions [151, 152].

Given their relative convenience, simplicity, and ease of use, oral pharmacotherapy in the form of PDE5 inhibitors (PDE5is) represent a first-line treatment option for ED [151]. Currently, three oral PDE5is comprise the mainstay of oral ED therapies: sildenafil, vardenafil, and tadalafil. Each of these oral agents blocks

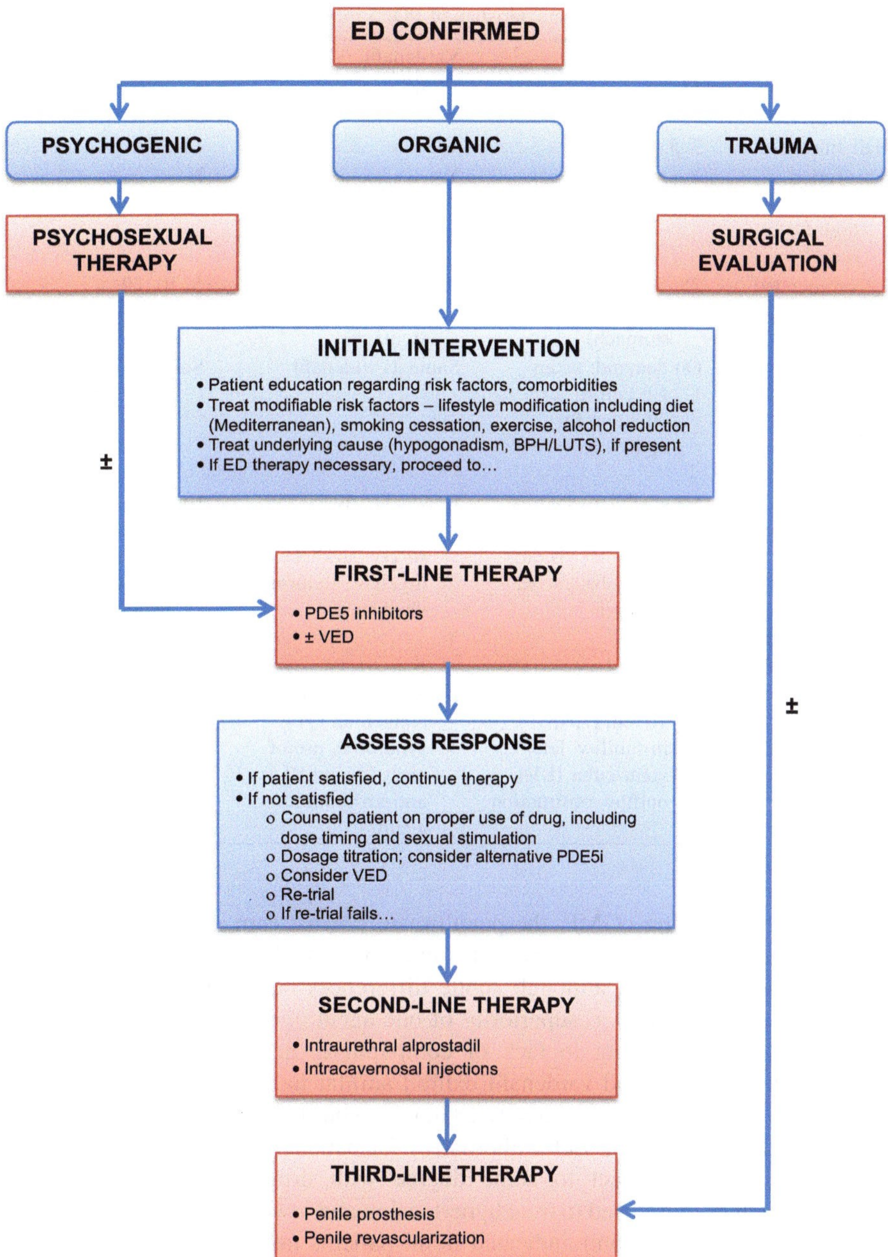

Fig. 6.3 Treatment algorithm for ED management

Table 6.4 Comparative clinical characteristics of PDE5 inhibitors for ED

Characteristic	Sildenafil	Vardenafil	Tadalafil
Onset of action (min)	15–60	15–60	15–120
Half-life (h)	3–5	4–5	17.5
Absorption reduced by high fat meal?	Y	Y	N
Recommended dosage (mg)	25, 50, 100 (on empty stomach)	5, 10, 20 (on empty stomach)	5, 10, 20
Dose timing	On demand: taken 1 h before sex; effective for up to 4 h	Same as sildenafil	Same as sildenafil *or* 2.5–5 mg dose may be taken routinely once daily
Side effects	Headache, dyspepsia, facial flushing, abnormal vision; *rarely* backache, myalgia	Headache, dyspepsia, facial flushing; *rarely* backache, myalgia, abnormal vision	Headache, dyspepsia, facial flushing, backache, myalgia; *rarely* abnormal vision
Contraindicated with nitrates?	Y	Y	Y
Precautions/ warnings	Autonomic nervous system (ANS) instability, left ventricular (LV) outflow obstruction	LV outflow obstruction, congenital QT syndrome, use of class IA and III anti-arrhythmic agents	ANS instability, LV outflow obstruction, avoid excessive alcohol consumption

PDE5 from degrading cGMP, the penultimate downstream mediator of corporal smooth muscle relaxation that mediates erection. All three PDE5is have similar efficacy and tolerability, although subtle differences between these three agents exist (Table 6.4). However, superiority of one agent over the others has not been established, mostly owing to lack of comparative, head-to-head clinical trials [36]. While sildenafil and vardenafil exhibit similar half-lives of 3–5 h, tadalafil possesses a half-life of approximately 18 h, which has led to a daily dosing protocol for tadalafil and may be a useful alternative for patients in select cases [153]. All three medications interact to some degree with drugs α-adrenergic receptor blockers, such as those used to treat hypertension and lower urinary tract symptoms (LUTS). Vardenafil is contraindicated in all patients taking α-blockers, and both sildenafil (50 and 100 mg doses) and tadalafil should be administered with caution to such patients. All three PDE5is are absolutely contraindicated in patients taking any form of nitrate medication [151].

Overall, PDE5is are effective, with successful sexual intercourse rates of approximately 70 %. However, these medications are not effective or sufficient in all patients [36]. In the event a patient fails a trial of PDE5is, the best next step is to reassess the therapeutic plan. Several modifiable factors influence the success or the failure of PDE5i therapy. For example, the timing of medication use is important. PDE5is should be taken on demand approximately 1 h before initiating sexual activity. This interval allows sufficient time for achievement of peak serum concentrations and peak efficacy. In addition, achieving an erection sufficient for intercourse also depends on the presence of adequate sexual stimulation. PDE5is inhibit degradation of nitric oxide (NO) by cGMP, but NO release is dependent on sexual stimulation and arousal. Insufficient stimulation may therefore result in suboptimal NO levels and diminished PDE5i efficacy. PDE5i efficacy may also be limited by high fat intake, and reduction of fat intake proximal to drug usage may improve PDE5i efficacy. The patient should also be aware that up to ten attempts with PDE5i may be necessary to achieve satisfactory erections, although high first-use response rates can occur [36, 154–157]. If treatment failure persists despite appropriate medication usage, the clinician may consider second-line options.

Second-line therapy for the treatment of ED consists of intracavernous injectable (ICI) agents or intraurethral suppositories [158]. Alprostadil, a synthetic formulation of the potent vasodilator prostaglandin E_1 (PGE1), is available as an intraurethral suppository, which is inserted through the urethral meatus to the distal urethra, from which the drug is absorbed through the urethral mucosa and into the corpora cavernosa, stimulating erection. Up to 56 % of men will engage in intercourse to completion in two of the three attempts using intraurethral alprostadil (IUA) [41]. However, other studies have shown lower success rates and a lack of consistency in treatment response [159, 160]. Clinicians must take care to present realistic expectations to patients in light of the variable data on outcomes with IUA. Of note, the efficacy of IUA may be supplemented with the use of an adjustable penile constriction band designed to prevent medication migration out of the corpora. PDE5is may also serve as an adjunct to patients using IUA, with combination therapy with PDE5is having improved efficacy than IUA alone [161–163]. The most common adverse events associated with IUA are penile or urethral pain, seen in upwards of 10 % of cases. Headache, dizziness, or minor bleeding are also associated with IUA usage but at much lower rates (between 1 and 10 %) [164].

Intracavernosal injection of vasoactive agents represents the most effective nonsurgical treatment for ED and is successful in otherwise normal men with ED as well as difficult-to-treat subgroups of men with ED, including those with diabetes, cardiovascular disease, and other chronic illnesses [164–166]. As the name suggests, ICI involves the direct injection of vasodilatory drug into the corpora cavernosa. Alprostadil, papaverine, and phentolamine are the three agents regularly used in clinical practice, and they may be administered either as a single agent or in combination. Success rates of up to 70–90 % have been reported with ICI, depending on the combination of agents used [167–171]. Possible side effects of ICI include pain at the injection site, penile pain with erection, penile fibrosis, and priapism [165, 172]. However, these side effects may be mitigated by using combination rather than monotherapy [171]. ICI is contraindicated in patients with a history of psychiatric disorder or mental instability, risk of priapism, coagulopathy, or cardiovascular disease or in those deemed unable to administer self-injections (e.g., poor manual dexterity, morbid obesity).

A brief note regarding vacuum erection devices (VED) is also warranted in this discussion, and this may be used as first-line ED therapy or as an adjunct to first- or second-line therapies [173]. VEDs are medical devices consisting of a cylindrical chamber into which the penis is inserted. Air is vacuumed from the chamber, creating negative pressure around the penis and drawing blood into the corpora, resulting in erection. An elastic constriction band is then placed around the base of the penis to prevent blood regress, and the device is removed [174, 175]. The constriction band should be left in place for no longer than 30 min, given the risk of cavernosal ischemia, and if the patient requires an erection lasting for more than 30 min, the band must be released, detumescence achieved, and the procedure repeated [176, 177]. Unlike medical therapies, VEDs do not activate or modulate a biochemical signaling pathway and, as such, do not produce a "physiologic" erection [174, 178]. Nevertheless, they are effective in generating erections sufficient for intercourse 60–90 % of the time. Unfortunately, patient satisfaction rates with VEDs are low overall, between 30 and 68 % [179–184]. Complications associated with VEDs are relatively infrequent, tend to decrease with continued use of the device, and include penile pain, petechiae, bruising, and difficultly with ejaculation given the physical obstruction of ejaculate passage [180, 185].

If a patient fails oral, intraurethral, or injectable therapy, third-line treatment for ED involves surgical management via implantation of a penile prosthesis or, in select cases, penile revascularization surgery [158, 186, 187]. However, an in-depth discussion of the surgical management of ED is beyond the scope of this chapter.

Erectile Dysfunction Treatment for Infertile Men

In the setting of male infertility, the algorithm for ED management does not deviate greatly from Fig. 6.3. However, the clinician should be aware that in the setting of male infertility, overall ED rates, as well as prevalence of psychogenic ED, may be higher than in the general population [116, 188]. This interplay has been discussed above, and in such cases, psychosexual therapy might be a valuable treatment option [189–191]. Unfortunately, the volume of evidence-based, well-controlled, and large-scale trials investigating the effectiveness of psychosexual therapy in ED treatment is lacking. That said, psychosexual therapy has shown benefit in men with ED, especially those who continued therapy for longer time intervals [191]. Dearth of evidence notwithstanding, consultation with a trained sexual therapist is an important treatment modality to consider in the infertile male, as integrated treatment plans combining psychosexual and medical therapy may aid the patient in achieving overall sexual well-being [190, 192].

The spectrum of ED treatments affects the male sexual response cycle and may therefore negatively impact male fertility. The effect of PDE5is on male fertility and seminal parameters is discussed elsewhere in this text, although no apparent negative effects have been reported.

Studies investigating the effects of IUA on semen parameters have reported no adverse effects on sperm motility, viability, or membrane integrity [193]. In contrast, phentolamine and other α1-receptor antagonists may negatively impact sperm quality and ejaculatory function. Andrade et al. showed a dose-dependent reduction in sperm motility in men using phentolamine, while Kobayashi et al. observed loss of seminal emission in 15 healthy male volunteers while on silodosin, an α1-receptor antagonist [194, 195]. The general association between α1-receptor antagonists, such as prazosin and phentolamine, and impaired ejaculation is also well established [196, 197]. However, consensus data regarding the effect of intracavernous phentolamine, specifically when delivered in combination with other ICI agents such as alprostadil and papaverine, on male fertility has not been established.

As mentioned previously, VEDs may cause difficulty with ejaculation and trapping of ejaculate due to urethral compression in 12–30 % of patients and may pose a problem for men seeking treatment for both infertility and ED [184].

Overall, the current evidence base examining the effects of ED therapies on infertility shows little detrimental effect on fertility apart from several specific drugs, supporting the use of most ED therapies in men with fertility concerns or difficulties.

Conclusion

Since the first successful delivery resulting from in IVF was reported in 1982, progress in the field of ART has been dramatic [198]. Consumer consumption and increased availability of ART, and consequently the number of babies born via these technologies, have significantly increased in recent years. An area of particular excitement in this new age of reproductive healthcare is that of male factor infertility. Couples who previously would have no recourse other than donor insemination or adoption due to the presence of a severe male factor or prior treatment failures may now achieve pregnancies thanks to the breakthroughs in ART. One area of future investigation in this realm is that of the relationship between male infertility and ED. While recent work describes clear relationships between ED and male infertility on numerous levels, including causes and treatments, numerous etiologies of both conditions, as well as cause-specific treatments, remain to be elucidated.

Ultimately, the clear association between ED and male infertility highlights the need to consider these entities together when evaluating the infertile male or the male with erectile difficulties and to target the evaluation and treatment approaches to afflicted men.

Financial Support None.

References

1. Tietze C, Guttmacher AF, Rubin S. Time required for conception in 1727 planned pregnancies. Fertil Steril. 1950;1(4):338–46.
2. Spira A. Epidemiology of human reproduction. Hum Reprod. 1986;1(2):111–5.
3. Thonneau P, Marchand S, Tallec A, et al. Incidence and main causes of infertility in a resident population (1,850,000) of three French regions (1988-1989). Hum Reprod. 1991;6(6):811–6.
4. Martinez GM, Chandra A, Abma JC, Jones J, Mosher WD. Fertility, contraception, and fatherhood: data on men and women from cycle 6 (2002) of the 2002 national survey of family growth. Vital Health Stat 23. 2006;26:1–142
5. Meacham RB, Joyce GF, Wise M, Kparker A, Niederberger C, Urologic Diseases in America Project. Male infertility. J Urol. 2007;177(6):2058–66. doi:10.1016/j.juro.2007.01.131.
6. Marketdata Enterprises I. U.S. fertility clinics & infertility services: an industry analysis. http://www.marketresearch.com/Marketdata-Enterprises-Inc-v416/Fertility-Clinics-Infertil ity-Services-2403343/. Accessed 1 Aug 2009.
7. Kolettis PN, Sabanegh ES. Significant medical pathology discovered during a male infertility evaluation. J Urol. 2001;166(1):178–80.
8. Eisenberg ML, Park Y, Hollenbeck AR, Lipshultz LI, Schatzkin A, Pletcher MJ. Fatherhood and the risk of cardiovascular mortality in the NIH-AARP diet and health study. Hum Reprod. 2011;26(12):3479–85. doi:10.1093/humrep/der305.
9. NIH Consensus Conference. Impotence. NIH consensus development panel on impotence. JAMA. 1993;270(1):83–90.
10. Rosen RC, Riley A, Wagner G, Osterloh IH, Kirkpatrick J, Mishra A. The international index of erectile function (IIEF): a multidimensional scale for assessment of erectile dysfunction. Urology. 1997;49(6):822–30.
11. Derogatis LR, Burnett AL. The epidemiology of sexual dysfunctions. J Sex Med. 2008;5 (2):289–300. doi:10.1111/j.1743-6109.2007.00668.x.
12. Ayta IA, McKinlay JB, Krane RJ. The likely worldwide increase in erectile dysfunction between 1995 and 2025 and some possible policy consequences. BJU Int. 1999;84(1):50–6.
13. Braun M, Wassmer G, Klotz T, Reifenrath B, Mathers M, Engelmann U. Epidemiology of erectile dysfunction: results of the 'cologne male survey'. Int J Impot Res. 2000;12 (6):305–11. doi:10.1038/sj.ijir.3900622.
14. Nicolosi A, Laumann EO, Glasser DB, et al. Sexual behavior and sexual dysfunctions after age 40: the global study of sexual attitudes and behaviors. Urology. 2004;64(5):991–7. doi:10.1016/j.urology.2004.06.055.
15. Rosen RC, Fisher WA, Eardley I, et al. The multinational men's attitudes to life events and sexuality (MALES) study: I. prevalence of erectile dysfunction and related health concerns in the general population. Curr Med Res Opin. 2004;20(5):607–17.
16. Saigal CS, Wessells H, Pace J, Schonlau M, Wilt TJ, Urologic Diseases in America Project. Predictors and prevalence of erectile dysfunction in a racially diverse population. Arch Intern Med. 2006;166(2):207–12. doi:10.1001/archinte.166.2.207.
17. Laumann EO, West S, Glasser D, Carson C, Rosen R, Kang JH. Prevalence and correlates of erectile dysfunction by race and ethnicity among men aged 40 or older in the United States: from the male attitudes regarding sexual health survey. J Sex Med. 2007;4(1):57–65. doi:10.1111/j.1743-6109.2006.00340.x.
18. Selvin E, Burnett AL, Platz EA. Prevalence and risk factors for erectile dysfunction in the US. Am J Med. 2007;120(2):151–7. doi:10.1016/j.amjmed.2006.06.010.
19. Litwin MS, Saigal CS, Yano EM, et al. Urologic diseases in America project: analytical methods and principal findings. J Urol. 2005;173(3):933–7. doi:10.1097/01.ju.0000152365.43125.3b.
20. Wessells H, Joyce GF, Wise M, Wilt TJ. Erectile dysfunction. J Urol. 2007;177(5):1675–81. doi:10.1016/j.juro.2007.01.057.

21. Schouten BW, Bohnen AM, Groeneveld FP, Dohle GR, Thomas S, Bosch JL. Erectile dysfunction in the community: trends over time in incidence, prevalence, GP consultation and medication use—the Krimpen study: trends in ED. J Sex Med. 2010;7(7):2547–53. doi:10.1111/j.1743-6109.2010.01849.x.
22. Ralph D, McNicholas T. UK management guidelines for erectile dysfunction. BMJ. 2000;321 (7259):499–503.
23. Seftel AD, Miner MM, Kloner RA, Althof SE. Office evaluation of male sexual dysfunction. Urol Clin North Am. 2007;34(4):463–82. doi:10.1016/j.ucl.2007.08.004.
24. Shabsigh R, Klein LT, Seidman S, Kaplan SA, Lehrhoff BJ, Ritter JS. Increased incidence of depressive symptoms in men with erectile dysfunction. Urology. 1998;52(5):848–52.
25. Araujo AB, Durante R, Feldman HA, Goldstein I, McKinlay JB. The relationship between depressive symptoms and male erectile dysfunction: cross-sectional results from the Massachusetts Male Aging Study. Psychosom Med. 1998;60(4):458–65.
26. Mannino DM, Klevens RM, Flanders WD. Cigarette smoking: an independent risk factor for impotence? Am J Epidemiol. 1994;140(11):1003–8.
27. Feldman HA, Johannes CB, Derby CA, et al. Erectile dysfunction and coronary risk factors: prospective results from the Massachusetts Male Aging Study. Prev Med. 2000;30(4):328–38. doi:10.1006/pmed.2000.0643.
28. Bacon CG, Mittleman MA, Kawachi I, Giovannucci E, Glasser DB, Rimm EB. A prospective study of risk factors for erectile dysfunction. J Urol. 2006;176(1):217–21. doi:10.1016/S0022-5347(06)00589-1.
29. Feldman HA, Goldstein I, Hatzichristou DG, Krane RJ, McKinlay JB. Impotence and its medical and psychosocial correlates: results of the Massachusetts Male Aging Study. J Urol. 1994;151(1):54–61.
30. Derby CA, Mohr BA, Goldstein I, Feldman HA, Johannes CB, McKinlay JB. Modifiable risk factors and erectile dysfunction: can lifestyle changes modify risk? Urology. 2000;56 (2):302–6.
31. Esposito K, Giugliano F, Di Palo C, et al. Effect of lifestyle changes on erectile dysfunction in obese men: a randomized controlled trial. JAMA. 2004;291(24):2978–84. doi:10.1001/jama.291.24.2978.
32. Esposito K, Ciotola M, Giugliano F, et al. Mediterranean diet improves erectile function in subjects with the metabolic syndrome. Int J Impot Res. 2006;18(4):405–10. doi:10.1038/sj.ijir.3901447.
33. Schrader SM, Breitenstein MJ, Lowe BD. Cutting off the nose to save the penis. J Sex Med. 2008;5(8):1932–40. doi:10.1111/j.1743-6109.2008.00867.x.
34. Rosen RC, Lane RM, Menza M. Effects of SSRIs on sexual function: a critical review. J Clin Psychopharmacol. 1999;19(1):67–85.
35. Nurnberg HG, Gelenberg A, Hargreave TB, Harrison WM, Siegel RL, Smith MD. Efficacy of sildenafil citrate for the treatment of erectile dysfunction in men taking serotonin reuptake inhibitors. Am J Psychiatry. 2001;158(11):1926–8.
36. Carson CC, Lue TF. Phosphodiesterase type 5 inhibitors for erectile dysfunction. BJU Int. 2005;96(3):257–80. doi:10.1111/j.1464-410X.2005.05614.x.
37. Linet OI, Neff LL. Intracavernous prostaglandin E1 in erectile dysfunction. Clin Investig. 1994;72(2):139–49.
38. Lakin MM, Montague DK, VanderBrug Medendorp S, Tesar L, Schover LR. Intracavernous injection therapy: analysis of results and complications. J Urol. 1990;143(6):1138–41.
39. Hellstrom WJ, Bennett AH, Gesundheit N, et al. A double-blind, placebo-controlled evaluation of the erectile response to transurethral alprostadil. Urology. 1996;48(6):851–6.
40. Padma-Nathan H, Hellstrom WJ, Kaiser FE, et al. Treatment of men with erectile dysfunction with transurethral alprostadil. Medicated Urethral System for Erection (MUSE) Study Group. N Engl J Med. 1997;336(1):1–7.
41. Guay AT, Perez JB, Velasquez E, Newton RA, Jacobson JP. Clinical experience with intraurethral alprostadil (MUSE) in the treatment of men with erectile dysfunction.

A retrospective study. Medicated urethral system for erection. Eur Urol. 2000;38(6):671–6. doi: 20360.
42. Hellstrom WJ, Montague DK, Moncada I, et al. Implants, mechanical devices, and vascular surgery for erectile dysfunction. J Sex Med. 2010;7(1 Pt 2):501–23. doi:10.1111/j.1743-6109.2009.01626.x.
43. Nagler HM. Varicocele. In: Lipshultz LI, editor. Infertility in the male. St. Louis: Mosby Year Book; 1997. p. 336–59.
44. Nieschlag E. Classification of andrological disorders. In: Nieschlag E, Behre H, Nieschlag S, editors. Andrology: male reproductive health and dysfunction. 2nd ed. Berlin: Springer; 1997. p. 83–7.
45. de Kretser D. Male infertility. Lancet. 1997;349(9054):787–90. doi:10.1016/S0140-6736(96)08341-9.
46. Badenoch DF, Waxman J, Boorman L, et al. Administration of a gonadotropin releasing hormone analogue in oligozoospermic infertile males. Acta Endocrinol (Copenh). 1988;117(2):265–7.
47. Crottaz B, Senn A, Reymond MJ, Rey F, Germond M, Gomez F. Follicle-stimulating hormone bioactivity in idiopathic normogonadotropic oligoasthenozoospermia: double-blind trial with gonadotropin-releasing hormone. Fertil Steril. 1992;57(5):1034–43.
48. Attia AM, Al-Inany HG, Proctor ML. Gonadotrophins for idiopathic male factor subfertility. Cochrane Database Syst Rev. 2006(1):CD005071. doi:10.1002/14651858.CD005071.pub2.
49. Ashkenazi J, Bar-Hava I, Farhi J, et al. The role of purified follicle stimulating hormone therapy in the male partner before intracytoplasmic sperm injection. Fertil Steril. 1999;72(4):670–3.
50. Baccetti B, Piomboni P, Bruni E, et al. Effect of follicle-stimulating hormone on sperm quality and pregnancy rate. Asian J Androl. 2004;6(2):133–7.
51. Micic S, Dotlic R. Evaluation of sperm parameters in clinical trial with clomiphene citrate of oligospermic men. J Urol. 1985;133(2):221–2.
52. Liu PY, Handelsman DJ. The present and future state of hormonal treatment for male infertility. Hum Reprod Update. 2003;9(1):9–23.
53. Pavlovich CP, King P, Goldstein M, Schlegel PN. Evidence of a treatable endocrinopathy in infertile men. J Urol. 2001;165(3):837–41.
54. Clark RV, Sherins RJ. Treatment of men with idiopathic oligozoospermic infertility using the aromatase inhibitor, testolactone. results of a double-blinded, randomized, placebo-controlled trial with crossover. J Androl. 1989;10(3):240–7.
55. Suleiman SA, Ali ME, Zaki ZM, el-Malik EM, Nasr MA. Lipid peroxidation and human sperm motility: protective role of vitamin E. J Androl. 1996;17(5):530–7.
56. Rolf C, Cooper TG, Yeung CH, Nieschlag E. Antioxidant treatment of patients with asthenozoospermia or moderate oligoasthenozoospermia with high-dose vitamin C and vitamin E: a randomized, placebo-controlled, double-blind study. Hum Reprod. 1999;14(4):1028–33.
57. Keskes-Ammar L, Feki-Chakroun N, Rebai T, et al. Sperm oxidative stress and the effect of an oral vitamin E and selenium supplement on semen quality in infertile men. Arch Androl. 2003;49(2):83–94.
58. Balercia G, Regoli F, Armeni T, Koverech A, Mantero F, Boscaro M. Placebo-controlled double-blind randomized trial on the use of L-carnitine, L-acetylcarnitine, or combined L-carnitine and L-acetylcarnitine in men with idiopathic asthenozoospermia. Fertil Steril. 2005;84(3):662–71. doi:10.1016/j.fertnstert.2005.03.064.
59. Sigman M, Glass S, Campagnone J, Pryor JL. Carnitine for the treatment of idiopathic asthenospermia: a randomized, double-blind, placebo-controlled trial. Fertil Steril. 2006;85(5):1409–14. doi:10.1016/j.fertnstert.2005.10.055.
60. Cohlen BJ. Should we continue performing intrauterine inseminations in the year 2004? Gynecol Obstet Invest. 2005;59(1):3–13. doi:10.1159/000080492.

61. Palermo GD, Neri QV, Takeuchi T, Rosenwaks Z. ICSI: where we have been and where we are going. Semin Reprod Med. 2009;27(2):191–201. doi:10.1055/s-0029-1202309.
62. Hwang K, Yatsenko AN, Jorgez CJ, et al. Mendelian genetics of male infertility. Ann N Y Acad Sci. 2010;1214(1):E1–17. doi:10.1111/j.1749-6632.2010.05917.x.
63. Lue TF. Erectile dysfunction. N Engl J Med. 2000;342(24):1802–13. doi:10.1056/NEJM200006153422407.
64. Hwang K, Walters RC, Lipshultz LI. Contemporary concepts in the evaluation and management of male infertility. Nat Rev Urol. 2011;8(2):86–94. doi:10.1038/nrurol.2010.230.
65. Mulligan T, Schmitt B. Testosterone for erectile failure. J Gen Intern Med. 1993;8(9):517–21.
66. Araujo AB, Esche GR, Kupelian V, et al. Prevalence of symptomatic androgen deficiency in men. J Clin Endocrinol Metab. 2007;92(11):4241–7. doi:10.1210/jc.2007-1245.
67. Pfeifer S, Fritz M, Goldberg J, et al. Diagnostic evaluation of the infertile male: a committee opinion. Fertil Steril. 2012;98(2):294–301. doi: 10.1016/j.fertnstert.2012.05.033.
68. Slag MF, Morley JE, Elson MK, et al. Impotence in medical clinic outpatients. JAMA. 1983;249(13):1736–40.
69. Spark RF, White RA, Connolly PB. Impotence is not always psychogenic. Newer insights into hypothalamic-pituitary-gonadal dysfunction. JAMA. 1980;243(8):750–5.
70. Buvat J, Lemaire A. Endocrine screening in 1,022 men with erectile dysfunction: clinical significance and cost-effective strategy. J Urol. 1997;158(5):1764–7.
71. Earle CM, Stuckey BG. Biochemical screening in the assessment of erectile dysfunction: what tests decide future therapy? Urology. 2003;62(4):727–31.
72. Kelly TM, Edwards CQ, Meikle AW, Kushner JP. Hypogonadism in hemochromatosis: reversal with iron depletion. Ann Intern Med. 1984;101(5):629–32.
73. Walton C, Kelly WF, Laing I, Bu'lock DE. Endocrine abnormalities in idiopathic haemochromatosis. Q J Med. 1983;52(205):99–110.
74. Schwanzel-Fukuda M, Bick D, Pfaff DW. Luteinizing hormone-releasing hormone (LHRH)-expressing cells do not migrate normally in an inherited hypogonadal (Kallmann) syndrome. Brain Res Mol Brain Res. 1989;6(4):311–26.
75. Carter JN, Tyson JE, Tolis G, Van Vliet S, Faiman C, Friesen HG. Prolactin-screening tumors and hypogonadism in 22 men. N Engl J Med. 1978;299(16):847–52. doi:10.1056/NEJM197810192991602.
76. Segal S, Yaffe H, Laufer N, Ben-David M. Male hyperprolactinemia: effects on fertility. Fertil Steril. 1979;32(5):556–61.
77. Melmed S, Casanueva FF, Hoffman AR, et al. Diagnosis and treatment of hyperprolactinemia: an endocrine society clinical practice guideline. J Clin Endocrinol Metab. 2011;96(2):273–88. doi:10.1210/jc.2010-1692.
78. Velazquez EM, Bellabarba Arata G. Effects of thyroid status on pituitary gonadotropin and testicular reserve in men. Arch Androl. 1997;38(1):85–92.
79. Abalovich M, Levalle O, Hermes R, et al. Hypothalamic-pituitary-testicular axis and seminal parameters in hyperthyroid males. Thyroid. 1999;9(9):857–63.
80. Krassas GE, Pontikides N, Deligianni V, Miras K. A prospective controlled study of the impact of hyperthyroidism on reproductive function in males. J Clin Endocrinol Metab. 2002;87(8):3667–71.
81. Corona G, Wu FCW, Forti G, et al. Thyroid hormones and male sexual function. Int J Androl. 2012;35(5):668–79. doi:10.1111/j.1365-2605.2012.01266.x.
82. Maggi M, Buvat J, Corona G, Guay A, Torres LO. Hormonal causes of male sexual dysfunctions and their management (hyperprolactinemia, thyroid disorders, GH disorders, and DHEA). J Sex Med. 2012. doi:10.1111/j.1743-6109.2012.02735.x.
83. Hendry WF. Iatrogenic damage to male reproductive function. J R Soc Med. 1995;88(10): P579–84.
84. Kedia KR, Markland C, Fraley EE. Sexual function after high retroperitoneal lymphadenectomy. Urol Clin North Am. 1977;4(3):523–8.

85. Nijman JM, Schraffordt Koops H, Oldhoff J, Kremer J, Sleijfer DT. Sexual function after surgery and combination chemotherapy in men with disseminated nonseminomatous testicular cancer. J Surg Oncol. 1988;38(3):182–6.
86. Schover LR. Sexuality and fertility in urologic cancer patients. Cancer. 1987;60 (3 Suppl):553–8.
87. Walsh PC, Donker PJ. Impotence following radical prostatectomy: insight into etiology and prevention. J Urol. 2002;167(2 Pt 2):1005–10.
88. Quinlan DM, Epstein JI, Carter BS, Walsh PC. Sexual function following radical prostatectomy: influence of preservation of neurovascular bundles. J Urol. 1991;145(5):998–1002.
89. Borchers H, Brehmer B, Kirschner-Hermanns R, Reineke T, Tietze L, Jakse G. Erectile function after non-nerve-sparing radical prostatectomy: fact or fiction? Urol Int. 2006;76 (3):213–6. doi:10.1159/000091621.
90. Weinstein M, Roberts M. Sexual potency following surgery for rectal carcinoma. A follow-up of 44 patients. Ann Surg. 1977;185(3):295–300.
91. Catalona WJ, Bigg SW. Nerve-sparing radical prostatectomy: evaluation of results after 250 patients. J Urol. 1990;143(3):538–43. discussion 544.
92. Liang JT, Lai HS, Lee PH, Chang KJ. Laparoscopic pelvic autonomic nerve-preserving surgery for sigmoid colon cancer. Ann Surg Oncol. 2008;15(6):1609–16. doi:10.1245/s10434-008-9861-x.
93. Schoenberg MP, Walsh PC, Breazeale DR, Marshall FF, Mostwin JL, Brendler CB. Local recurrence and survival following nerve sparing radical cystoprostatectomy for bladder cancer: 10-year follow-up. J Urol. 1996;155(2):490–4.
94. Sica DA. Pharmacokinetics and pharmacodynamics of mineralocorticoid blocking agents and their effects on potassium homeostasis. Heart Fail Rev. 2005;10(1):23–9. doi:10.1007/s10741-005-2345-1.
95. Griffin JE, Wilson JD. Disorders of the testes and male reproductive tract. In: Wilson JD, editor. Williams textbook of endocrinology. 10th ed. Philadelphia: Saunders; 2003. p. 709–69.
96. Harrison WM, Rabkin JG, Ehrhardt AA, et al. Effects of antidepressant medication on sexual function: a controlled study. J Clin Psychopharmacol. 1986;6(3):144–9.
97. Monteiro WO, Noshirvani HF, Marks IM, Lelliott PT. Anorgasmia from clomipramine in obsessive-compulsive disorder. A controlled trial. Br J Psychiatry. 1987;151:107–12.
98. Keltner NL, McAfee KM, Taylor CL. Mechanisms and treatments of SSRI-induced sexual dysfunction. Perspect Psychiatr Care. 2002;38(3):111–6.
99. Sullivan G, Lukoff D. Sexual side effects of antipsychotic medication: evaluation and interventions. Hosp Community Psychiatry. 1990;41(11):1238–41.
100. Nudell DM, Monoski MM, Lipshultz LI. Common medications and drugs: how they affect male fertility. Urol Clin North Am. 2002;29(4):965–73.
101. Giuliano F. Impact of medical treatments for benign prostatic hyperplasia on sexual function. BJU Int. 2006;97 Suppl 2:34–8. doi:10.1111/j.1464-410X.2006.06104.x. discussion 44–5.
102. Traish AM, Hassani J, Guay AT, Zitzmann M, Hansen ML. Adverse side effects of 5alpha-reductase inhibitors therapy: persistent diminished libido and erectile dysfunction and depression in a subset of patients. J Sex Med. 2011;8(3):872–84. doi:10.1111/j.1743-6109.2010.02157.x.
103. Roehrborn CG, Siami P, Barkin J, et al. The effects of dutasteride, tamsulosin and combination therapy on lower urinary tract symptoms in men with benign prostatic hyperplasia and prostatic enlargement: 2-year results from the CombAT study. J Urol. 2008;179(2):616–21. doi:10.1016/j.juro.2007.09.084. discussion 621.
104. Amory JK, Anawalt BD, Matsumoto AM, et al. The effect of 5alpha-reductase inhibition with dutasteride and finasteride on bone mineral density, serum lipoproteins, hemoglobin, prostate specific antigen and sexual function in healthy young men. J Urol. 2008;179(6):2333–8. doi:10.1016/j.juro.2008.01.145.

105. AUA Practice Guidelines Committee. AUA guideline on management of benign prostatic hyperplasia (2003). Chapter 1: diagnosis and treatment recommendations. J Urol. 2003;170 (2 Pt 1):530–47. doi:10.1097/01.ju.0000078083.38675.79.
106. Marberger M, Roehrborn CG, Marks LS, Wilson T, Rittmaster RS. Relationship among serum testosterone, sexual function, and response to treatment in men receiving dutasteride for benign prostatic hyperplasia. J Clin Endocrinol Metab. 2006;91(4):1323–8. doi:10.1210/jc.2005-1947.
107. Hsieh TC, Pastuszak AW, Hwang K, Lipshultz LI. Concomitant intramuscular human chorionic gonadotropin preserves spermatogenesis in men undergoing testosterone replacement therapy. J Urol. 2012. doi:10.1016/j.juro.2012.09.043.
108. Zacharin M, Sabin MA, Nair VV, Dagabdhao P. Addition of recombinant follicle-stimulating hormone to human chorionic gonadotropin treatment in adolescents and young adults with hypogonadotropic hypogonadism promotes normal testicular growth and may promote early spermatogenesis. Fertil Steril. 2012;98(4):836–42. doi:10.1016/j.fertnstert.2012.06.022.
109. Wischmann T, Stammer H, Scherg H, Gerhard I, Verres R. Psychosocial characteristics of infertile couples: a study by the 'Heidelberg fertility consultation service'. Hum Reprod. 2001;16(8):1753–61.
110. Kedem P, Mikulincer M, Nathanson YE, Bartoov B. Psychological aspects of male infertility. Br J Med Psychol. 1990;63(Pt 1):73–80.
111. Shindel AW, Nelson CJ, Naughton CK, Ohebshalom M, Mulhall JP. Sexual function and quality of life in the male partner of infertile couples: prevalence and correlates of dysfunction. J Urol. 2008;179(3):1056–9. doi:10.1016/j.juro.2007.10.069.
112. Monga M, Alexandrescu B, Katz SE, Stein M, Ganiats T. Impact of infertility on quality of life, marital adjustment, and sexual function. Urology. 2004;63(1):126–30.
113. Jain K, Radhakrishnan G, Agrawal P. Infertility and psychosexual disorders: relationship in infertile couples. Indian J Med Sci. 2000;54(1):1–7.
114. Benazon N, Wright J, Sabourin S. Stress, sexual satisfaction, and marital adjustment in infertile couples. J Sex Marital Ther. 1992;18(4):273–84. doi:10.1080/00926239208412852.
115. Slade P, Raval H, Buck P, Lieberman BE. A 3-year follow-up of emotional, marital and sexual functioning in couples who were infertile. J Reprod Inf Psychol. 1992;10(4):233–43. doi:10.1080/02646839208403956.
116. O'Brien JH, Lazarou S, Deane L, Jarvi K, Zini A. Erectile dysfunction and andropause symptoms in infertile men. J Urol. 2005;174(5):1932–4. doi:10.1097/01.ju.0000177453.14334.a2. discussion 1934.
117. Mahlstedt PP. The psychological component of infertility. Fertil Steril. 1985;43(3):335–46.
118. Glover L, Gannon K, Sherr L, Abel PD. Psychological distress before and immediately after attendance at a male sub-fertility clinic. J R Soc Med. 1994;87(8):448–9.
119. Keye Jr WR. Psychosexual responses to infertility. Clin Obstet Gynecol. 1984;27(3):760–6.
120. Sigg C. Sexuality and sterility. Ther Umsch. 1994;51(2):115–9.
121. Gurkan L, Raynor MC, Hellstrom WJ. Sex and the infertile male. Semin Reprod Med. 2009;27(2):186–90. doi:10.1055/s-0029-1202308.
122. Saleh RA, Ranga GM, Raina R, Nelson DR, Agarwal A. Sexual dysfunction in men undergoing infertility evaluation: a cohort observational study. Fertil Steril. 2003;79 (4):909–12.
123. Nachtigall RD, Becker G, Wozny M. The effects of gender-specific diagnosis on men's and women's response to infertility. Fertil Steril. 1992;57(1):113–21.
124. Drake TS, Grunert GM. A cyclic pattern of sexual dysfunction in the infertility investigation. Fertil Steril. 1979;32(5):542–5.
125. Burns LH. Psychiatric aspects of infertility and infertility treatments. Psychiatr Clin North Am. 2007;30(4):689–716. doi:10.1016/j.psc.2007.08.001.
126. Lue TF. Impotence: a patient's goal-directed approach to treatment. World J Urol. 1990;8 (2):67–74.

127. Lue TF. A patient's goal-directed approach to erectile dysfunction and Peyronie's disease. Can J Urol. 1995;2(Supp 1):13–7.
128. Hatzichristou D, Rosen RC, Broderick G, et al. Clinical evaluation and management strategy for sexual dysfunction in men and women. J Sex Med. 2004;1(1):49–57. doi:10.1111/j.1743-6109.2004.10108.x.
129. Hatzichristou D, Rosen RC, Derogatis LR, et al. Recommendations for the clinical evaluation of men and women with sexual dysfunction. J Sex Med. 2010;7(1 pt 2):337–48. doi:10.1111/j.1743-6109.2009.01619.x.
130. Jarow JP, Nana-Sinkam P, Sabbagh M, Eskew A. Outcome analysis of goal directed therapy for impotence. J Urol. 1996;155(5):1609–12.
131. Hanash KA. Comparative results of goal oriented therapy for erectile dysfunction. J Urol. 1997;157(6):2135–8.
132. Jardin A, Wagner G, Khoury S, Giuliano F, Padma-Nathan H, Rosen R. Recommendations of the international scientific committee on the evaluation and treatment of erectile dysfunction. 2000.
133. Lue TF, Giuliano F, Montorsi F, et al. Original research: summary of the recommendations on sexual dysfunctions in men. J Sex Med. 2004;1(1):6–23. doi:10.1111/j.1743-6109.2004.10104.x.
134. Montorsi F, Adaikan G, Becher E, et al. Summary of the recommendations on sexual dysfunctions in men. J Sex Med. 2010;7(11):3572–88. doi:10.1111/j.1743-6109.2010.02062.x.
135. Lewis JM, Osbourne AL, O'Leary MP. Erectile dysfunction. J Med Liban. 2004;52(4):213–6.
136. Nusbaum MR, Hamilton CD. The proactive sexual health history. Am Fam Physician. 2002;66(9):1705–12.
137. Burnett AL. Erectile dysfunction: a practical approach for primary care. Geriatrics. 1998;53(2):34. http://search.ebscohost.com/login.aspx?direct=true&db=rzh&AN=1998040346&site=ehost-live.
138. Davis-Joseph B, Tiefer L, Melman A. Accuracy of the initial history and physical examination to establish the etiology of erectile dysfunction. Urology. 1995;45(3):498–502.
139. Martin-Morales A, Sanchez-Cruz JJ, Saenz de Tejada I, Rodriguez-Vela L, Jimenez-Cruz JF, Burgos-Rodriguez R. Prevalence and independent risk factors for erectile dysfunction in Spain: results of the epidemiologia de la disfuncion erectil masculina study. J Urol. 2001;166(2):569–74. discussion 574–5.
140. Kostis JB, Jackson G, Rosen R, et al. Sexual dysfunction and cardiac risk (the Second Princeton Consensus Conference). Am J Cardiol. 2005;96((12, Supplement 2)):85–93. doi:10.1016/j.amjcard.2005.12.018.
141. Kingsberg SA. Taking a sexual history. Obstet Gynecol Clin North Am. 2006;33(4):535–47. doi:10.1016/j.ogc.2006.09.002.
142. Fisher WA, Eardley I, McCabe M, Sand M. Original research? Couples' sexual Dysfunctions: erectile dysfunction (ED) is a shared sexual concern of couples I: couple conceptions of ED. J Sex Med. 2009;6(10):2746–60. doi:10.1111/j.1743-6109.2009.01457.x.
143. Rosen RC, Cappelleri JC, Smith MD, Lipsky J, Pena BM. Development and evaluation of an abridged, 5-item version of the international index of erectile function (IIEF-5) as a diagnostic tool for erectile dysfunction. Int J Impot Res. 1999;11(6):319–26.
144. Sun P, Swindle R. Are men with erectile dysfunction more likely to have hypertension than men without erectile dysfunction? A naturalistic national cohort study. J Urol. 2005;174(1):244–8. doi:10.1097/01.ju.0000162050.84946.86.
145. Zonszein J. Diagnosis and management of endocrine disorders of erectile dysfunction. Urol Clin North Am. 1995;22(4):789–802.
146. Ghanem HM, Salonia A, Martin-Morales A. Physical examination and laboratory testing for men with ED. J Sex Med. 2012. doi:10.1111/j.1743-6109.2012.02671.x

147. Ghanem HM, Salonia A, Martin-Morales A. SOP: physical examination and laboratory testing for men with erectile dysfunction. J Sex Med. 2013;10(1):108–10. doi:10.1111/j.1743-6109.2012.02734.x.
148. Wing RR, Rosen RC, Fava JL, et al. Effects of weight loss intervention on erectile function in older men with type 2 diabetes in the look AHEAD trial. J Sex Med. 2010;7(1 Pt 1):156–65. doi:10.1111/j.1743-6109.2009.01458.x.
149. Lamina S, Okoye CG, Dagogo TT. Therapeutic effect of an interval exercise training program in the management of erectile dysfunction in hypertensive patients. J Clin Hypertens (Greenwich). 2009;11(3):125–9. doi:10.1111/j.1751-7176.2009.00086.x.
150. Gupta BP, Murad MH, Clifton MM, Prokop L, Nehra A, Kopecky SL. The effect of lifestyle modification and cardiovascular risk factor reduction on erectile dysfunction: a systematic review and meta-analysis. Arch Intern Med. 2011;171(20):1797–803. doi:10.1001/archinternmed.2011.440.
151. Montague DK, Jarow JP, Broderick GA, et al. Chapter 1: the management of erectile dysfunction: an AUA update. J Urol. 2005;174(1):230–9. doi:10.1097/01.ju.0000164463.19239.19.
152. Esposito K, Giugliano D. Lifestyle for erectile dysfunction: a good choice. Arch Intern Med. 2012;172(3):295–6. doi:10.1001/archinternmed.2011.785. author reply 296.
153. Shabsigh R, Donatucci C, Costabile R, et al. Reliability of efficacy in men with erectile dysfunction treated with tadalafil once daily after initial success. Int J Impot Res. 2010;22(1):1–8. doi:10.1038/ijir.2009.29.
154. Montorsi F, Padma-Nathan H, Buvat J, et al. Earliest time to onset of action leading to successful intercourse with vardenafil determined in an at-home setting: a randomized, double-blind, placebo-controlled trial. J Sex Med. 2004;1(2):168–78. doi:10.1111/j.1743-6109.2004.04025.x.
155. Padma-Nathan H, Stecher VJ, Sweeney M, Orazem J, Tseng LJ, Deriesthal H. Minimal time to successful intercourse after sildenafil citrate: results of a randomized, double-blind, placebo-controlled trial. Urology. 2003;62(3):400–3.
156. Carson CC. Erectile dysfunction in the 21st century: whom we can treat, whom we cannot treat and patient education. Int J Impot Res. 2002;14 Suppl 1:S29–34. doi:10.1038/sj.ijir.3900804.
157. Rajagopalan P, Mazzu A, Xia C, Dawkins R, Sundaresan P. Effect of high-fat breakfast and moderate-fat evening meal on the pharmacokinetics of vardenafil, an oral phosphodiesterase-5 inhibitor for the treatment of erectile dysfunction. J Clin Pharmacol. 2003;43(3):260–7.
158. Wespes E, Amar E, Hatzichristou D, et al. EAU guidelines on erectile dysfunction: an update. Eur Urol. 2006;49(5):806–15. doi:10.1016/j.eururo.2006.01.028.
159. Fulgham PF, Cochran JS, Denman JL, et al. Disappointing initial results with transurethral alprostadil for erectile dysfunction in a urology practice setting. J Urol. 1998;160(6 Pt 1):2041–6.
160. Mulhall JP, Jahoda AE, Ahmed A, Parker M. Analysis of the consistency of intraurethral prostaglandin E(1) (MUSE) during at-home use. Urology. 2001;58(2):262–6.
161. Nehra A, Blute ML, Barrett DM, Moreland RB. Rationale for combination therapy of intraurethral prostaglandin E(1) and sildenafil in the salvage of erectile dysfunction patients desiring noninvasive therapy. Int J Impot Res. 2002;14 Suppl 1:S38–42. doi:10.1038/sj.ijir.3900795.
162. Mydlo JH, Volpe MA, MacChia RJ. Results from different patient populations using combined therapy with alprostadil and sildenafil: predictors of satisfaction. BJU Int. 2000;86(4):469–73.
163. Lewis RW. Intraurethral and topical agents. Drugs Today (Barc). 2000;36(2–3):113–9.
164. Costa P, Potempa AJ. Intraurethral alprostadil for erectile dysfunction: a review of the literature. Drugs. 2012;72(17):2243–54. doi:10.2165/11641380-000000000-00000.

165. Linet OI, Ogrinc FG. Efficacy and safety of intracavernosal alprostadil in men with erectile dysfunction. The Alprostadil Study Group. N Engl J Med. 1996;334(14):873–7. doi:10.1056/NEJM199604043341401.
166. Heaton JP, Lording D, Liu SN, et al. Intracavernosal alprostadil is effective for the treatment of erectile dysfunction in diabetic men. Int J Impot Res. 2001;13(6):317–21.
167. Sidi AA, Cameron JS, Duffy LM, Lange PH. Intracavernous drug-induced erections in the management of male erectile dysfunction: experience with 100 patients. J Urol. 1986;135(4):704–6.
168. Zorgniotti AW, Lefleur RS. Auto-injection of the corpus cavernosum with a vasoactive drug combination for vasculogenic impotence. J Urol. 1985;133(1):39–41.
169. Robinette MA, Moffat MJ. Intracorporal injection of papaverine and phentolamine in the management of impotence. Br J Urol. 1986;58(6):692–5.
170. Porst H. The rationale for prostaglandin E1 in erectile failure: a survey of worldwide experience. J Urol. 1996;155(3):802–15.
171. Bennett AH, Carpenter AJ, Barada JH. An improved vasoactive drug combination for a pharmacological erection program. J Urol. 1991;146(6):1564–5.
172. Moemen MN, Hamed HA, Kamel II, Shamloul RM, Ghanem HM. Clinical and sonographic assessment of the side effects of intracavernous injection of vasoactive substances. Int J Impot Res. 2004;16(2):143–5. doi:10.1038/sj.ijir.3901194.
173. Hackett G, Kell P, Ralph D, et al. British society for sexual medicine guidelines on the management of erectile dysfunction. J Sex Med. 2008;5(8):1841–65. doi:10.1111/j.1743-6109.2008.00773.x.
174. Broderick GA, McGahan JP, Stone AR, White RD. The hemodynamics of vacuum constriction erections: assessment by color Doppler ultrasound. J Urol. 1992;147(1):57–61.
175. McMahon CG. Nonsurgical treatment of cavernosal venous leakage. Urology. 1997;49(1):97–100. doi:10.1016/S0090-4295(96)00389-5.
176. Witherington R. Vacuum constriction device for management of erectile impotence. J Urol. 1989;141(2):320–2.
177. Sidi AA, Becher EF, Zhang G, Lewis JH. Patient acceptance of and satisfaction with an external negative pressure device for impotence. J Urol. 1990;144(5):1154–6.
178. Nadig PW, Ware JC, Blumoff R. Noninvasive device to produce and maintain an erection-like state. Urology. 1986;27(2):126–31.
179. Vrijhof HJ, Delaere KP. Vacuum constriction devices in erectile dysfunction: acceptance and effectiveness in patients with impotence of organic or mixed aetiology. Br J Urol. 1994;74(1):102–5.
180. Dutta TC, Eid JF. Vacuum constriction devices for erectile dysfunction: a long-term, prospective study of patients with mild, moderate, and severe dysfunction. Urology. 1999;54(5):891–3.
181. Blackard CE, Borkon WD, Lima JS, Nelson J. Use of vacuum tumescence device for impotence secondary to venous leakage. Urology. 1993;41(3):225–30.
182. Baltaci S, Aydos K, Kosar A, Anafarta K. Treating erectile dysfunction with a vacuum tumescence device: a retrospective analysis of acceptance and satisfaction. Br J Urol. 1995;76(6):757–60.
183. Turner LA, Althof SE, Levine SB, et al. Treating erectile dysfunction with external vacuum devices: impact upon sexual, psychological and marital functioning. J Urol. 1990;144(1):79–82.
184. Turner LA, Althof SE, Levine SB, Bodner DR, Kursh ED, Resnick MI. External vacuum devices in the treatment of erectile dysfunction: a one-year study of sexual and psychosocial impact. J Sex Marital Ther. 1991;17(2):81–93. doi:10.1080/00926239108404950.
185. Cookson MS, Nadig PW. Long-term results with vacuum constriction device. J Urol. 1993;149(2):290–4.
186. Montague DK, Angermeier KW. Penile prosthesis implantation. Urol Clin North Am. 2001;28(2):355–61. x.

187. Montague DK, Angermeier KW. Contemporary aspects of penile prosthesis implantation. Urol Int. 2003;70(2):141–6. doi: 68189.
188. Lotti F, Corona G, Rastrelli G, Forti G, Jannini EA, Maggi M. Clinical correlates of erectile dysfunction and premature ejaculation in men with couple infertility. J Sex Med. 2012;9(10):2698–707. doi:10.1111/j.1743-6109.2012.02872.x.
189. Rosen RC. Psychogenic erectile dysfunction. Classification and management. Urol Clin North Am. 2001;28(2):269–78.
190. McCabe M, Althof SE, Assalian P, et al. Psychological and interpersonal dimensions of sexual function and dysfunction. J Sex Med. 2010;7(1 Pt 2):327–36. doi:10.1111/j.1743-6109.2009.01618.x.
191. Wylie KR. Treatment outcome of brief couple therapy in psychogenic male erectile disorder. Arch Sex Behav. 1997;26(5):527–45.
192. Hawton K. Integration of treatments for male erectile dysfunction. Lancet. 1998;351(9095):7–8. doi:10.1016/S0140-6736(05)78097-1.
193. Hellstrom WJ, Wang R, Peterson CA, Varady JC, Gesundheit N, Sikka SC. Effects of alprostadil and prazosin on motility, viability and membrane integrity of human sperm. J Urol. 1998;159(5):1559–62. doi:10.1097/00005392-199805000-00041.
194. Kobayashi K, Masumori N, Hisasue S, et al. Inhibition of seminal emission is the main cause of anejaculation induced by a new highly selective alpha1A-blocker in normal volunteers. J Sex Med. 2008;5(9):2185–90. doi:10.1111/j.1743-6109.2008.00779.x.
195. Andrade JR, Traboulsi A, Hussain A, Dubin NH. In vitro effects of sildenafil and phentolamine, drugs used for erectile dysfunction, on human sperm motility. Am J Obstet Gynecol. 2000;182(5):1093–5.
196. Tillem SM, Mellinger BC. Azoospermia due to aperistalsis of the vas deferens: successful treatment with pseudoephedrine. Urology. 1999;53(2):417–9.
197. Smith JF, Walsh TJ, Turek PJ. Ejaculatory duct obstruction. Urol Clin North Am. 2008;35(2):221–7. doi:10.1016/j.ucl.2008.01.011. viii.
198. Jones Jr HW, Jones GS, Andrews MC, et al. The program for in vitro fertilization at Norfolk. Fertil Steril. 1982;38(1):14–21.

Chapter 7
Anejaculation, Retrograde Ejaculation, and Anorgasmia

Peter J. Stahl and Doron S. Stember

Introduction

Antegrade transit of sperm through the male genital ductal system and ultimately out the anterior urethra is among the most basic and essential biological processes for male reproduction. Neither natural conception nor assisted reproduction is possible unless sperm-containing semen can be delivered into the female reproductive tract or to the embryology laboratory. Disorders that impair semen delivery should be broadly categorized as either anorgasmia or absence of antegrade ejaculation, which may result from retrograde ejaculation or anejaculation. Anorgasmia, as the term suggests, refers to inability to achieve climactic pleasure during sexual activity. Retrograde ejaculation refers to the absence of antegrade ejaculate but presence of sperm in a postorgasmic urinalysis. Anejaculation refers to absence of antegrade or retrograde ejaculate despite achievement of orgasm. Anorgasmia, retrograde ejaculation, and anejaculation are pathophysiologically distinct disorders that warrant specific diagnostic and therapeutic approaches.

Physiology

Basic understanding of the male sexual response cycle provides an essential framework for conceptualizing and treating disorders of orgasm and ejaculation in men. Desire and arousal comprise the first two phases of the male sexual response cycle and are critical for normal male reproductive function [1]. Desire depends upon cortical processing of environmental factors, partner factors, and prior sexual

P.J. Stahl (✉)
Department of Urology, Columbia University Medical Center, New York, NY 10032, USA
e-mail: ps2192@columbia.edu

J.P. Mulhall and W. Hsiao (eds.), *Men's Sexual Health and Fertility*,
DOI 10.1007/978-1-4939-0425-9_7,

experiences. Though incompletely understood, serotoninergic, dopaminergic, and sex steroid signaling play integral roles [2].

In the arousal phase, peripheral afferent genital and nongenital tactile, auditory, visual, and olfactory stimuli are integrated and centrally processed. The main genital tactile input is derived from receptors and free nerve endings located in the glans of the penis, the penile shaft skin, and the scrotum. Sensory information from the penis is carried by the paired dorsal penile nerves (sensory branches of the pudendal nerves) to the sacral segments of the spinal cord.

Penile tumescence results from both a spinal reflex arc and higher-order efferent central signals, which may be excitatory but are tonically inhibitory. Increased rigidity of the corpora cavernosa during erection enables higher levels of sexual stimulation (i.e., through penetrative sexual activity) and pushes free nerve endings within the penile skin closer to the surface, thereby increasing the level of afferent input. However, it should be noted that erection is not required for orgasm or ejaculation. Ultimately a threshold of arousal is reached that triggers the orgasmic and ejaculatory responses, which constitute the effector phase of the male sexual response cycle that in normal cases results in passage of semen out the urethral meatus. Orgasm and ejaculation are integrated but incompletely interdependent processes, as orgasm may occur in the absence of ejaculation (but not vice versa). This is commonly the case after surgical removal of the prostate and seminal vesicles for prostate cancer.

Ejaculation consists of two distinct phases: emission and expulsion. Seminal emission refers to deposition of seminal fluid, prostatic fluid, and sperm into the posterior urethra. Emission is mediated by sympathetic fibers that originate in the thoracic spinal cord at levels T10–L2, course through the paraspinal sympathetic ganglia that comprise the sympathetic chains, and ultimately travel to the prostate, seminal vesicles, vasa deferentia, and epididymis as the pelvic nerves. Alpha-1 receptor signaling is critical for emission.

Expulsion refers to rhythmic, forcible contractions of striated periurethral muscles including the bulbospongiosus muscle while the bladder neck is closed, resulting in projectile expulsion of semen out the urethral meatus. The bulbocavernosus and other periurethral muscles are innervated by the pudendal nerve, which is therefore thought to be integral for the expulsive phase. It is important to note that contraction of the bladder neck is necessary to prevent retrograde ejaculation during expulsion.

Effective ejaculation of semen requires precise regulatory coordination of emission and expulsion that occurs at the spinal level. A neural circuit known as the ejaculatory central pattern generator (CPG) integrates supraspinal modulatory input with peripheral sensory input and initiates coordinated action of the many effectors of the ejaculatory response, including the prostate, seminal vesicles, vasa deferentia, epididymis, bladder neck, and periurethral muscles [3]. It is important to note that supraspinal input is modulatory and not required, as men with complete spinal cord injuries above T10 can ejaculate in response to vibratory stimulation.

Orgasm is a distinct supraspinal, higher-order cognitive event that occurs after a threshold level of arousal is attained. The neurobiological basis of orgasm remains incompletely understood. It may require central integration of ascending signaling from the ejaculatory CPG or may be the result of central processing of proprioceptive input derived from the rhythmic contractions of the periurethral and bulbocavernosus muscles during the expulsive phase of ejaculation.

Pathophysiology

Conceptualization of anorgasmia, retrograde ejaculation, and anejaculation within the framework of the male sexual response cycle enables logical formulation of differential diagnoses, informs selection of diagnostic tests, and ultimately guides therapeutic intervention. Disorders that inhibit the desire and arousal phases result in anorgasmia, whereas anejaculation results from failure of emission and/or expulsion, and retrograde ejaculation results from disordered expulsion. Table 7.1 lists physiologic drivers and facilitators of each phase of the male sexual response cycle and commonly clinically encountered factors that disrupt each phase. Though in-depth discussion of each clinical disruptor is beyond the scope of this chapter, most cases of absent antegrade ejaculate result from several common clinical scenarios.

Pharmacologic Disruptors

Medications are among the most commonly encountered causes of orgasmic and ejaculatory dysfunction. Any pharmacotherapy that interferes with dopaminergic, serotoninergic, adrenergic, or gamma aminobutyric acid (GABA) signaling can impair the desire, arousal, or ejaculatory phases of the male sexual response cycle. Antidepressant medications that disrupt serotoninergic signaling affect all three phases of male sexual response, though in men the desire and orgasm phases seem to be preferentially disrupted [4]. The selective serotonin reuptake inhibitors (SSRIs) and the serotonin-norepinephrine reuptake inhibitors (SNRIs) are the most commonly implicated agents. Antipsychotic medications predominantly target dopaminergic signaling and may impair sexual arousal or orgasm in up to 70 % of patients [5]. Alpha-1 adrenoreceptor antagonists inhibit contracture of the bladder neck and thus may cause retrograde ejaculation through interference with the expulsion phase of ejaculation, though these agents may also exert peripheral or central effects that impair emission and thus result in anejaculation [6]. Antiepileptic drugs and neuromodulatory agents including gabapentin have also been implicated in ejaculatory and orgasmic dysfunction [7].

Table 7.1 Conceptual framework for disorders of absent antegrade ejaculation

Phase of male sexual response	Physiologic drivers/ facilitators	Clinical disruptors	Result
Desire	Environment Sex steroid signaling Dopamine signaling Serotonin signaling	Stress/anxiety Endocrine disorders Antipsychotic drugs SSRIs Brain disorders Depression	Anorgasmia
Arousal	Dorsal penile nerves Pudendal nerves Central processing Erection	Peripheral neuropathy (DM) Brain disorders Depression Erectile dysfunction Spinal cord injury	Anorgasmia
Emission	Sympathetic chain Pelvic nerves Alpha adrenergic signaling	Peripheral neuropathy Sympathetic nerve injury (RPLND, radiation) Spinal cord injury Multiple sclerosis Alpha-blockers Ejaculatory duct obstruction	Anejaculation
Expulsion	Bladder neck Pudendal nerve	Bladder neck surgery Peripheral neuropathy (DM) Spinal cord Injury Pelvic nerve injury (RPLND, radiation) Antipsychotic drugs Alpha-blockers	Anejaculation Retrograde ejaculation

Neurogenic Disruptors

Spinal cord injury is a commonly encountered etiology of orgasmic and ejaculatory dysfunction. Most spinal cord-injured men are unable to ejaculate without therapeutic intervention [8]. Complete or partial injury at any level usually results in multiphase disruption of the male sexual response cycle. Low self-esteem and psychosocial dysfunction may impair sexual desire. Absent or reduced afferent sensory input affects arousal. Disruption of the spinal ejaculatory CPG and spinal reflex arcs that control emission and expulsion can result in anejaculation or retrograde ejaculation.

Retroperitoneal lymph node dissection (RPLND) is an integral component of multimodality treatment for testicular cancer and a common cause of neurogenic ejaculatory dysfunction. Retroperitoneal lymph nodes near the aorta, vena cava, and iliac blood vessels are excised to remove any sites of potential retroperitoneal nodal metastases. During RPLND the sympathetic chains, the postganglionic branches of the thoracolumbar sympathetic nerves, and the autonomic nerves of the pelvis are at risk of injury or excision. Injury to these structures can result in complete failure of emission with resultant anejaculation or in discoordination of emission and bladder neck closure with resultant retrograde ejaculation. The development of limited operative templates and nerve-sparing procedures has greatly reduced the incidence of ejaculatory dysfunction after RPLND to under 5 % [9]. However, nerve sparing is difficult in some clinical scenarios (i.e., after chemotherapy), and RPLND remains a common cause of ejaculatory dysfunction [10].

Diabetes mellitus is a common cause of peripheral and autonomic neuropathy that may interfere with orgasm and ejaculation. Decreased genital and nongenital sensation from loss of afferent sensory fibers may inhibit arousal and orgasm. Autonomic neuropathy may affect emission, bladder neck closure, or both. Affected men often progress from decreased semen volume to complete absence of antegrade ejaculation, which usually reflects either retrograde ejaculation or more commonly complete failure of emission [11].

Mechanical Disruptors

Mechanical disruption of the bladder neck or prostate from prior surgery is yet another cause of ejaculatory dysfunction. Transurethral resection of the prostate and reconstruction of the bladder neck for outlet obstruction are common acquired causes of retrograde ejaculation, as these surgeries often render the bladder neck partially incompetent and unable to fully close during the expulsive phase of ejaculation. Up to 30–40 % of men report retrograde ejaculation after transurethral prostate surgery [12].

Clinical Evaluation

History

The clinical evaluation should begin with a focused history. The initial focus should be to distinguish anorgasmia from absence of antegrade ejaculation by direct questioning about whether or not the patient is able to achieve a climactic pleasurable experience during sexual activity. This may be difficult in patients with limited sexual awareness or experience. It is important to determine if absence of antegrade ejaculate is a lifelong or acquired problem. Patients should be queried about whether or not there is any situational variability in their ability to produce antegrade ejaculate and if nocturnal emissions are present. Situational variability in orgasmic function suggests a disorder of desire or arousal, as opposed to a pharmacologically induced or neurogenic failure of emission or expulsion. Patients should be screened for signs and symptoms of hypogonadism (i.e., low energy, low libido), erectile dysfunction, diabetes (i.e., polyuria), psychiatric illness (i.e., depression), and neurological disease (i.e., sensory abnormalities, bowel or bladder dysfunction). Obtaining detailed sexual, medical, and surgical histories is critically important, as is identification of all prescribed medications.

Physical Examination

The focused physical examination should include examination of the penis and scrotum for assessment of the location of the urethral meatus, penile development, testicular size, and presence of the vasa deferentia and a full neurological exam. Body habitus, gynecomastia, and/or thyroid abnormalities may indicate the presence of endocrinopathy and should be noted. Assessment of penile vibratory sensory thresholds with biothesiometry is a useful adjunct that may be helpful to identify decreased penile sensation [13].

Additional Testing

Additional testing should be directed by findings in the history and physical examination. There should be a low threshold for serum testing to screen patients for diabetes (hemoglobin A1c), hypogonadism (early morning total testosterone), or hypothyroidism (thyroxine- and thyroid-stimulating hormone). Postorgasm urinalysis should be performed in all patients who are able to achieve orgasm to distinguish anejaculation from retrograde ejaculation. The diagnosis of retrograde ejaculation can be made if sperm, fructose, or seminal fluid are observed in the postorgasm voided urine sample [14]. Postorgasm urinalysis should be performed after at least 2 days of ejaculatory abstinence. The patient should first empty his bladder, after which he should perform self-stimulation to achieve orgasm. Any antegrade ejaculate is collected in its own specimen container. The patient should then be instructed to void after waiting 15–20 min. The postorgasm urine sample is then centrifuged, and the derived pellet is microscopically examined for the presence and quantity of sperm.

Medical Management

Withdrawal of Disruptive Medications

The first step in the medical management of anejaculation is cessation or adjustment of medications that interfere with the emission or expulsion phases of

Table 7.2 Drug classes implicated in orgasmic and ejaculatory dysfunction

Drug class	Phase of male sexual response affected
Antidepressants	Desire, arousal, orgasm
Antipsychotics	Arousal, orgasm
Alpha-blockers	Orgasm, emission, expulsion
Antiepileptics	Anorgasmia
Neuromodulators	Anorgasmia

ejaculation (Table 7.2). In patients on alpha-blockers who cannot discontinue alpha-blocker therapy, switching to the highly selective agent alfuzosin may be beneficial [15].

Sympathomimetic Therapy

In some patients, therapy with oral sympathomimetic agents may improve bladder neck contraction during the expulsive phase of ejaculation and thereby convert retrograde ejaculation to antegrade ejaculation [16]. In some cases sympathomimetic therapy is effective for anejaculatory patients and results in either induction of retrograde or antegrade ejaculation. Commonly used sympathomimetic agents include the tricyclic antidepressant imipramine (25–75 mg daily), pseudoephedrine (60 mg four times daily), and midodrine (7.5–30 mg daily) [17].

Sperm Harvesting from Postorgasm Urine

Collection of sperm from a postorgasm voided urine sample can be considered for acquisition of sperm to be used for assisted reproduction techniques. The urine is typically alkalinized with sodium bicarbonate (50 mg 12 and 2 h prior to sperm harvest) to minimize the toxic effect of acidic urine on sperm. The bladder is catheterized or the patient is asked to void immediately prior to orgasm to minimize the volume of urine in the bladder. After orgasm the voided or catheterized urine is centrifuged for collection of sperm, which are then resuspended in appropriate media for use in assisted reproduction [18].

Assisted Ejaculation Procedures

Assisted ejaculation procedures can be used to obtain sperm for assisted reproduction in anorgasmic and anejaculatory men. Surgical sperm retrieval from the seminal vesicles, epididymis, or testes is another option that may be considered, though discussion of these techniques is outside the scope of this chapter. Two assisted ejaculation procedures are available: penile vibratory stimulation and electroejaculation.

Penile vibratory stimulation (PVS) refers to use of a vibrator applied to the frenular surface of the penis to induce ejaculation. PVS activates an ejaculatory reflex arc that results in a normal ejaculation when all components of the reflex arc are intact and descending cortical inhibitory input is absent. The reflex arc begins with afferent sensory input from the dorsal penile nerves that travels through the pudendal nerve to enter the sacral spinal cord (S2–S4) and travels through spinal interneurons to the thoracolumbar spinal cord (T10–L2). There is then simultaneous sympathetic outflow from T10–L2 to the effector organs of emission (the prostate, seminal vesicles, vas deferens, epididymis, and bladder neck) and efferent motor outflow from S2 to S4 via the pudendal nerve to the periurethral muscles, which mediate expulsion.

The best candidates for PVS are those men with a complete spinal cord injury above the level of T9–T10 in whom the ejaculation reflex arc is intact and inhibitory cortical input is disrupted. Optimal vibration parameters are 2.5 mm amplitude and 100 Hz frequency [19], though simple vibrators without adjustable amplitudes and frequencies may also be used effectively. PVS may also be used in non-spinal cord-injured patients with idiopathic anorgasmia or peripheral neuropathy, though reported experience in such patients is limited. Possible side effects of PVS include abrasions of the penile skin and autonomic dysreflexia in at-risk spinal cord-injured men. Such men should be treated prophylactically with nifedipine (10–20 mg) prior to the procedure. Ejaculated sperm retrieved via PVS have been used successfully for in vitro fertilization, intrauterine insemination, and intravaginal insemination [8].

Electroejaculation (EEJ) is a more invasive assisted ejaculation procedure in which a specialized transrectal probe is used to deliver rhythmic electrostimulation directly to the prostate and seminal vesicles. EEJ is effective for inducing ejaculation in the vast majority of men with anejaculation or anorgasmia of any etiology [20]. It may be performed in the office in spinal cord-injured men but requires general anesthesia for those with intact sensation. Pre-procedure bladder catheterization is performed to empty the bladder, after which sperm transport media is instilled through the catheter. Rectoscopy is recommended before and after EEJ to identify rectal pathology that might preclude or result from the procedure. EEJ should be aborted if rectal ulcerations or other mucosal abnormalities are identified. After rectoscopy the EEJ probe is inserted and held firmly against the prostate and seminal vesicles. An escalating amplitude of rhythmic electrostimulation is administered until ejaculation is achieved, which may be retrograde or antegrade and is collected for use in assisted reproduction. As is the case for PVS, patients at risk for autonomic dysreflexia should receive prophylactic nifedipine prior to EEJ. Sperm harvested during EEJ have been used to successfully achieve pregnancy via intrauterine insemination and in vitro fertilization [21].

Conclusion

Failure of the male sexual response cycle at various points may result in anorgasmia, retrograde ejaculation, and anejaculation. These disorders each present with absence of antegrade ejaculation. However, each is a pathophysiologically distinct disorder that warrants a specific diagnostic and therapeutic approach. An informed, logical multimodal approach to affected men is successful in the majority of cases.

References

1. Rowland D, McMahon CG, Abdo C, Chen J, Jannini E, Waldinger MD, et al. Disorders of orgasm and ejaculation in men. J Sex Med. 2010;7(4 Pt 2):1668–86.
2. Giuliano F. Neurophysiology of erection and ejaculation. J Sex Med. 2011;8 Suppl 4:310–5.
3. Allard J, Truitt WA, McKenna KE, Coolen LM. Spinal cord control of ejaculation. World J Urol. 2005;23(2):119–26.
4. Serretti A, Chiesa A. Sexual side effects of pharmacological treatment of psychiatric diseases. Clin Pharmacol Ther. 2011;89(1):142–7.
5. Baggaley M. Sexual dysfunction in schizophrenia: focus on recent evidence. Hum Psychopharmacol. 2008;23(3):201–9.
6. Kobayashi K, Masumori N, Hisasue S, Kato R, Hashimoto K, Itoh N, et al. Inhibition of seminal emission is the main cause of anejaculation induced by a new highly selective alpha1A-blocker in normal volunteers. J Sex Med. 2008;5(9):2185–90.
7. Labbate LA, Rubey RN. Gabapentin-induced ejaculatory failure and anorgasmia. Am J Psychiatry. 1999;156(6):972.
8. Ohl DA, Quallich SA, Sonksen J, Brackett NL, Lynne CM. Anejaculation: an electrifying approach. Semin Reprod Med. 2009;27(2):179–85.
9. Beck SD, Bey AL, Bihrle R, Foster RS. Ejaculatory status and fertility rates after primary retroperitoneal lymph node dissection. J Urol. 2010;184(5):2078–80.
10. Coogan CL, Hejase MJ, Wahle GR, Foster RS, Rowland RG, Bihrle R, et al. Nerve sparing post-chemotherapy retroperitoneal lymph node dissection for advanced testicular cancer. J Urol. 1996;156(5):1656–8.
11. Dunsmuir WD, Holmes SA. The aetiology and management of erectile, ejaculatory, and fertility problems in men with diabetes mellitus. Diabet Med. 1996;13(8):700–8.
12. Hill B, Belville W, Bruskewitz R, Issa M, Perez-Marrero R, Roehrborn C, et al. Transurethral needle ablation versus transurethral resection of the prostate for the treatment of symptomatic benign prostatic hyperplasia: 5-year results of a prospective, randomized, multicenter clinical trial. J Urol. 2004;171(6 Pt 1):2336–40.
13. Breda G, Xausa D, Giunta A, Tamai A, Silvestre P, Gherardi L. Nomogram for penile biothesiometry. Eur Urol. 1991;20(1):67–9.
14. Colpi G, Weidner W, Jungwirth A, Pomerol J, Papp G, Hargreave T, et al. EAU guidelines on ejaculatory dysfunction. Eur Urol. 2004;46(5):555–8.
15. Hellstrom WJ, Sikka SC. Effects of acute treatment with tamsulosin versus alfuzosin on ejaculatory function in normal volunteers. J Urol. 2006;176(4 Pt 1):1529–33.
16. Ohl DA, Quallich SA, Sonksen J, Brackett NL, Lynne CM. Anejaculation and retrograde ejaculation. Urol Clin North Am. 2008;35(2):211–20. viii.
17. Kamischke A, Nieschlag E. Update on medical treatment of ejaculatory disorders. Int J Androl. 2002;25(6):333–44.

18. Jefferys A, Siassakos D, Wardle P. The management of retrograde ejaculation: a systematic review and update. Fertil Steril. 2012;97(2):306–12.
19. Sonksen J, Biering-Sorensen F, Kristensen JK. Ejaculation induced by penile vibratory stimulation in men with spinal cord injuries. The importance of the vibratory amplitude. Paraplegia. 1994;32(10):651–60.
20. Brackett NL, Ibrahim E, Iremashvili V, Aballa TC, Lynne CM. Treatment for ejaculatory dysfunction in men with spinal cord injury: an 18-year single center experience. J Urol. 2010;183(6):2304–8.
21. Brackett NL, Lynne CM, Ibrahim E, Ohl DA, Sonksen J. Treatment of infertility in men with spinal cord injury. Nat Rev Urol. 2010;7(3):162–72.

Chapter 8
Premature Ejaculation

Patrick E. Teloken and John P. Mulhall

Abbreviation

APA	American Psychiatric Association
AUA	American Urological Association
ED	Erectile dysfunction
EMLA	Eutectic mixture of local anesthetics
ICD	International Classification of Diseases
IELT	Intravaginal ejaculatory latency time
ISSM	International Society for Sexual Medicine
PDE5	Phosphodiesterase type 5
PE	Premature ejaculation
PRN	Pro re nata; as needed
SSRI	Selective serotonin reuptake inhibitor
WHO	World Health Organization

Introduction

Premature ejaculation (PE) is a male sexual disorder characterized by (a) ejaculation which always or nearly always occurs before or within about 1 min of vaginal penetration, (b) the inability to delay ejaculation on all or nearly all vaginal penetrations, and (c) negative personal consequences such as distress, bother, frustration, and/or the avoidance of sexual intimacy. While the complaint of ejaculating more rapidly than desired is common, in isolation this is not diagnostic of the disorder. Two types of PE have been described: lifelong, which occurs from

J.P. Mulhall (✉)
Department of Urology, Memorial Sloan Kettering Cancer Center, 1275 York Avenue, Box 435, New York, NY 10065, USA
e-mail: mulhalj1@mskcc.org

J.P. Mulhall and W. Hsiao (eds.), *Men's Sexual Health and Fertility*, DOI 10.1007/978-1-4939-0425-9_8, © Springer Science+Business Media New York 2014 the first sexual encounter, and acquired, which ensues after a period of normal sexual function. This disorder is associated with low self-esteem, anxiety, depression, and relationship strain. Lack of awareness about the condition and its treatable nature represent barriers for seeking treatment, leaving many patients unattended. There are multiple options for the management of PE, including behavioral therapy, topical, and oral medications. Some of the treatments for PE can have a negative impact on seminal parameters, and care must be taken in patients trying to conceive. Particularly in couples who are under significant stress due to fertility difficulties, PE can represent a significant added burden. Successful treatment of PE has the potential to significantly improve the quality of life and well-being of patients and their partners.

Definition of Premature Ejaculation

The two definitions for premature ejaculation (PE) that had been utilized most often come from the American Psychiatric Association [1] and the World Health Organization [2] (Table 8.1). Definitions were derived by expert panels and were devoid of any evidence-based support of definitions.

When studying PE, an endpoint commonly used in studies and clinical practice is the intravaginal ejaculatory latency time (IELT, also known as IVELT). The IELT is the time from the first moment of vaginal penetration to ejaculation and orgasm. However, in the absence of patient and/or partner distress, IELT should not be used to characterize sexual dysfunction. On the hand the complaint of "ejaculating prematurely" is frequent even among men with normal IELT [3]. Thereby, no single factor adequately defines PE, and its definition should include multiple factors [4].

The International Society for Sexual Medicine (ISSM) first convened a panel of experts in 2007 to review the current medical literature and to arrive at a functional definition for lifelong PE [5][6]. The panel defined PE as having three components: (a) ejaculation which always or nearly always occurs before or within about 1 min of vaginal penetration, (b) the inability to delay ejaculation on all or nearly all vaginal penetrations, and (c) negative personal consequences such as distress, bother, frustration, and/or the avoidance of sexual intimacy. Lifelong PE is characterized by onset from the very first sexual encounter and is persistent, whereas acquired PE starts after a period of normal ejaculatory latency and is associated with milder reductions in IELT.

In an attempt to create a classification that has better clinical utility, Waldinger proposed to categorize PE into four subtypes: lifelong, acquired, natural variable, and premature-like ejaculatory dysfunction (Table 8.2) [4]. While it may seem a subtle change, this subcategorization has clinical utility because this system categorizes nearly all patients seen in clinical practice. The class with natural variable PE consists of men who only occasionally suffer from rapid ejaculation, which in

Table 8.1 Definitions of premature ejaculation

Organization	Year	Definition
APA—DSM-V	2013	• Ejaculation within approximately 1 min following vaginal penetration and before the individual wishes • Present for at least 6 months and experienced in almost all or all occasions (75–100 %) • Causes significant distress to the individual • Not better explained by another disorder or stressor
ISSM	2008	• Ejaculation within about a minute • Inability to delay ejaculation • All or nearly all vaginal penetrations • Negative personal consequences
AUA	2004	• Ejaculation occurring sooner than desired • Ejaculation before or shortly after penetration • Causes distress to one/both partners
APA—DSM-IV	2000	• Persistent or recurrent ejaculation with minimal sexual stimulation before, on, or shortly after penetration • Ejaculation before the person wishes it
ICD-10 (WHO)	1993	• Inability to delay ejaculation sufficiently to enjoy intercourse • Ejaculation before/very soon after beginning of intercourse (within 15 s) or in the absence of sufficient erection for penetration • Not due to prolonged sexual abstinence

APA American Psychiatric Association, *WHO* World Health Organization, *ISSM* International Society for Sexual Medicine, *AUA* American Urological Association, *ICD* International Classification of Diseases

this schema is considered normal. Finally, men with premature-like ejaculatory dysfunction complain of rapid ejaculation but have normal or even prolonged IELT.

The fifth edition of the Diagnostic and Statistical Manual of Mental Disorders (DSM-V) definition now more closely matches that of the ISSM requiring (a) a persistent or recurrent pattern of ejaculation during partnered sexual activity within approximately 1 min following vaginal penetration and before the individual wishes; (b) present for at least 6 months and experienced in almost all or all occasions; (c) causes significant distress to the individual; and (d) not better explained by a nonsexual mental disorder or as a consequence of a severe relationship distress or other significant stressors and is not attributable to the effects of a substance or another medical condition [7].

Epidemiology

Premature ejaculation (PE) is different from other sexual dysfunctions as it is highly dependent on the cultural context, is self-identified, and is self-rated in terms of severity. In the Multicountry Concept Evaluation and Assessment of Premature

Table 8.2 Variations of premature ejaculation (adapted from Waldinger)

Type	Features
Lifelong	• PE at all or nearly all intercourse attempts • With all or nearly all women • In majority of cases within 1 min • Consistent during life
Acquired	• Rapid ejaculation occurring at some point in life • Normal ejaculation prior to onset of PE • Source of problem often identifiable (organic, psychological)
Natural variable	• Rapid ejaculation inconsistent and irregular
Premature-like ejaculatory dysfunction	• Subjective perception of rapid ejaculation • IELT in normal range • Preoccupation with imagined rapid ejaculation • Preoccupation with poor control of ejaculation • Preoccupation not accounted for by another mental disorder

Ejaculation (MCCA-PE) study, the perception of average time a man to ejaculate varied greatly from 7 to 14 min [8].

Over the past 5 years, our understanding of the epidemiology of PE has been expanded significantly by several prospective studies (Table 8.3). One of the first large-scale prospective studies to assess the prevalence of PE was the National Health and Social Life Survey [9]. One of the major aims of this study was the assessment of the variation of timing and sequence of individual sex activity in response to the life course events and changes in social and cultural environment. This study was interview-based and used a probability sample of 3,442 men aged 19–59 years. Subjects were questioned regarding "climaxing too early" over the course of the preceding 12 months. Using this definition, the prevalence of PE in the study was 29 %. Of note, there appeared to be no significant impact of age on the PE prevalence.

Patrick et al. in 2005 conducted an industry-sponsored, 4-week multicenter observational study in heterosexual men in a stable monogamous relationship for more than 6 months [10]. PE was defined according to DSM-IV criteria. The study couples were required to engage in sexual intercourse at least twice weekly and record IELT with a partner-held stopwatch. 1,587 subjects were enrolled in the study, and the prevalence of premature ejaculation was 13 %. Demographic characteristics were similar between PE and non-PE groups. Subjects in the PE group had significantly shorter IELT compared to subjects in the non-PE group. The median IELT values were 1.8 and 7.3 min, respectively, for the PE and non-PE group. However, significant overlap existed in the distribution of IELT values between the two groups. 95 % of subjects in the non-PE group had IELT values of at least 2 min, while only 50 % of subjects in a PE group met that threshold, further supporting that IELT alone cannot adequately define PE.

Table 8.3 Prospective prevalence studies

Author	Year	Number of patients	Definition of PE	Methods	Prevalence	Comments
Giuliano	2007	1,115	DSM-IV	• Prospective, 8-week observational study at 44 centers in five European countries • Stopwatch IELT • PRO measures	18 %	• PE group: IELT ≤ 2 and ≤ 4 min in 75 and 56 %, respectively • Non-PE group: IELT ≤ 2 and ≤ 4 min in 25 and 12 %, respectively
Porst (PEPA)	2006	12,133	Two proprietary questions regarding ejaculatory control and bother	Web-based survey conducted in three countries (USA, Germany, Italy)	22.7 %	• No variation between countries • No variation with age • Men with PE more likely to have other sexual dysfunctions
Fasolo	2005	12,558	DSM-IV	Screening at 186 Italian sexual medicine clinics	21.2 %	• PE prevalence decreased with age • 70 % had acquired PE
Laumann (GSSAB)	2005	13,618	Single question regarding achieving orgasm too quickly	Interviews/questionnaire to men in 29 countries	20–30 %	• Geographical variation
Patrick	2005	1,587	DSM-IV	• Prospective, 4-week observational study at 42 US centers • Stopwatch IELT • PRO measures	13 %	• Median IELT 1.8 vs. 7.3 min in PE and non-PE groups • Significant overlap in IELT values between groups • PE group with lower mean rating on PRO questions
Laumann (NHSLS)	1994	3,442	Single question regarding climaxing too early	• Population-based survey • Interview-based • Population 19–59 years old	29 %	• Representative of the general US population

In the *Global Study of Sexual Attitudes and Behaviors (GSSAB)*, Laumann et al. conducted an international poll of 13,618 male subjects in 29 countries [11]. Subjects were questioned in either face-to-face or telephone interviews and in certain countries by mailed questionnaires. The prevalence of PE, which in this analysis was defined using a single question regarding "achieving orgasm too quickly," ranged between 20 and 30 % with significant geographical variation. Fasolo et al. analyzed 12,558 men presenting to 186 sexual medicine clinics and found a prevalence of PE using DSM-IV criteria at 21 % [12]. Interestingly, in this analysis 70 % of the PE patients had acquired PE, indicating that lifelong PE is of much lower prevalence than acquired PE.

Porst et al. in the *Premature Ejaculation Prevalence and Attitudes (PEPA)* study recruited 12,133 men using a web-based survey conducted in three countries (USA, Germany, Italy) [13]. PE in this study was defined using two proprietary questions, one regarding ejaculatory control and the other bother. The prevalence of PE in this analysis was 23 %. Approximately half of men had lifelong premature ejaculation, and nearly one third reported that they had acquired PE, while the remaining 15 % of men indicated that PE had been present when they first began having sex and then went away and returned again more recently.

Giuliano et al. performed an industry-sponsored, prospective, 8-week observational study at 44 centers in five European countries [14]. Stopwatch IELT was used as the endpoint in 1,115 men. Using DSM-IV criteria, the prevalence of PE was 18 %. In the PE group, mean IELT values less than 2 min and less than 4 min were observed in 75 and 56 % of the group, respectively. In the non-PE group, mean IELT values less than 2 min and less than 4 min occurred in 25 and 12 % of this group, respectively. In summary, the prevalence of PE is approximately 20–30 %, and when adjusted for the presence of ED (and secondary acquired PE), it is more common in younger men.

Recent studies have clearly shown wide variations in the prevalence of PE when different definitions are used. Lee et al. studied 2,081 patients (1,035 had stopwatch-recorded IELT) and found that the prevalence of PE according to self-report, premature ejaculation diagnostic tool (PEDT), and IELT <1 min was 19.5, 11.3, and 3 %, respectively [15]. Of note, the PEDT is a self-administered questionnaire developed to capture the factors described on the outdated DSM-IV-TR definition. A study of 3,016 Chinese men found that 25.8 % complained of ejaculating more rapidly than desired. When the complaint was further characterized to match the clinical syndromes described by Waldinger, only 4.5 % fitted the definition of acquired and 3 % the definition of lifelong PE [16]. The Global Online Sexuality Survey (GOSS) accrued results from 1,133 patients in the USA and found PE prevalences of 6.3 % according to the using the ISSM definition and 49.6 % if the PEDT was used [17]. These studies stress the importance of strict definitions for the diagnosis of PE as a disorder, since many men with complaints ejaculating more rapidly than desired do not meet the diagnostic criteria.

Impact of PE on Behavior and Quality of Life

Due to the embarrassing nature of and the lack of a simple screening tool for PE, most men do not discuss it with their physicians, nor do physicians generally assess their male patients for PE [13, 18–20]. These factors may be, at least in part, why most men with PE do not seek treatment for the condition, despite the distress it causes them. In subfertile couples this might be another factor contributing to individual and relationship stress. A lack of awareness that the condition is treatable and the fact that currently only one over-the-counter agent is approved by the US Food and Drug Administration (FDA) its treatment may also contribute.

PE can lower a man's sexual self-confidence and self-esteem. Its impact can extend to the sexual partner, with resultant effects on the sexual relationship and the relationship as a whole [10, 13, 18, 21]. For example, men have reported that their PE made them reluctant to establish new relationships [18], caused them anxiety about having intercourse [21], and even decreased their frequency of having intercourse [21, 22]. This can pose another obstacle to subfertile couples trying to conceive. Lower sexual satisfaction of female partners was found to be related to PE as well [23]. Thus, PE represents a significant unmet medical need.

Current Management of PE

Behavioral Therapy

Historically, PE was considered to be a psychological rather than a physiological problem, and it was treated with behavioral therapy and psychotherapy. Semans [24] employed the start–stop technique, and Masters and Johnson [25] added psychotherapy to complement this technique. However, these forms of non-pharmacologic therapy require time and commitment from both the individual with PE and his partner and thus may be difficult to implement and adhere to. These techniques also focus on distraction and reduction of excitement or stimulation, which may detract from overall sexual satisfaction. Although behavioral techniques have been shown to have success rates of 45–65 %, benefits are generally short-lived, and patients usually relapse [26–28]. Hawton et al. found that after 3 years of follow-up, 75 % of men with PE showed no lasting improvement [27]. De Amicis et al. also found that although men treated for PE via couples therapy experienced significant immediate benefits, these gains were not sustained when measured at a follow-up visit 3 years later [28].

Pharmacotherapy

SSRI Agents

Increasing evidence now suggests that the etiology of PE involves a strong physiological component. Preclinical research has identified a distinct ejaculation-related neural circuit in the central nervous system [29]. Psychopharmacologic studies suggest that PE may be related, at least in part, to diminished serotonergic neurotransmission; thus, pharmacologic agents might be utilized to modulate the 5-HT receptor system [30–32]. In support of the neurophysiological findings, delayed ejaculation is commonly reported as a side effect of antidepressant therapy with selective serotonin reuptake inhibitors (SSRIs) [33, 34]. In a multicenter study conducted to assess the incidence of sexual dysfunctions associated with SSRI treatment for depression, a group of 12 male patients with depression who suffered from PE before SSRI administration showed a high tolerance to the side effect of delayed ejaculation [33]. After treatment, their sexual satisfaction and that of their partners improved (treatment was with fluoxetine in five patients, paroxetine in three patients, sertraline in two patients, and fluvoxamine in two patients).

These results, along with the findings of others [31, 35–42], form some of the basis for SSRI use in the treatment of PE. The exact mechanism by which SSRI effect improved IELT is still unknown, but a variety of mechanisms have been proposed (Fig. 8.1).

SSRIs, other antidepressants, and other PDE5 inhibitors are commonly used in the treatment of PE, but these agents were not designed for the treatment of PE and are not approved for this indication by the FDA. When used for PE, they are dosed differently from their approved uses, and no large-scale, randomized, placebo-controlled clinical trials have been conducted to determine their efficacy and safety in PE. Table 8.4 contains examples of the types of trials that have been conducted in PE and illustrates, for antidepressants, that studies to date have been small (all under 100 subjects and most under 50 subjects) and have used varying definitions and evaluations of PE. As a result, conclusions regarding the efficacy and safety of these agents in men with PE are limited [20].

With regard to dosing regimens in PE treatment, as shown in Table 8.4, daily dosing and on-demand (PRN) dosing of antidepressants are often used; however, there is some evidence that a period of daily dosing is typically required prior to PRN dosing for better efficacy compared with PRN dosing alone. McMahon and Touma showed that the effect of paroxetine on prolongation of IELT after 6 weeks of treatment was significantly better if patients were treated initially with and had responded to 20 mg paroxetine daily for 2 weeks, followed by 4 weeks of PRN dosing with 20 mg, compared with patients who commenced on PRN dosing with 20 mg alone [38]. To date, studies of PRN dosing of antidepressants in men with PE have determined that these agents must be taken 3–4 h prior to intercourse to be effective. PRN dosing seems to be becoming more common than daily dosing for PE [20]; however, antidepressants were designed for continuous use and have been

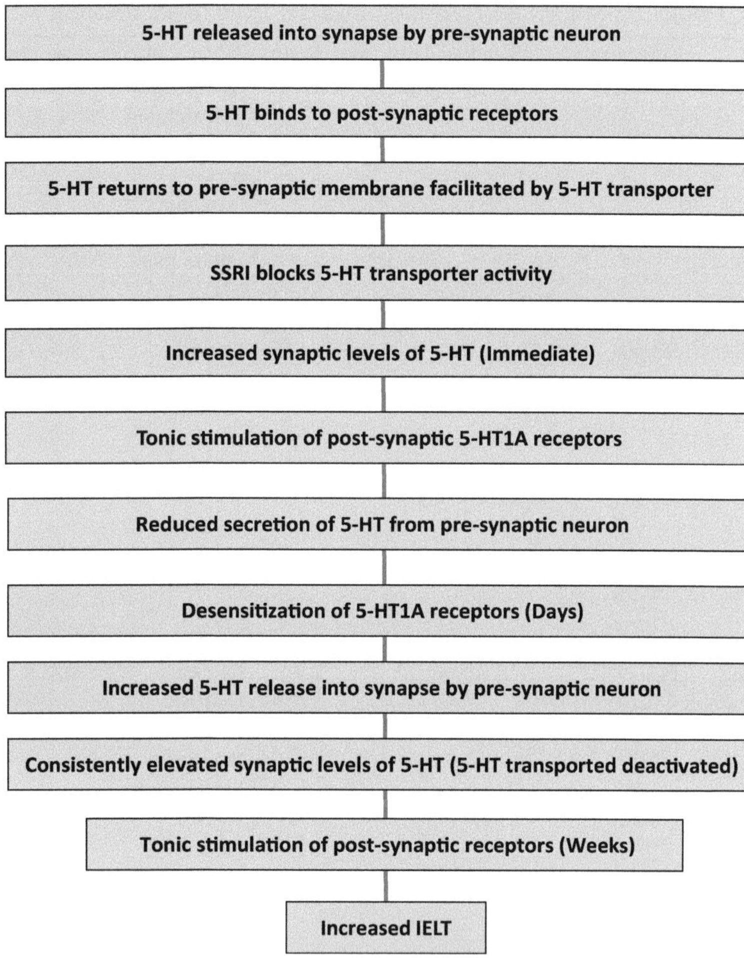

Fig. 8.1 Incidence of sexual dysfunction induced by SSRIs used for the treatment of depression ($N = 344$). Sexual dysfunction included decreased libido, delay of orgasm or ejaculation, anorgasmia or no ejaculation, and erectile dysfunction. Reprinted with permission from Montejo-González AL, Llorca G, Izquierdo JA, et al: J Sex Marital Ther 23: 176–194, 1997

shown to provide better activity in the management of PE following daily administration than following PRN dosing [38].

Daily administration of SSRIs, along with the associated side effects, may reduce patient compliance with antidepressants when used to treat PE. Compounding these factors are the findings that the onset of effect of most SSRIs in men with PE is typically 2–4 weeks [38, 41]. Manasia et al. demonstrated that administration of 90 mg fluoxetine once weekly for 3 months was more efficacious in prolonging end-of-study IELT than 20 mg fluoxetine daily in

Table 8.4 Characteristics of the most commonly used oral agents for PE treatment

Agent	Trade name	Standard daily dose	$T\frac{1}{2}$ (h)	Adverse effects	Contraindication
Clomipramine	Anafranil	25–50 mg/day	19–37	Dry mouth Constipation	MAOI
Fluoxetine	Prozac Sarafem	5–20 mg/day	36	Nausea Anxiety Insomnia Anhidrosis Libido loss ED	MAOI
Paroxetine	Paxil Seroxat Pexeva	10–40 mg/day	21	Nausea Anxiety Insomnia Anhidrosis Libido loss ED	MAOI
Sertraline	Zoloft	25–200 mg/day	26	Nausea Anxiety Insomnia Anhidrosis Libido loss ED	MAOI
Dapoxetine[a]	Priligy	15–60 mg	1.5	Nausea Diarrhea Headache Dizziness Somnolence	MAOI
Tramadol	Ultram	25–50 mg	5–7	Nausea Dizziness Insomnia Dyspepsia Seizures	MAOI SSRI TCA

[a]Not currently FDA approved but approved in Europe

*T*½ half-life, *SSRI* selective serotonin reuptake inhibitor, *MAOI* monoamine oxidase inhibitor, *TCA* tricyclic antidepressants

80 patients with PE [41]. One drawback associated with the once-weekly schedule was that the onset of effect was prolonged to 6 weeks.

As shown in Table 8.1, SSRIs used in the treatment of PE include paroxetine (Paxil©, GlaxoSmithKline, Research Triangle Park, NC), fluoxetine (Prozac©, Eli Lilly and Company, Indianapolis, IN), and sertraline (Zoloft©, Pfizer Inc., New York, NY). In comparative studies and a recent meta-analysis, paroxetine has been shown to be more effective in prolonging IELT than other SSRIs [39, 42]. The tricyclic antidepressant clomipramine (Anafranil©, Mallinckrodt Pharmaceuticals, St. Louis, MO) has also been used to treat PE in small-scale trials [35, 37, 43]. Adverse effects of antidepressants for the treatment of PE have not been carefully studied; however, the frequency and type of side effects are expected to be similar to those seen in patients taking these drugs for depression. Nausea, dry mouth, drowsiness, anejaculation, inhibited orgasm, and decreased libido have been commonly reported in studies to date [35]. Pharmacodynamic interactions may occur with concomitant use of monoamine oxidase inhibitors, lithium, sumatriptan, or tryptophan, as well as with concomitant use of drugs metabolized by cytochrome p450 isozymes or extensively bound to plasma proteins. Adverse effects may vary with dosing schedule (daily or PRN). Collectively, trials of antidepressants in the treatment of PE show that while some benefit on IELT is achieved by most men, the required dosing schedules, time to onset of effect, and incidence and nature of side effects limit their widespread usefulness and acceptance by patients for this condition.

Few studies have investigated the effects of SSRIs on semen parameters and fertility. An in vitro study found that all five tested SSRIs (fluoxetine, sertraline, fluvoxamine, paroxetine, and citalopram) exhibited spermicidal activity, with minimum effective concentration ranging from 0.05 to 0.5 % [44]. A case–control study of patients receiving an SSRI for depression found that these men had lower sperm counts, lower motility, higher morphological abnormality, and higher sperm DNA damage than age-matched controls [45]. Moreover, SSRI treatment duration was associated with greater compromise in seminal parameters.

Tanrikut et al. performed seminal analyses in 35 healthy volunteers at baseline and after 5 weeks of treatment with paroxetine. While there was no significant change in usual seminal parameters, abnormal sperm DNA fragmentation increased from 9.7 to 50 % [46]. Also, there was a significant decrease in serum testosterone and estradiol. The disruption of hormonal homeostasis could be mediated via stimulation of 5-HT receptors, which may increase prolactin secretion [47].

Koyuncu et al. studied 25 men with lifelong PE using the ISSM definition and normal seminal parameter. After daily escitalopram 10 mg for 3 months, there was a significant decrease in sperm concentration, motility, and normal morphology [48]. These studies suggest a negative impact of daily SSRI use on seminal parameters. The clinical implications of these findings are yet to be established. Also, on-demand treatment has not been studied.

Topical Therapies

Topical anesthetics have also been used for the treatment of PE, in an effort to decrease penile stimulation to delay time to ejaculation. Application of lidocaine 2.5 %/prilocaine 2.5 % cream (EMLA Cream, AstraZeneca Pharmaceuticals, Wilmington, DE) to the penis prior to covering it with a condom 20–30 min before intercourse delayed ejaculation in men ($N = 40$) with PE (defined as IELT $\leq$ 1 min) [49]. However, prolonged application (30–45 min) prior to intercourse resulted in loss of erection. In addition, others have found that a reduction in genital sensitivity of both partners may limit repeated use of topical anesthetics [50].

A recently published randomized, double-blind, placebo-controlled study in 42 men aged 18–50 years with PE showed that lidocaine/prilocaine cream used over a period of 30–60 days significantly increased mean IELT (as measured by a stopwatch) from a baseline value of 1.49 min to an end-of-study value of 8.45 min ($P < 0.001$) [51]. In contrast, the placebo cream did not achieve a significant increase (1.67 min at baseline, 1.95 min at the end of the study, $P > 0.05$). In this study, men were defined as having PE based on the satisfaction of the couple with their sex life rather than by IELT. Prior to the study, six participants (three in the lidocaine/prilocaine group and three in the placebo group) had received treatment with SSRIs but had discontinued due to side effects. Side effects of topical anesthetic application included retarded ejaculation >30 min (two subjects), decreased penile sensitivity (two subjects), penile irritation (two subjects), and decreased vaginal sensitivity (one partner) [51]. These adverse events, along with the disruption of spontaneity inherent to this method, may make it an unpalatable option for men with PE and their partners. There is no data to suggest that EMLA adversely affects fertility.

Promescent is a new eutectic formulation of unionized lidocaine without prilocaine that was approved by the FDA to be sold over the counter. Its main differentiation points are the absence of prilocaine and the more rapid absorption, with onset in 10 min. Theoretically, condom use is not necessary because the rapid absorption would not cause reduced genital sensitivity in the female partner. However, clinical studies of efficacy, safety, and side-effect profiles are lacking.

PDE5 Inhibitors

Medications indicated for ED have also been studied for their efficacy in PE. In men with IELTs <1 min, PRN administration of 50 mg sildenafil combined with 20 mg paroxetine (1 h before planned sexual intercourse) after 21 days of daily administration of 10 mg paroxetine alone showed superiority to daily administration of 10 mg paroxetine for 21 days and PRN dosing of 20 mg paroxetine 3–4 h prior to intercourse [52]. Differences in treatment arms were significant after 3 and 6 months of treatment ($P < 0.01$). Patients in the sildenafil group had a higher incidence of headache and flushing (20 and 15 %, respectively) compared to those in the paroxetine-only group (10 and 0 %, respectively). In another study, men with PE who were dissatisfied with 5 % lidocaine ointment were given 20 mg paroxetine daily for 30 days and 20 mg paroxetine combined with 25–100 mg sildenafil 7 h before intercourse. Psychological and behavioral counseling was also provided throughout the study. Sildenafil combined with paroxetine and psychological and behavioral counseling significantly increased IELT and decreased the frequency of patient-reported episodes of premature ejaculation, being considered satisfactory by 56 of 58 patients [53]. By demonstrating improved efficacy through combining pharmacotherapy with non-pharmacologic therapy, this study raises the possibility that the maximum effect of any pharmacologic therapy may be enhanced by adding behavioral and psychological therapy to the treatment protocol.

Shindel et al. investigated the prevalence of complaints of ejaculating more rapidly than desired among couples presenting to an infertility clinic. This complaint was observed in 50 % of men, but less than half of their partners corroborated the complaint. This was associated with lower scores on the Self-Esteem and Relationship Quality (SEAR) scale [54].

Lotti et al. investigated the occurrence of PE in 244 men with couple infertility using the premature ejaculation diagnostic tool (PEDT), a self-administered questionnaire developed to capture the factors on the outdated PE definition of the DSM-IV-TR. Overall, 15.6 % of patients had PEDT scores consistent with PE, and higher scores were associated with phobic anxiety [55].

In a case–control study of 1,468 infertile and 942 fertile men, Gao et al. found that the infertile patients had significantly higher prevalences of PE, anxiety, and depression. Moreover, lower IELT and higher scores on the PEDT were associated with worse score in self-rated anxiety and depression scales [56]. Fertility issues are known to cause significant stress and anxiety to couples, which might cause or exacerbate PE. Because these studies have utilized outdated definitions, the prevalence of PE, as per the current definition, in subfertile patients/couples is unknown.

Summary and Conclusions

PE is a common problem that may be distressing to individuals and their partners. PE is a treatable condition. However, more effective methods of treatment are needed. Off-label uses of antidepressants, topical anesthetics, and PDE5 inhibitors have shown some efficacy in the treatment of PE, but because the studies assessing these agents have been small, we do not have a clear understanding of their efficacy, safety, and tolerability for the treatment of PE. Furthermore, undesirable features are associated with each of these methods. Antidepressants have a long onset of action, must be taken daily for maximum efficacy, can depress libido, can cause ED, and often carry an associated stigma. Topical anesthetics may interfere with spontaneity and cause genital numbness in the man and his partner. Behavioral therapies require extensive time and commitment and continued use/practice from the man and his partner to be successful.

In conclusion, there is a need for improved treatment approaches for PE. While support and education of both the man and his partner are an integral part of therapy, PE has a physiological basis and should not be considered purely a psychological problem. Thus, medications specifically developed for PE, those that not only increase ejaculatory latency, improve control over ejaculation, and increase satisfaction with sexual intercourse but also have more convenient dosing schedules and a lower incidence of sexual side effects than existing options, will find a ready place in the pharmacologic armamentarium of the urologist, sexual medicine physician, and primary care physician. Effective treatment for PE has the potential to improve self-esteem, well-being, and relationship satisfaction. Particularly in couples facing fertility issues, it can represent removing an added burden to an already stressful situation.

An ideal pharmacologic agent should be an on-demand-dosed treatment with high rates of efficacy on early doses, have a short onset of action, not interfere with sexual spontaneity, and not have sexual side effects. In addition to providing effective treatment for PE, availability of such an agent will likely prompt dialogue between men with PE and their physicians and men with PE and their partners.

References

1. American Psychiatric Association. Diagnostic and statistical manual of mental disorders, 4th edn, Text Revision (DSM-IV-TR). Arlington, VA: American Psychiatric Association; 2000.
2. WHO. The ICD-10 classification of mental and behavioural disorders: diagnostic criteria for research. Geneva: WHO; 1993.
3. Waldinger MD, Schweitzer DH. The DSM-IV-TR Is an inadequate diagnostic tool for premature ejaculation. J Sex Med. 2007;4(3):822–3.
4. Waldinger MD. Premature ejaculation: state of the art. Urol Clin N Am. 2007;34(4):591–9. vii–viii.
5. McMahon CG, Althof SE, Waldinger MD, Porst H, Dean J, Sharlip ID, et al. An evidence-based definition of lifelong premature ejaculation: report of the International Society for Sexual Medici (ISSM) ad hoc committee for the definition of premature ejaculation. J Sex Med. 2008;5(7):1590–606.
6. Althof SE, Abdo CHN, Dean J, Hackett G, McCabe M, McMahon CG, et al. International Society for Sexual Medicine's guidelines for the diagnosis and treatment of premature ejaculation. J Sex Med. 2010;7(9):2947–69.
7. American Psychiatric Association (2013) Diagnostic and statistical manual of mental disorders, 5th edn (DSM-V). Arlington, VA: American Psychiatric Association; 2013.
8. Montorsi F. Prevalence of premature ejaculation: a global and regional perspective. J Sex Med. 2005;2 Suppl 2:96–102.
9. Laumann EO, Paik A, Rosen RC. Sexual dysfunction in the United States: prevalence and predictors. JAMA. 1999;281(6):537–44.
10. Patrick DL, Althof SE, Pryor JL, Rosen R, Rowland DL, Ho KF, et al. Premature ejaculation: an observational study of men and their partners. J Sex Med. 2005;2(3):358–67.
11. Laumann EO, Nicolosi A, Glasser DB, Paik A, Gingell C, Moreira E, et al. Sexual problems among women and men aged 40–80 y: prevalence and correlates identified in the Global Study of Sexual Attitudes and Behaviors. Int J Impot Res. 2005;17(1):39–57.
12. Basile Fasolo C, Mirone V, Gentile V, Parazzini F, Ricci E. Premature ejaculation: prevalence and associated conditions in a sample of 12,558 men attending the andrology prevention week 2001 – a study of the Italian Society of Andrology (SIA). J Sex Med. 2005;2(3):376–82.
13. Porst H, Montorsi F, Rosen RC, Gaynor L, Grupe S, Alexander J. The premature ejaculation prevalence and attitudes (PEPA) survey: prevalence, comorbidities, and professional help-seeking. Eur Urol. 2007;51(3):816–23. discussion 824.
14. Giuliano F, Patrick DL, Porst H, La Pera G, Kokoszka A, Merchant S, et al. Premature ejaculation: results from a five-country European observational study. Eur Urol. 2008;53(5):1048–57.
15. Lee SW, Lee JH, Sung HH, Park HJ, Park JK, Choi SK, et al. The prevalence of premature ejaculation and its clinical characteristics in Korean men according to different definitions. Int J Impot Res. 2013;25(1):12–7.
16. Gao J, Zhang X, Su P, Liu J, Xia L, Yang J, et al. Prevalence and factors associated with the complaint of premature ejaculation and the four premature ejaculation syndromes: a large observational study in China. J Sex Med. 2013;10(7):1874–81.

17. Shaeer O. The global online sexuality survey (GOSS): The United States of America in 2011 Chapter III – Premature ejaculation among English-speaking male Internet users. J Sex Med. 2013;10(7):1882–8.
18. Symonds T, Roblin D, Hart K, Althof S. How does premature ejaculation impact a man's life? J Sex Marital Ther. 2003;29(5):361–70.
19. Aschka C, Himmel W, Ittner E, Kochen MM. Sexual problems of male patients in family practice. J Fam Pract. 2001;50(9):773–8.
20. Montague DK, Jarow J, Broderick GA, Dmochowski RR, Heaton JPW, Lue TF, et al. AUA guideline on the pharmacologic management of premature ejaculation. J Urol. 2004;172 (1):290–4.
21. Rowland D, Perelman M, Althof S, Barada J, McCullough A, Bull S, et al. Self-reported premature ejaculation and aspects of sexual functioning and satisfaction. J Sex Med. 2004;1 (2):225–32.
22. Spiess WF, Geer JH, O'Donohue WT. Premature ejaculation: investigation of factors in ejaculatory latency. J Abnorm Psychol. 1984;93(2):242–5.
23. Byers ES, Grenier G. Premature or rapid ejaculation: heterosexual couples' perceptions of men's ejaculatory behavior. Arch Sex Behav. 2003;32(3):261–70.
24. Semans JH. Premature ejaculation: a new approach. South Med J. 1956;49(4):353–8.
25. Masters W, Johnson V. Human sexual inadequacy. New York: Little Brown and Company; 1970.
26. St Lawrence JS, Madakasira S. Evaluation and treatment of premature ejaculation: a critical review. Int J Psychiatry Med. 1992;22(1):77–97.
27. Hawton K, Catalan J, Martin P, Fagg J. Long-term outcome of sex therapy. Behav Res Ther. 1986;24(6):665–75.
28. De Amicis LA, Goldberg DC, LoPiccolo J, Friedman J, Davies L. Clinical follow-up of couples treated for sexual dysfunction. Arch Sex Behav. 1985;14(6):467–89.
29. Truitt WA, Coolen LM. Identification of a potential ejaculation generator in the spinal cord. Science. 2002;297(5586):1566–9.
30. Waldinger MD, Berendsen HH, Blok BF, Olivier B, Holstege G. Premature ejaculation and serotonergic antidepressants-induced delayed ejaculation: the involvement of the serotonergic system. Behav Brain Res. 1998;92(2):111–8.
31. Waldinger MD, Olivier B. Selective serotonin reuptake inhibitor-induced sexual dysfunction: clinical and research considerations. Int Clin Psychopharmacol. 1998;13 Suppl 6:S27–33.
32. Waldinger MD. The neurobiological approach to premature ejaculation. J Urol. 2002;168 (6):2359–67.
33. Montejo-González AL, Llorca G, Izquierdo JA, Ledesma A, Bousoño M, Calcedo A, et al. SSRI-induced sexual dysfunction: fluoxetine, paroxetine, sertraline, and fluvoxamine in a prospective, multicenter, and descriptive clinical study of 344 patients. J Sex Marital Ther. 1997;23(3):176–94.
34. Rosen RC, Lane RM, Menza M. Effects of SSRIs on sexual function: a critical review. J Clin Psychopharmacol. 1999;19(1):67–85.
35. Althof SE, Levine SB, Corty EW, Risen CB, Stern EB, Kurit DM. A double-blind crossover trial of clomipramine for rapid ejaculation in 15 couples. J Clin Psychiatry. 1995;56(9):402–7.
36. Waldinger MD, Hengeveld MW, Zwinderman AH. Ejaculation-retarding properties of paroxetine in patients with primary premature ejaculation: a double-blind, randomized, dose-response study. Br J Urol. 1997;79(4):592–5.
37. Kim SC, Seo KK. Efficacy and safety of fluoxetine, sertraline and clomipramine in patients with premature ejaculation: a double-blind, placebo controlled study. J Urol. 1998;159 (2):425–7.
38. McMahon CG, Touma K. Treatment of premature ejaculation with paroxetine hydrochloride as needed: 2 single-blind placebo controlled crossover studies. J Urol. 1999;161(6):1826–30.

39. Waldinger MD, Hengeveld MW, Zwinderman AH, Olivier B. Effect of SSRI antidepressants on ejaculation: a double-blind, randomized, placebo-controlled study with fluoxetine, fluvoxamine, paroxetine, and sertraline. J Clin Psychopharmacol. 1998;18(4):274–81.
40. Kara H, Aydin S, Yücel M, Agargün MY, Odabaş O, Yilmaz Y. The efficacy of fluoxetine in the treatment of premature ejaculation: a double-blind placebo controlled study. J Urol. 1996;156(5):1631–2.
41. Manasia P, Pomerol J, Ribè N. Gutierrez del Pozo R, Alcover Garcia J. Comparison of the efficacy and safety of 90 mg versus 20 mg fluoxetine in the treatment of premature ejaculation. J Urol. 2003;170(1):164–5.
42. Waldinger MD, Zwinderman AH, Schweitzer DH, Olivier B. Relevance of methodological design for the interpretation of efficacy of drug treatment of premature ejaculation: a systematic review and meta-analysis. Int J Impot Res. 2004;16(4):369–81.
43. Haensel SM, Rowland DL, Kallan KT. Clomipramine and sexual function in men with premature ejaculation and controls. J Urol. 1996;156(4):1310–5.
44. Kumar VSK, Sharma VL, Tiwari P, Singh D, Maikhuri JP, Gupta G, et al. The spermicidal and antitrichomonas activities of SSRI antidepressants. Bioorg Med Chem Lett. 2006;16(9):2509–12.
45. Safarinejad MR. Sperm DNA, damage and semen quality impairment after treatment with selective serotonin reuptake inhibitors detected using semen analysis and sperm chromatin structure assay. J Urol. 2008;180(5):2124–8.
46. Tanrikut C, Feldman AS, Altemus M, Paduch DA, Schlegel PN. Adverse effect of paroxetine on sperm. Fertil Steril. 2010;94(3):1021–6.
47. Meltzer H, Bastani B, Jayathilake K, Maes M. Fluoxetine, but not tricyclic antidepressants, potentiates the 5-hydroxytryptophan-mediated increase in plasma cortisol and prolactin secretion in subjects with major depression or with obsessive compulsive disorder. Neuropsychopharmacology. 1997;17(1):1–11.
48. Koyuncu H, Serefoglu EC, Yencilek E, Atalay H, Akbas NB, Sarıca K. Escitalopram treatment for premature ejaculation has a negative effect on semen parameters. Int J Impot Res. 2011;23(6):257–61.
49. Atikeler MK, Gecit I, Senol FA. Optimum usage of prilocaine-lidocaine cream in premature ejaculation. Andrologia. 2002;34(6):356–9.
50. Sahin H, Bircan MK. Re: Efficacy of prilocaine-lidocaine cream in the treatment of premature ejaculation. J Urol. 1996;156(5):1783–4.
51. Busato W, Galindo CC. Topical anaesthetic use for treating premature ejaculation: a double-blind, randomized, placebo-controlled study. BJU Int. 2004;93(7):1018–21.
52. Salonia A, Maga T, Colombo R, Scattoni V, Briganti A, Cestari A, et al. A prospective study comparing paroxetine alone versus paroxetine plus sildenafil in patients with premature ejaculation. J Urol. 2002;168(6):2486–9.
53. Chen J, Mabjeesh NJ, Matzkin H, Greenstein A. Efficacy of sildenafil as adjuvant therapy to selective serotonin reuptake inhibitor in alleviating premature ejaculation. Urology. 2003;61(1):197–200.
54. Shindel AW, Nelson CJ, Naughton CK, Mulhall JP. Premature ejaculation in infertile couples: prevalence and correlates. J Sex Med. 2008;5(2):485–91.
55. Lotti F, Corona G, Rastrelli G, Forti G, Jannini EA, Maggi M. Clinical correlates of erectile dysfunction and premature ejaculation in men with couple infertility. J Sex Med. 2012;9(10):2698–707.
56. Gao J, Zhang X, Su P, Liu J, Shi K, Hao Z, et al. Relationship between sexual dysfunction and psychological burden in men with infertility: a large observational study in China. J Sex Med. 2013;10(8):1935–42.

Chapter 9
Delayed Ejaculation and Orgasm

Christian J. Nelson, Dylan Brock, and Robert C. Dean

Introduction

Delayed ejaculation is a condition characterized by difficulty achieving orgasm and extended ejaculatory latency. When comparing delayed ejaculation to other male sexual dysfunctions, it is one of the most poorly understood and pharmacologically resistant dysfunctions. While seldom recognized or addressed clinically, reports indicate that delayed ejaculation affects more than 8 % of men and up to one-third of men taking SSRIs [1]. For many men and their partners, this condition results in a significant reduction in sexual satisfaction and psychological well-being, contributing to anxiety, distress, poor confidence, and low self-esteem, among other issues. The concerns are compounded in couples, where impaired sexual functioning may disrupt relationship intimacy and frustrate couples' attempts to conceive.

Terminology

The term *delayed ejaculation* is often used synonymously with delayed orgasm, inhibited ejaculation, retarded ejaculation/orgasm, and ejaculatory incompetence to describe delayed or absent orgasmic and/or ejaculatory response in men. Increasingly, the terms retarded ejaculation and ejaculatory incompetence are avoided because of their negative and potentially stigmatizing associations [2, 3]. Following the International Society for Sexual Medicine's (ISSM) lead on the subject, *delayed ejaculation* will serve as the preferred term for the condition herein [3]. However,

C.J. Nelson (✉)
Department of Psychiatry and Behavioral Sciences, Memorial Sloan-Kettering Cancer Center, 641 Lexington Ave., 7th Floor, New York, NY 10022, USA
e-mail: nelsonc@mskcc.org

J.P. Mulhall and W. Hsiao (eds.), *Men's Sexual Health and Fertility*, DOI 10.1007/978-1-4939-0425-9_9, © Springer Science+Business Media New York 2014 this terminological imprecision provides some indication of the difficulty involved in garnering wide acceptance for diagnostic criteria and treatment guidelines for the condition. This is perhaps because, of all the male sexual disorders, the literature on delayed ejaculation relies mostly on case studies and anecdotal observations for its diagnosis and treatment.

The most widely cited clinical definition of delayed ejaculation, provided by the American Psychiatric Association's (APA) DSM-IV-TR, describes the condition as:

1. The persistent or recurrent delay in, or absence of, orgasm following a normal sexual excitement phase during sexual activity that the clinician, taking into account the person's age, judges to be adequate in focus, intensity, and duration.
2. The disturbance causes marked distress or interpersonal difficulty.
3. The orgasmic dysfunction is not better accounted for by another Axis I disorder (except another sexual dysfunction) and is not due exclusively to the direct physiological effects of a substance (e.g., a drug of abuse, a medication) or a general medical condition [4].

Likewise, the defining features of delayed ejaculation according to the World Health Organization include "the persistent or recurrent difficulty, delay in, or absence of attaining orgasm after sufficient sexual stimulation, which causes personal distress" [5].

Primary delayed ejaculation characterizes a lifelong condition, wherein ejaculation during intercourse has rarely or never occurred. The prevalence of primary delayed ejaculation is rare, estimated at 1–2 % of all men, and representing only one-quarter of men suffering from delayed ejaculation [6, 7]. The majority of men with primary delayed ejaculation are still able to ejaculate from masturbation and/or manual or oral stimulation. Such cases, in which ejaculation is restricted to one form of sexual stimulation (e.g., intercourse), are further classified as *situational*. In contrast, delayed ejaculation may be experienced *globally*, or during all forms of sexual activity. *Secondary* or "acquired" delayed ejaculation appears after a period of relatively normal sexual functioning and is much more common, representing up to 75 % of all cases [3, 6]. As is true of primary delayed ejaculation, a large majority of men can still reach orgasm through masturbation. *Anejaculation* or *anorgasmia* is the most severe form of this condition and is characterized by the inability to ejaculate or achieve an orgasm.

While the *DSM-IV-TR* has a separate classification for delayed ejaculation when it is caused by medication or drug abuse (i.e., substance-induced sexual dysfunction with impaired orgasm), or when secondary to a medical condition, in practice, many sex therapists and urologists use the term delayed ejaculation to refer to all male-inhibited orgasmic or delayed ejaculatory disorders regardless of etiology [8]. Drug side effects, prior pelvic or spinal surgery, and underlying medical conditions are routinely cited in the literature as common causes of delayed ejaculation.

Incidence and Prevalence

Most texts indicate that delayed ejaculation is rare; however, the condition has yet to be systematically studied or described, such that the true prevalence of delayed ejaculation is unclear. Historically, the reported incidence rates of delayed ejaculation have been relatively low, with rates between 1 and 4 % of the general population [9–12]. Largely consistent with these reports, a more recent 2003 cross-sectional study of men attending London general practitioners reported a prevalence rate of 2.5 % for "inhibited orgasm," defined as the inability to "ejaculate 75 % of the time or more often" [13]. Employing a more liberal standard in a large, nationally representative sample of 18- to 59-year-old men, the National Health and Social Life Survey found that 8 % of men endorsed "inability achieving climax or ejaculation" as posing a problem for two months in the last year [1]. Still, such findings may be conservative in their own right, as they likely underreport the true rates of "delayed" ejaculation.

Importantly, over the past decade clinicians have identified an increase in these rates with the use of selective serotonin reuptake inhibitors (SSRIs) [14–17]. The side effects of these medications may be useful in treating premature ejaculation by extending intervaginal ejaculatory latencies [18]; however, they also have the potential to prolong ejaculatory latency in men with normal ejaculation latencies, contributing to difficulty attaining orgasm and delayed ejaculation [15, 17]. For those taking SSRI medications, rates of delayed ejaculation range from 16 to 37 % [19, 20].

Delayed ejaculation is also related to age and may arise from aging-related physiological and psychosocial changes or medical comorbidities [6, 21]. Often with aging comes an increase in the rates of chronic illness and medication use, each of which may impair sexual functioning. Alterations in circulation, diminished penile sensation, degeneration of ejaculatory reflexes, reduced testosterone levels, and poor erection quality can all occur as men age [22]. In concert with other factors, these age-related processes may adversely impact sexual functioning and contribute to difficulty achieving orgasm and delay ejaculation [2]. The Multinational Survey of the Aging Male found that ejaculatory dysfunctions were directly correlated to both age and severity of lower urinary tract symptoms and/or benign prostatic hyperplasia (BPH) [23, 24].

Impact

Clinical reports have suggested that men with delayed ejaculation report high levels of relationship distress, sexual dissatisfaction, shame, and apprehension over their performance, negatively impacting overall psychological well-being and contributing to anxiety and depression [12, 25, 26]. For men with delayed ejaculation, there can be feelings of inadequacy both in sexual function and in self-image

[27]. Due to frustration and low self-esteem, a man may avoid intimacy and problem solving with his partner, and many years may elapse before seeking help [28]. For many men, this dysfunction results in the complete inability to achieve an orgasm during sexual relations. Masters and Johnson observed that men with this condition may seek partners who can accommodate a minimal sexual lifestyle [29]. Jannini and colleagues suggest that delayed ejaculation can have significant deleterious effects on a man's sexual satisfaction and a couple's relationship [12, 28].

Etiology of Delayed Ejaculation

The etiologies of delayed ejaculation are diverse and frequently multifactorial, originating from a network of biological, psychological, pharmacological, interpersonal, and individual factors [7, 30]. Most reports classify the major causes of delayed ejaculation as either pathophysiological or psychological. Clinically, if medication side effects have been ruled out, the primary etiologies of this condition are, broadly speaking, either neurological or psychological. The primary causes of delayed ejaculation are described below (also see Table 9.1).

Neurogenic: Potential neurological causes for delayed ejaculation include spinal cord injury, multiple sclerosis, and diabetes [31–33]. Most of the research examining the association between neurological disorders and ejaculatory problems has investigated patients with spinal cord injuries, which is considered the main neurological cause of delayed ejaculation. Multiple sclerosis is associated with a variety of sexual dysfunctions, including ejaculatory disorders, difficulty achieving orgasm, and erectile dysfunction [31]. Survey studies indicate that 35–45 % of men with multiple sclerosis report difficulty achieving ejaculation [34]. Likewise, sexual dysfunctions, including delayed ejaculation, are well-documented complications of severe diabetes and related autonomic neuropathy [35]. Additionally, some researchers hypothesize that delayed ejaculation is caused, at least in part, by slower bulbocavernous reflexes, less sensitivity in the penis, and a too-high penile sensory threshold [12, 36]. Some of these factors may underlie the age-related prevalence of delayed ejaculation. Penile biothesiometry may be one way to determine if penile sensitivity is a root cause of delayed ejaculation. Penile biothesiometry uses electromagnetic vibration to help gauge the level of sensitivity or potential nerve damage.

Endocrine: Like most aspects of male reproduction, ejaculation and ejaculatory latency are regulated by a "hormonal milieu" [37]. As such, another key set of physiological mechanisms underlying delayed ejaculation involves the endocrine system, particularly gonadal, thyroid, and pituitary hormones. Testosterone, thyroid-stimulating hormone (TSH), and prolactin have received most of the attention [37–40].

Studies indicate that low testosterone is associated with delayed ejaculation. Androgen receptors are found throughout the central nervous system, including

Table 9.1 Causes of delayed ejaculation (Adapted from Rowland [3])

Age
Pathophysiological
• Neurogenic causes
– Spinal cord injury
– Diabetic autonomic neuropathy
• Anatomical and congenital
– Duct cyst
– Mullerian duct
• Infection
– Urethritis
– Genitourinary tuberculosis
Medication
• Selective serotonin reuptake inhibitors (SSRI)
Endocrine factors
• Testosterone
• Thyroid hormones
• Prolactin
Psychosexual and relationship factors
• Disconnect between arousal and sexual situation
• Masturbation style
• Psychic conflict

several areas important to ejaculation such as the medial preoptic area, the bed of the nucleus of the stria terminalis, the median amygdala, and the posterior thalamus [41]. Moreover, pelvic floor muscles (e.g., bulbocavernosus, ischiocavernosus, and levator ani) may be androgen dependent [42]. The NO-PDE5 system, important for contractility of the male genital tract, is also testosterone mediated [37]. Low testosterone levels may also negatively impact arousal, which in turn may impair control over ejaculation [40].

Elevated TSH and prolactin levels have also been associated with delayed ejaculation [37]. There is a well-documented relationship between hypothyroidism and delayed ejaculation [38] and, conversely, hyperthyroidism with premature ejaculation [38, 43]. Some authors have argued that delayed ejaculation and premature ejaculation can be considered two sides of a single continuum under endocrine control [44], a theory that recently received empirical support [37]. Thyroid hormones may regulate seminal vesicle contraction frequency and bulbospongiosus muscle contractile activity, impacting emission and expulsion during ejaculation [45]. Reduced thyroid function and low thyroid hormone levels, then, may underlie forms of delayed ejaculation. This is largely consistent with findings demonstrating that elevated TSH levels and hypothyroidism are both correlated with delayed ejaculation [38]. Given the negative relationship between TSH and thyroid function, these results are both expected and supportive of the importance of thyroid hormones for maintaining normal ejaculatory function. Additionally, recent evidence suggests that prolactin mirrors serotonergic activity and may serve as a useful clinical proxy for serotonergic tone [45]. In fact, some authors have suggested that prolactin assessment be performed on all patients with ejaculatory dysfunctions [45].

Anatomical and surgical: Common congenital abnormalities associated with delayed ejaculation include persistent Mullerian duct remnants (contributing to duct cyst formation), Wolffian duct malformation (affecting the ejaculatory duct, vas deferens, and seminal vesicle), and prune belly syndrome [21, 46, 47]. There also may be abnormalities due to pelvic trauma or surgery, such as following correction of an imperforate anus in infancy. Common surgical procedures that have been associated with delayed orgasm or ejaculation are transurethral resection of the prostate and bladder neck surgery [46].

Medication side effects: Prolonged ejaculatory latency and delayed ejaculation are frequent side effects of commonly prescribed pharmaceuticals. Examples of medications that can impact ejaculatory latency are antidepressants, antiadrenergics, antihypertensives, alpha-adrenergic antagonists (alpha-blockers), antipsychotics, and anticholinergics [32, 48].

The evidence for psychopharmacologic-induced delayed ejaculation is perhaps strongest for antidepressants. At rates of 16–37 %, delayed ejaculation is of the most commonly reported side effect of SSRIs [15, 49]. In studies using multivariable models predicting delayed ejaculation, SSRI use is reported to be the most important factor explaining ejaculatory latency variance (Corona 2009). Substantial evidence indicates that the use of SSRIs delays ejaculation via their effect on central serotonergic tone and 5HT2C receptor activation [44, 50]. Clinically, this effect is the main drive controlling ejaculation [15, 50]. Accordingly, the ejaculation-delaying effects of some SSRIs are currently used therapeutically to treat premature ejaculation [50, 51]. Of importance is that bupropion is the only currently available antidepressant that has not been linked to ejaculatory dysfunction.

Psychosexual and relational: Despite the numerous physical and pathophysiological causes of delayed ejaculation, a considerable share of men with delayed ejaculation exhibit no obvious organic factors that account for the disorder [8]. In most cases, relational difficulties, psychosexual difficulties, or idiosyncratic masturbation styles account for the ejaculatory dysfunction. Cultural factors or religious beliefs may limit sexual experience and increase guilt and impact sexual functioning [29]. Unfortunately, carefully controlled research on these factors is limited [52].

A number of theories have suggested that when a man is experiencing delayed ejaculation, his sexual arousal is disconnected from the sexual experience. Recent studies, primarily performed by Rowland and colleagues (2005), seeking to differentiate men with delayed ejaculation using psychophysiological assessment, found that men with delayed ejaculation report lower subjective sexual arousal, relationship satisfaction, and attractiveness to partner and higher fear of failure as compared to men with normal sexual functioning [53]. The authors hypothesize that there exists a disconnection between sexual experience and sexual arousal. In line with this theory, other experts highlight sexual performance anxiety, noting that anxiety related to orgasm distracts from arousal and contributes to delayed ejaculation [21, 54]. Another similar theory suggests these men may have a subtle desire disorder. This has been characterized as men who have an "autosexual" orientation, may be able to sustain an erection without sexual arousal, and may find the touch of their partner inhibiting [52]. In addition, there may also be a disparity between partner and fantasy [55, 56]. The lack of sexual excitement may be related to a disconnect between sexual fantasy during masturbation and sexual relations with a partner [21]. It is important to note that the lack of sexual excitement can also be associated with the use of penile injections, of penile implants, and, to some extent, of PDE-5 inhibitors. These medications produce a situation where a man may sustain an erection in the midst of only being marginally sexual excited. As a result, the man (and the partner) may incorrectly interpret the erection as a sign of sexual excitement and then become concerned when ejaculation time is extended.

An important cause of delayed ejaculation also includes the use of a unique masturbation style. Perelman suggests that idiosyncratic masturbation style may be a primary cause of delayed ejaculation [21]. Essentially, any masturbation style that produces sensations that cannot be duplicated with a partner or vaginal intercourse may cause delayed ejaculation. Masturbation that includes excessive speed, pressure, duration, or intensity may be problematic [21] and may include a masturbation position (i.e., lying on his stomach) that produces truly unique sensations.

Finally, some men with idiopathic delayed ejaculation will show no overt etiology, physical or psychological that would account for the extended ejaculation latency. Regardless, a thorough assessment of the individual's psychosocial development, major life events, cultural and religious beliefs related to sexual attitudes and functioning, body image, self-esteem, gender identity, and history of relationships is advised [7, 57].

Assessment

Considering the multiple potential causes of delayed ejaculation, it is important to take a biopsychosocial approach when assessing a patient who reports delayed ejaculation. The first consideration should be the potential biological causes. Obvious neurological, anatomical, and surgical causes should be ruled out first. Considering the large impact SSRIs have on ejaculation latency time, the use of SSRIs should be explored. If these reasons are ruled out, then penile sensitivity by biothesiometry and testosterone, TSH, and prolactin should be assessed. Lastly, psychosexual factors should be assessed. The clinician should discuss masturbation style, the presence of a subtle desire disorder, or a disconnection between the patient's sexual experience and arousal. In a recent presentation, Toloken et al. [58] reported that of 157 men diagnosed with delayed orgasm, 34 % had SSRI-associated delayed orgasm, 35 % had abnormal penile sensation, 15 % had low testosterone, and 16 % were diagnosed with psychogenic delayed orgasm.

Treatment

Clinicians treating delayed ejaculation must recognize that delayed ejaculation is a multifactorial problem often involving interpersonal discord [52], underlying physiological and psychosexual problems, and/or pharmacological factors [59]. Proposed treatments for this disorder include changing or modifying SSRI use, testosterone replacement therapy, off-label use of specific medications, cognitive behavioral therapy, and penile vibratory stimulation (PVS) [60]. Treatment interventions should be selected according to the patient's presenting characteristics. When significant relationship distress is present, the problem may be best addressed as a couple's issue and require the presence of both the man and his partner; in other circumstances, it may be advantageous to see the patient alone. The paucity of systematic outcomes research and lack of treatment consensus, together with the diagnostic complexity involved, make for a clinical picture requiring an *eclectic approach* to treatment [52, 57].

Pharmacological: Past therapies have included medications principally for SSRI-induced delayed ejaculation. The most advantageous treatment for SSRI-induced delayed ejaculation is working with the patient's psychiatrist either to modify the treatment for depression to a non-SSRI medication or to reduce the dose of the SSRI.

To date, no pharmacological therapy has demonstrated consistent efficacy in managing delayed ejaculation unrelated to medication side effects; however, there are some promising pharmacological agents under current study. Common targets of pharmacological therapies include serotonergic modulation, dopaminergic (D2 specifically) tone enhancement, and hormone therapy [61]. Additionally, amantadine, cyproheptadine, yohimbine, bupropion, bethanechol, and buspirone have all been used with varying degrees of success, but none of the studies were placebo-controlled stopwatch studies [57].

Yohimbine: Researchers have explored the effects of yohimbine and cyproheptadine (Periactin) on male ejaculatory functioning with some success. In general, however, this research has been confined to animal experiments, and researchers have not systematically investigated the impact these mediations have on ejaculation time in humans [62]. Research in animals has shown yohimbine to trigger ejaculatory response after ejaculatory exhaustion [63, 64]. Yohimbine is an alkaloid and alpha-2 antagonist available as an over-the-counter dietary supplement usually taken for sexual dysfunction and decreased libido. In humans, yohimbine was shown to reverse clomipramine-induced anorgasmia [62] and, in a separate placebo-controlled study of 15 patients with fluoxetine-induced anorgasmia, was found to have a 73 % response rate with a delayed effect of up to eight weeks when taken 90 minutes before coitus [65]. In a large-scale retrospective study of men with SSRI-induced sexual dysfunction, it was shown that yohimbine, cyproheptadine, and amantadine were effective as an antidote, with yohimbine significantly more effective than the two alternatives [66]. More recently, a study of 29 men with anorgasmia given a dosage of 20 mg (up to 50 mg), reported 16 (55.2 %) could reach ejaculation by masturbation or coitus [67].

Cyproheptadine: Cyproheptadine has been tested in rats and demonstrated moderate effectiveness in facilitating male sexual activity [68]. In addition to its classic antihistaminic (H1 antagonist) properties, cyproheptadine also acts as a competitive serotonin receptor-blocking agent and is believed to increase central serotonin levels. Anecdotal case reports and some studies suggest that cyproheptadine may be efficacious in reversing SSRI-induced anorgasmia [66].

Amantadine (Symmetrel): The antiviral and antiparkinsonian drug, amantadine enhances dopaminergic tone centrally and peripherally through its properties as a weak NMDA receptor antagonist. In animals, amantadine is reported to stimulate sexual behavior, ejaculation, and sexual reflexes. Case reports indicate that amantadine, like yohimbine and cyproheptadine, can reverse SSRI-induced anorgasmia [69].

Cabergoline (Dostinex): A dopamine agonist with high affinity for D2 receptors and used in Parkinson patients and hyperprolactinemic disorders, it has been demonstrated to increase penile erection and orgasm in patients with Parkinson's disease [70]. Cabergoline's effect may not be limited to delayed ejaculation or orgasm, as research suggests that it may help modulate healthy men's sex drive and function [71] or improve men with psychogenic erectile dysfunction [72].

Apomorphine: Apomorphine, a central and peripheral DA2 receptor agonist, has been demonstrated to induce early ejaculation and improve erectile function in animal models. However, oral administration is not effective.

Buspirone (Buspar): The anxiolytic buspirone functions as a 5-HT1A receptor partial agonist and mild presynaptic DA2 receptor antagonist. While traditionally used in the treatment of generalized anxiety disorder and depression, buspirone was shown to increase sexual function in eight out of ten men with GAD [73]. In a larger controlled trial of 117 patients (men and women) with SSRI-induced sexual dysfunction, 58 % of buspirone-treated patients demonstrated sexual function improvement after four weeks of therapy, with a more pronounced response in women [74].

Bupropion (Wellbutrin, Zyban): Bupropion, with dopamine reuptake inhibitor activity used to treat depression, nicotine addiction, and neuropathic pain, remains the only approved antidepressant on the market without significant sexual side effects. The therapeutic role of bupropion, a non-tricyclic antidepressant, comes largely in the context of SSRI-induced delayed ejaculation, specifically its utility in reversing these sexual side effects (up to 66 % of patients) while acting as an effective antidepressant alternative [75]. Clinical studies have also supported the use of bupropion in the treatment of general sexual and orgasmic dysfunctions in both men and women, in cancer survivors, and in nondepressed cohorts [76–79].

Other possible medical therapies include pramipexole (D3), oxytocin, ropinirole (D3), quinelorane, midodrine (SCI), and flibanserin (5-HT1A).

Psychological: A number of authors have argued that cognitive behavioral sex therapy is a primary treatment for restoring orgasm during sexual relations [21, 59, 80]. This therapy may include a number of components to address the potential psychological causes of delayed ejaculation. In the past, psychological therapy has included meditative relaxation, increased sexual play, behavioral therapy with increased manual stimulation or vibratory stimulation to the penis, and increased sensory awareness, self-awareness, and partner communication [52]. The "sexual tipping point," devised by Perelman in the treatment of delayed ejaculation, suggests an integrated treatment combining systemic, psychodynamic, and cognitive behavioral modalities described by Hartmann and Waldinger and the integration of couples therapy and psychosexual skills training advocated by Metz and McCarthy [7, 81]. The available evidence on the effectiveness of these treatments is rather limited. Moreover, there are no research studies comparing the use of medication treatment with the use of psychotherapy treatment in delayed ejaculation. Both successful and unsuccessful case reports have been cited [82]. Although these types of reports are useful to help conceptualize the issues, they are limited in their scope and often overemphasize a single case instead of basing conclusions on a representative sample with empirical data [52].

If a unique masturbation style is present, masturbation retraining may be an aspect of therapy. Although this retraining may take a few months, patients have reported success in altering their masturbation style. This retraining can focus both on the physical technique (i.e., position, speed, force) and on the sexual fantasies during self-stimulation. The general idea is to produce physical sensations and fantasies that are more congruent with the sexual experience with a partner. Regardless of the presence of a unique masturbation style, having the patient withhold masturbation is an important element of this therapy. The use of sensate focus techniques, which can remove the anxiety of achieving an orgasm, can be used to help the patient explore the enjoyment of the sensations and help coach the partner on types of touch or sensations that are most enjoyable.

Penile vibratory stimulation (PVS): The use of penile vibratory stimulation has the strongest outcomes research in this area; however, the research does not meet the highest standard of evidence-based medicine (i.e., randomized, controlled trials). PVS utilizes a commercially available vibrator which patients apply to the frenular area of the penis for three 1 minutes periods separated by 1-min rest periods [36]. The available evidence indicates that the mechanism of action for PVS helps initiate a normal ejaculatory reflex in these men by stimulating the afferent nerves [83]. In a single-arm study, 36 men reported delayed ejaculation and no neurological damage, and 72 % of the men had restoration of their orgasm during sexual intercourse with PVS [36]. As stated above, PVS may be a viable option to integrate into cognitive behavioral techniques.

Conclusion

Delayed ejaculation can have significant quality of life implications for the patient and his partner. Historically, the prevalence has always been discussed as very low; however, there is evidence that the prevalence may be higher than previously documented and this is specifically true for those taking SSRIs. It is important to take a biopsychosocial perspective when diagnosing and treating delayed ejaculation. It is essential to consider a number of different possible causes of this disorder which include overt physical causes, SSRI use, hormonal imbalance, masturbation style, relationship difficulties, and other psychosocial possibilities. As a whole, the research in this area is characterized primarily of case reports and lacks consistent systematic research and controlled trials. The paucity of research signals an important opportunity for those interested in exploring the mechanisms and treatments for delayed ejaculation.

Conflicts of Interest None.

References

1. Laumann EO, Paik A, Rosen RC. Sexual dysfunction in the United States: prevalence and predictors. JAMA. 1999;281(6):537–44.
2. Perelman M, Rowland DL. Retarded and inhibited ejaculation. In: Rowland DL, Incrocci L, editors. Handbook of sexual and gender identity disorders. New York: Wiley; 2008. p. 100–21.
3. Rowland D et al. Disorders of orgasm and ejaculation in men. J Sex Med. 2010;7(4 Pt 2):1668–86.
4. APA. Male orgasmic disorder. Diagnostic and statistical manual of mental disorders, 4th edn, DSM-IV-TR®. New York: American Psychiatric Association; 2000.
5. McMahon CG et al. An evidence-based definition of lifelong premature ejaculation: report of the International Society for Sexual Medicine (ISSM) ad hoc committee for the definition of premature ejaculation. J Sex Med. 2008;5(7):1590–606.
6. Perelman M. Retarded ejaculation. Curr Sex Health Rep 2004 1(3)
7. Metz ME, McCarthy BW. Ejaculatory problems. In: VandeCreek L, Peterson FL, Bley JW, editors. Innovations in clinical practice: focus on sexual health. Sarasota, FL: Professional Resource Press; 2007. p. 135–47.
8. Shull GR, Sprenkle DH. Retarded ejaculation reconceptualization and implications for treatment. J Sex Marital Ther. 1980;6(4):234–46.
9. Lindal E, Stefansson JG. The lifetime prevalence of psychosexual dysfunction among 55 to 57-year-olds in Iceland. Soc Psychiatry Psychiatr Epidemiol. 1993;28(2):91–5.
10. Fugl-Meyer AR, Sjögren Fugl-Meyer K. Sexual disabilities, problems and satisfaction in 18–74 year old Swedes. Scand J Sexol. 1999;3:79–105.
11. Solstad K, Hertoft P. Frequency of sexual problems and sexual dysfunction in middle-aged Danish men. Arch Sex Behav. 1993;22(1):51–8.
12. Jannini EA, Simonelli C, Lenzi A. Disorders of ejaculation. J Endocrinol Invest. 2002;25 (11):1006–19.
13. Nazareth I, Boynton P, King M. Problems with sexual function in people attending London general practitioners: cross sectional study. BMJ. 2003;327(7412):423.
14. Burton TD, Liday C. The comparison of combination SSRI and PDE-5 inhibitor therapy to SSRI monotherapy in men with premature ejaculation. Ann Pharmacother. 2011;45(7–8):1000–4.
15. Corona G et al. Selective serotonin reuptake inhibitor-induced sexual dysfunction. J Sex Med. 2009;6(5):1259–69.
16. Kennedy SH et al. Antidepressant-induced sexual dysfunction during treatment with moclobemide, paroxetine, sertraline, and venlafaxine. J Clin Psychiatry. 2000;61(4):276–81.
17. Madeo B et al. The effects of citalopram and fluoxetine on sexual behavior in healthy men: evidence of delayed ejaculation and unaffected sexual desire. A randomized, placebo-

controlled, double-blind, double-dummy, parallel group study. J Sex Med. 2008;5(10):2431–41.
18. Porst H. An overview of pharmacotherapy in premature ejaculation. J Sex Med. 2011;8 Suppl 4:335–41.
19. Kiev A, Feiger A. A double-blind comparison of fluvoxamine and paroxetine in the treatment of depressed outpatients. J Clin Psychiatr. 1997;58(4):146–52.
20. Rosen RC et al. The international index of erectile function (IIEF): a multidimensional scale for assessment of erectile dysfunction. Urology. 1997;49(6):822–30.
21. Perelman MA, Rowland DL. Retarded ejaculation. World J Urol. 2006;24(6):645–52.
22. Rowland DL, Cooper SE, Slob AK. The treatment of premature ejaculation: psychological and biological strategies. Drugs Today (Barc). 1998;34(10):879–99.
23. Rosen R et al. Lower urinary tract symptoms and male sexual dysfunction: the multinational survey of the aging male (MSAM-7). Eur Urol. 2003;44(6):637–49.
24. Rosen RC. Prevalence and risk factors of sexual dysfunction in men and women. Curr Psychiatry Rep. 2000;2(3):189–95.
25. Montorsi F et al. Summary of the recommendations on sexual dysfunctions in men. J Sex Med. 2010;7(11):3572–88.
26. Abdel-Hamid IA, Salehel S. Primary lifelong delayed ejaculation: characteristics and response to bupropion. J Sex Med. 2011;8(6):1772–9.
27. Zilbergeld B. The new male sexuality. Revth ed. New York: Bantam Books; 1999. p. 414. Xvi.
28. Jannini EA, Simonelli C, Lenzi A. Sexological approach to ejaculatory dysfunction. Int J Androl. 2002;25(6):317–23.
29. Masters WH, Johnson VE. Human sexual inadequacy. London: Churchill; 1970. p. 467. xi.
30. Foley S. The complex etiology of delayed ejaculation: assessment and treatment implication. J Fam Psychother. 2009;20:261–82.
31. DasGupta R, Fowler CJ. Sexual and urological dysfunction in multiple sclerosis: better understanding and improved therapies. Curr Opin Neurol. 2002;15(3):271–8.
32. Richardson D, Goldmeier D. Recommendations for the management of retarded ejaculation: BASHH Special Interest Group for Sexual Dysfunction. Int J STD AIDS. 2006;17(1):7–13.
33. Schuster TG, Ohl DA. Diagnosis and treatment of ejaculatory dysfunction. Urol Clin North Am. 2002;29(4):939–48.
34. Minderhoud JM et al. Sexual disturbances arising from multiple sclerosis. Acta Neurol Scand. 1984;70(4):299–306.
35. Enzlin P et al. Prevalence and predictors of sexual dysfunction in patients with type 1 diabetes. Diabetes Care. 2003;26(2):409–14.
36. Nelson CJ et al. Assessment of penile vibratory stimulation as a management strategy in men with secondary retarded orgasm. Urology. 2007;69(3):552–5. discussion 555-6.
37. Corona G et al. Different testosterone levels are associated with ejaculatory dysfunction. J Sex Med. 2008;5(8):1991–8.
38. Carani C et al. Multicenter study on the prevalence of sexual symptoms in male hypo- and hyperthyroid patients. J Clin Endocrinol Metab. 2005;90(12):6472–9.
39. Jannini EA, Lenzi A. Ejaculatory disorders: epidemiology and current approaches to definition, classification and subtyping. World J Urol. 2005;23(2):68–75.
40. Corona G et al. Psychobiological correlates of delayed ejaculation in male patients with sexual dysfunctions. J Androl. 2006;27(3):453–8.
41. Swaab DF. Sexual differentiation of the brain and behavior. Best Pract Res Clin Endocrinol Metab. 2007;21(3):431–44.
42. Kicman AT. Pharmacology of anabolic steroids. Br J Pharmacol. 2008;154(3):502–21.
43. Cihan A et al. The relationship between premature ejaculation and hyperthyroidism. J Urol. 2009;181(3):1273–80.
44. Waldinger MD. The neurobiological approach to premature ejaculation. J Urol. 2002;168 (6):2359–67.

45. Corona G et al. Sexual dysfunction in subjects with Klinefelter's syndrome. Int J Androl. 2010;33(4):574–80.
46. Hendry WF. Disorders of ejaculation: congenital, acquired and functional. Br J Urol. 1998;82 (3):331–41.
47. Schlegel PN, Shin D, Goldstein M. Urogenital anomalies in men with congenital absence of the vas deferens. J Urol. 1996;155(5):1644–8.
48. Segraves RT. Antidepressant-induced orgasm disorder. J Sex Marital Ther. 1995;21(3):192–201.
49. Kiev A, Feiger A. A double-blind comparison of fluvoxamine and paroxetine in the treatment of depressed outpatients. J Clin Psychiatry. 1997;58(4):146–52.
50. Waldinger MD. Premature ejaculation: state of the art. Urol Clin North Am. 2007;34(4):591–9. vii–viii.
51. Buvat J et al. Dapoxetine for the treatment of premature ejaculation: results from a randomized, double-blind, placebo-controlled phase 3 trial in 22 countries. Eur Urol. 2009;55(4):957–67.
52. Althof SE. Psychological interventions for delayed ejaculation/orgasm. Int J Impot Res. 2012;24(4):131–6.
53. Rowland D et al. Psychosexual factors that differentiate men with inhibited ejaculation from men with no dysfunction or another sexual dysfunction. J Sex Med. 2005;2(3):383–9.
54. Althof SE, Wieder M. Psychotherapy for erectile dysfunction: now more relevant than ever. Endocrine. 2004;23(2–3):131–4.
55. Perelman MA. Idiosyncratic masturbation patterns: a key unexplored variable in the treatment of retarded ejaculation by the practicing urologist. J Urol. 2005;173(4):340.
56. Perelman MA. Unveiling retarded ejaculation. J Urol. 2006;175(4):430.
57. Richardson D et al. Recommendations for the management of premature ejaculation: BASHH Special Interest Group for Sexual Dysfunction. Int J STD AIDS. 2006;17(1):1–6.
58. Toloken P, Nelson CJ, Mulhall JP. Proposed clinical pathways for secondary delayed orgasm. Abstract Presented at the American Urological Meeting; 2012.
59. Perelman MA. Regarding ejaculation, delayed and otherwise. J Androl. 2003;24(4):496.
60. Master VA, Turek PJ. Ejaculatory physiology and dysfunction. Urol Clin N Am. 2001;28 (2):363–75.
61. Wolters JP, Hellstrom WJ. Current concepts in ejaculatory dysfunction. Rev Urol. 2006;8 Suppl 4:S18–25.
62. Cappiello A et al. Yohimbine augmentation of fluvoxamine in refractory depression: a single-blind study. Biol Psychiatry. 1995;38(11):765–7.
63. Carro-Juareza M, Rodriguez-Manzo G. Yohimbine reverses the exhaustion of the coital reflex in spinal male rats. Behav Brain Res. 2003;141(1):43–50.
64. Smith ER, Davidson JM. Yohimbine attenuates aging-induced sexual deficiencies in male rats. Physiol Behav. 1990;47(4):631–4.
65. Jacobsen FM. Fluoxetine-induced sexual dysfunction and an open trial of yohimbine. J Clin Psychiatry. 1992;53(4):119–22.
66. Keller Ashton A, Hamer R, Rosen RC. Serotonin reuptake inhibitor-induced sexual dysfunction and its treatment: a large-scale retrospective study of 596 psychiatric outpatients. J Sex Marital Ther. 1997;23(3):165–75.
67. Adeniyi AA et al. Yohimbine in the treatment of orgasmic dysfunction. Asian J Androl. 2007;9 (3):403–7.
68. Menendez Abraham E et al. Modifications of the sexual activity in male rats following administration of antiserotoninergic drugs. Behav Brain Res. 1988;30(3):251–8.
69. Balon R. Intermittent amantadine for fluoxetine-induced anorgasmia. J Sex Marital Ther. 1996;22(4):290–2.
70. Wittstock M, Benecke R, Dressler D. Cabergoline can increase penile erections and libido. Neurology. 2002;58(5):831.

71. Kruger TH et al. Effects of acute prolactin manipulation on sexual drive and function in males. J Endocrinol. 2003;179(3):357–65.
72. Nickel M et al. Cabergoline treatment in men with psychogenic erectile dysfunction: a randomized, double-blind, placebo-controlled study. Int J Impot Res. 2007;19(1):104–7.
73. Othmer E, Othmer SC. Effect of buspirone on sexual dysfunction in patients with generalized anxiety disorder. J Clin Psychiatry. 1987;48(5):201–3.
74. Landen M et al. Effect of buspirone on sexual dysfunction in depressed patients treated with selective serotonin reuptake inhibitors. J Clin Psychopharmacol. 1999;19(3):268–71.
75. Ashton AK, Rosen RC. Bupropion as an antidote for serotonin reuptake inhibitor-induced sexual dysfunction. J Clin Psychiatry. 1998;59(3):112–5.
76. Crenshaw TL, Goldberg JP, Stern WC. Pharmacologic modification of psychosexual dysfunction. J Sex Marital Ther. 1987;13(4):239–52.
77. Segraves RT et al. Bupropion sustained release (SR) for the treatment of hypoactive sexual desire disorder (HSDD) in nondepressed women. J Sex Marital Ther. 2001;27(3):303–16.
78. Mathias C et al. An open-label, fixed-dose study of bupropion effect on sexual function scores in women treated for breast cancer. Ann Oncol. 2006;17(12):1792–6.
79. Modell JG, May RS, Katholi CR. Effect of bupropion-SR on orgasmic dysfunction in nondepressed subjects: a pilot study. J Sex Marital Ther. 2000;26(3):231–40.
80. Masters WH, Johnson VE. Human sexual inadequacy. Boston, MA: Little, Brown and Company; 1970.
81. Hartmann U, Waldinger MD. Ejaculatory disorders. World J Urol. 2005;23(2):67.
82. Apfelbaum B. Retarded ejaculation; a much-misunderstood syndrome. In: Lieblum SR, Rosen RC, editors. Principles and practice of sex therapy. New York: Guiford Press; 2000. p. 205–41.
83. Sonksen J, Ohl DA, Wedemeyer G. Sphincteric events during penile vibratory ejaculation and electroejaculation in men with spinal cord injuries. J Urol. 2001;165(2):426–9.

Chapter 10
Hypogonadism and Infertility

Geoffrey S. Gaunay, Seth D. Cohen, Peter J. Stahl, and Doron S. Stember

Introduction

The Practice Committee of the American Society has defined infertility for Reproductive Medicine (ASRM) as a failure to conceive after 12 or more months of regular unprotected intercourse [1]. Studies have related 20 % of cases of infertility to purely male factor etiology, while an additional 30–40 % involve both male and female factor pathology [2]. Newer studies have shown little change in this distribution with more than 50 % attributable to male factor, despite advances in the diagnosis and management of infertility [3, 4]. Men with impaired fertility commonly also manifest serum low testosterone (T), or hypogonadism (HG).

Current recommendations by the Practice Committees of the American Urological Association (AUA) and ASRM recommend a couple undergo an infertility evaluation before 1 year if (1) male infertility risk factors (e.g., history of bilateral cryptorchidism) are known to be present, (2) female infertility risk factors including advanced female age (i.e., older than 35 years) are suspected, or (3) the couple questions the male partner's fertility potential [5]. A thorough history and physical exam is the primary initial step in the diagnosis and treatment of male infertility. In most cases, the etiology of subfertility or the need for adjunctive diagnostic testing can be readily ascertained from the history, physical examination, and semen analysis [6]. The basic evaluation for male infertility also requires serum follicle-stimulating hormone (FSH) and T levels.

The term HG describes a diminished T level and, by definition, one or more symptoms from a constellation that includes decreased libido, energy, overall sense of well-being, and erectile function. HG may be secondary to disruption of the hypothalamic-pituitary axis or primary testicular failure. Testicular failure is, in

D.S. Stember (✉)
Department of Urology, Beth Israel Medical Center, Mount Sinai Health System,
10 Union Square East, Suite 3A, New York, NY 10002, USA
e-mail: dstember@chpnet.org

J.P. Mulhall and W. Hsiao (eds.), *Men's Sexual Health and Fertility*,
DOI 10.1007/978-1-4939-0425-9_10,

turn, characterized by impairment of either, or both, the endocrine production of T or exocrine production of sperm.

We herein review the relationship of HG with male factor infertility and review therapeutic management options that address both conditions.

The Male Reproductive-Hormonal Axis

An intact hypothalamic-pituitary-gonadal axis is critically important for normal sperm production. The hypothalamus secretes gonadotropin-releasing hormone (GnRH), also known as luteinizing hormone-releasing hormone (LHRH), in a pulsatile fashion. GnRH stimulates the release of the gonadotropin FSH and luteinizing hormone (LH) from the anterior pituitary gland [6].

Testicular function is dependent upon both FSH and LH. Whereas LH stimulates Leydig cells in the testicular interstitium to synthesize and secrete T (approximately 5–10 mg per day), spermatogenesis is maintained by the action of FSH on testicular Sertoli cells [6, 7]. T is then secreted both into systemic circulation and diffuses into the seminiferous tubules that surround the Leydig cells. This latter paracrine distribution of T results in highly concentrated levels that are needed to support spermatogenesis in the germinal epithelium and sperm maturation in the epididymis. Concentrations within the testes are 50–100 times higher than serum [8, 9].

T exerts negative feedback effects on LH secretion both directly and indirectly (via conversion to estradiol (E2) in the brain) [10]. T is converted to E2 in peripheral adipose tissue by the enzyme aromatase. When serum T/E2 ratios are low, usually <10, feedback central inhibition may negatively impact spermatogenesis. When sperm production is impaired, feedback inhibition of FSH release is diminished and serum FSH levels are usually elevated (>8 IU/L) [6].

It is extremely important for clinicians to understand these physiologic effects. The message is that men who are interested in fertility should not be treated with T replacement therapy (TRT), particularly for the diagnosis of infertility. TRT will produce a robust serum T level but will also cause intratesticular T concentration to sharply decline, for the reasons stated above, with results deleterious to spermatogenesis.

Evaluation of Hypogonadism and Infertility

The diagnosis of HG begins with clinical suspicion for the condition based on history and physical examination. Endocrine evaluation is indicated in men with (1) an abnormally low sperm concentration, typically defined as lower than 20 million/mL; (2) impaired sexual function; or (3) other clinical findings suggestive of endocrinopathies, such as marked reduction in testicular size or gynecomastia [5]. Although it is a rare cause of male infertility, up to 3 % of infertile men will have an underlying endocrinopathy [8]. Initial endocrine evaluation in those with indications for testing (i.e., subfertile men with abnormal semen analysis) should include serum follicle-stimulating hormone (FSH) and morning serum T measurements [5]. Morning T specimens are preferred over afternoon blood draws, as a method of standardization, due to a normal physiologic decline in T levels that occurs throughout the day. When T levels are low, FSH levels help provide information to suggest whether the disturbance is central, hypothalamic or pituitary, or testicular. Obstructive azoospermia is usually associated with normal gonadotropin and T levels. Elevated serum gonadotropins can be indicative of hypergonadotropic hypogonadism, or primary HG, with associated testicular disturbances in spermatogenesis, although normal FSH levels do not rule out spermatogenic failure [11].

In men with low serum T, FSH, and LH levels, serum prolactin should be measured, as well as in any man with decreased libido, sexual dysfunction, gynecomastia, or galactorrhea to screen for prolactinoma. Brain magnetic resonance imaging (MRI) may be indicated to characterize a prolactinoma, if prolactin is elevated, or rule out a pituitary or hypothalamic mass, should the prolactin be within normal limits [6]. Serum E2 levels should be measured whenever gynecomastia or a testicular mass is present and can also play a role in the selection of hormonal treatment when such therapy is indicated [12].

Classification of Hypogonadism

HG is characterized by a low T level (typically below 300 or 350 ng/dL) and a wide range of associated symptoms that can be significantly bothersome and physiologically detrimental to patients. In adults, the symptoms of HG can include sexual dysfunction, cognitive impairment, decreased energy, depressed mood, increased fat mass, loss of muscle mass and strength, and reduced bone mineral density (BMD) [9]. Classification of HG is determined by the location of the primary hormonal defect.

Primary HG is characterized by organ dysfunction at the level of the testes and results in decreased serum T and impaired spermatogenesis. Increased serum GnRH and gonadotropins typically result from lack of negative feedback on the hypothalamus and anterior pituitary. Primary testicular failure may result from many clinical conditions including gonadotoxin exposure (e.g., chemotherapeutic agents, radiation, nicotine, alcohol), atrophic or undescended testes, and genetic abnormalities such as Klinefelter syndrome (KS) or Noonan syndrome. In most cases, however, a distinct etiology is not identifiable and HG is classified as idiopathic primary testicular failure.

In men with primary testicular failure of unknown etiology, a karyotype to exclude KS should be obtained, especially in men with testicular volume less than 6 mL [13]. KS is the most common chromosomal disorder in men with testicular dysgenesis syndrome (TDS) and is definitively diagnosed by demonstration of an extra X chromosome demonstrated via karyotype (47, XXY). KS has an estimated prevalence of 0.2 % in the general population, 3 % among infertile men, and up to 11 % in men with nonobstructive azoospermia (NOA) [14].

Despite the wide variability in clinical presentation, all patients with KS suffer from absolute or relative HG, small testicular size, and impaired spermatogenesis. Sclerosis of the seminiferous tubules is typically observed on scrotal exploration [15]. The goal of TRT in adolescents with KS is to promote linear growth, increase muscle mass, preserve bone density, and allow for the development of secondary sexual characteristics [16].

Although T supplementation in KS has a beneficial effect on semen volume, exogenous T administration may also have an inadvertently detrimental impact on spermatogenesis by further suppressing testicular function overall [16]. Successful pregnancies in couples in which the male suffers from KS have been occasionally achieved using ejaculated sperm and assisted reproductive techniques. However, surgical sperm retrieval and intracytoplasmic sperm injection (ICSI) have dramatically improved the fertility potential of men with KS. This is particularly true when surgical exploration to harvest sperm is performed at a younger patient age (following puberty) since seminiferous tubules progressively lose function in a duration-dependent fashion in males with KS [17, 18]. Recent studies of men with KS, some concurrently treated with aromatase inhibitors, showed success rates of 66–72 % per testicular sperm extraction (TESE) with 69 % of men having sperm suitable for ICSI [18, 19]. Although no trials have specifically studied TRT and sperm retrieval rates, it is logical to assume TRT would lead to lower TESE yields. Studies have indicated that KS patients with higher baseline T, or those who best responded to medical therapy to correct T (as opposed to exogenous T), had more successful sperm retrieval [19].

Hypogonadotropic hypogonadism (HH) is a condition caused by insufficient or absent production of gonadotropin-releasing hormone (GnRH). In the absence of GnRH serum, FSH and LH will be low in addition to T. There are numerous identified causes of HH. HH in the presence of midline defects, such as anosmia, is defined as Kallmann's syndrome. Genetic causes like Prader-Willi syndrome (PWS) and Laurence-Moon-Bardet-Biedl syndrome may include a constellation of abnormalities, such as the mental retardation and physical defects associated with PWS. HH may result from a prolactin-secreting pituitary adenoma or iatrogenic causes, such as radiation or neurosurgical procedures, administration of opioids, anabolic steroids, or exogenous T. Regardless of the underlying cause, both T levels (due to low T) and sperm production (due to low T and FSH) are negatively affected [20]. Careful history is essential in ruling out iatrogenic causes, and adverse oral agents should be immediately discontinued.

Fertility potential can frequently be restored, with appropriate hormonal stimulation, in patients with HH. Men with primary testicular failure, on the other hand, cannot usually be successfully treated with medication alone. Fertility options for men in this group are limited to the use of donor sperm, adoption, or, in some patients, TESE to harvest sperm to be used with in vitro fertilization (IVF) and ICSI [18, 21].

Varicocele

The presence of varicocele, or dilated pampiniform plexus of the spermatic cord, can be identified in 15 % of the general population and in 35–40 % of subfertile men [22, 23]. Palpable varicoceles have been associated with decreased fertility and surgical varicocelectomy has been demonstrated to improve semen quality and pregnancy rates [22, 24, 25]. More recent studies have shown that varicoceles are also associated with HG and may be an independent risk factor for androgen deficiency [25]. The pathogenesis for this effect is not well understood but it has been speculated that increased intratesticular temperature in the presence of a varicocele may impair the enzyme 17 α-hydroxyprogesterone aldolase, which plays an important role in T production [27]. Surgical repair of varicoceles in men with low T has recently been shown to provide significant subsequent T level increases in the majority of study patients [26, 28]. The concept of varicocele as a risk factor for HG is covered in more detail in Chap. 11.

Effect of Exogenous T on Male Fertility

Therapeutic options to treat symptomatic HG are available in multiple forms. These include T replacement by intramuscular injections, patches, topically applied gels, and subcutaneous T pellet administration [13]. All of these options, however, have the effect of impairing spermatogenesis even while normalizing serum T levels. Iatrogenic androgens inhibit spermatogenesis due to direct feedback inhibition of gonadotropin secretion at the level of the hypothalamus and pituitary. This ultimately results in low intratesticular levels of T that are inadequate for maintenance of spermatogenesis. In fact, the effect on sperm production is so significant that there is a growing body of research exploring TRT as a potential male contraceptive medication [29].

Anabolic steroid users represent a distinct subpopulation of men with subfertility. As opposed to organically hypogonadal men who become subfertile due to TRT, steroid users typically have normal or high T levels initially. After one or more cycles of steroid use, native T production by Leydig cells declines and produces similar effects to those seen in men who undergo TRT. Studies of semen quality in athletes using high doses of anabolic steroids revealed severe impairment of sperm concentration, motility, and morphology [30]. Although cessation of use allowed normalization of seminal parameters in an average of 4 months, cases of persistent azoospermia have been reported occurring more than 1 year later [29].

Medical Treatment of Men with Hypogonadism and Infertility

As noted previously, patients with HH or primary testicular failure often require ARTs, such as IVF/ICSI, in order to achieve conception. This procedure may be performed using either ejaculated sperm or sperm obtained by percutaneous (TESA) or open testis biopsy (TESE) [17, 18]. Some potential benefit may be derived with use of recombinant FSH before IVF/ICSI in patients with testis failure, but this has not been conclusively established [31].

More medical options are available to men with HH who desire fertility. These therapies may be combined with assisted reproductive technologies such as IVF with ICSI, which may allow pregnancy to occur with very low numbers of sperm [32]. The medications are outlined below and summarized in Table 10.1.

Gonadotropin-Releasing Hormone (GnRH)

In patients with hypothalamic dysfunction underlying HH, the treatment goal is to increase GnRH or its downstream effectors. Although it may seem intuitive to simply administer GnRH, in practice, it is largely impractical and logistically difficult. GnRH is administered subcutaneously through the abdominal wall over 90–120 min intervals, thus mimicking gonadotropin pulsatility. GnRH has been shown to improve testis volume and serum T, but gonadotropin levels typically remain low, making it a poor choice for those with pituitary causes of HG [33–35].

Multiple studies have shown non-superiority of GnRH versus gonadotropin therapy for the induction of spermatogenesis or rate of pregnancies [36–38]. In addition to the high financial cost and impractical nature of this treatment, there also exists potential for infusion site infection [39]. Given these drawbacks, GnRH is usually utilized only after all other treatment options have failed to induce spermatogenesis.

Estrogen Receptor Modulators

Perhaps the most commonly used agents for hypothalamic hypogonadotropic HG are the antiestrogen agents clomiphene, tamoxifen, and enclomiphene. These estrogen receptor modulators raise T indirectly by blocking the coupling of estradiol with its receptors. The subsequent lack of negative feedback results in upregulation of LH and T [40]. Typical starting doses are 25–50 mg of clomiphene citrate taken every other day and are extremely well tolerated.

Increasing testicular T production has the benefit of normalizing serum T levels via an increase in intratesticular T production. Increasing T concentration within

Table 10.1 Medical therapies for men with hypogonadism and impaired fertility

Category	Formulation	Standard dosage	Benefits	Disadvantages
Gonadotropin therapy	Human chorionic gonadotropin (hCG)	1,000–2,000 International Units (IU) 2–3 times per week	– Financially inexpensive—may restore spermatogenesis in men with HH as a single agent	Requires intramuscular (IM) injection
Gonadotropin therapy	Human menopausal gonadotropin (HMG)	25–75 IU, 3 times per week	– May induce spermatogenesis when added to hCG – May be discontinued after spermatogenesis induced (patient can be maintained on hCG alone)	Requires IM injection
Gonadotropin therapy	Follicle-stimulating hormone (FSH)	– 1.5 IU/kg weekly × 18 months (urinary FSH) – 450 IU weekly × 12 months (recombinant FSH)	– May induce spermatogenesis when added to hCG	– Limited availability – Financially expensive – Requires IM injection
Physiological gonadotropin-releasing hormone (GnRH) replacement	GnRH	100–600 ng/kg per pulse, pulses given at approximately 2-h intervals, pumps worn for up to a year	– May be effective even if all other modalities have failed	– Financially expensive – Requires subcutaneous administration via portable abdominal wall infusion pumps for weeks or months – May result in pump site infections
Estrogen receptor modulator	Clomiphene citrate	25–50 mg daily or 25–50 mg every other day	– Easily tolerated – Oral convenience	– Potential side effects include breast tenderness, gynecomastia, and headache – 25 mg dose is not commercially available; 50 mg pills must be split in

(continued)

Table 10.1 (continued)

Category	Formulation	Standard dosage	Benefits	Disadvantages
				half to achieve that dose
Aromatase inhibitor	Anastrozole	1 mg daily	– Easily tolerated – Oral convenience	– Potential side effects include gastrointestinal distress, muscle aches, headache, and hypertension
Aromatase inhibitor	Testolactone	100–200 mg daily, taken orally	– Easily tolerated – Oral convenience	– Not available in the United States – Potential side effects include gastrointestinal distress, hypertension, edema, and paresthesias

the testes facilitates seminiferous tubule sperm production, which is in direct contradistinction to the decreased local testicular environment that results from exogenous T administration. Since antiestrogens work by raising LH levels, the candidates most likely to respond are patients with low to normal starting LH levels.

Supporting studies have shown normalized T levels and improved semen analyses in patients treated with clomiphene [41, 42]. However, a Cochrane meta-analysis of 738 men combining ten randomized controlled studies of the effects of short-term clomiphene and tamoxifen on men with oligoasthenozoospermia failed to show significant difference improvements in pregnancy rates when compared with controls [43]. Similar randomized controlled trials using tamoxifen therapy have not conclusively supported efficacy in either improved semen parameters or pregnancy rates [44].

Gonadotropin Therapy

Agents used for induction of spermatogenesis in HH include human chorionic gonadotropin (hCG), human menopausal gonadotropin (hMG), and FSH.

hCG binds to the same Leydig cell receptor as LH and mimics its action, stimulating the production of T. As intratesticular levels of T rise, often up to 100 times that of serum, spermatogenesis may be stimulated [45]. hCG alone can often restore spermatogenesis in men with adult onset of HH. Treatment is usually initiated with hCG but without FSH, since hCG has the ability to stimulate and maintain spermatogenesis alone at a fraction of the cost of FSH [46, 47].

In cases where hCG alone does not prove sufficient to stimulate spermatogenesis, FSH or hMG may be added to the regimen [47]. FSH or hMG preparations, which contain FSH, are administered after a suitable course of hCG. hCG is typically given as a 1,000–2,000 IU dose two to three times weekly for 18–24 weeks and is injected intramuscularly to the deltoid. hMG may be considered once serum T normalizes and semen analysis findings plateau [12].

hMG dosing (75 IU two to three times weekly) is typically continued until through the first 3 months of pregnancy after which the patient is maintained solely with hCG [48]. Combination hCG/hMG therapy may also induce virilization in hypogonadal prepubertal males and lead to testicular growth [36, 49, 50]. Urinary purified FSH (uFSH) and recombinant FSH (rFSH) have the added benefit of greater specific activity compared with hMG. The dose is 1.5 IU/kg weekly for 18 months and 450 IU weekly for 12 months, respectively [51, 52].

Aromatase Inhibitors

It has been observed that men with NOA or oligospermia frequently have low T and elevated E2, suggesting that increased aromatase activity is responsible for excessive conversion of T and subsequently lower serum levels [53]. These patients may therefore benefit from treatment with an aromatase inhibitor to prevent the conversion of T to E2, resulting in increased T and decreased E2 levels.

Treatment is comprised of anastrozole 1 mg taken orally daily. Anastrozole is an inexpensive medication with a favorable side effect profile. Testolactone 100–200 mg oral daily has been shown to be particularly effective in men with KS but this formulation is not available in the United States [54]. The effect of aromatase inhibitors is similar to that of antiestrogens, with resultant indirect increases in gonadotropins and T level.

Aromatase inhibitors are most effective in improving spermatogenesis in patients with serum T:E2 ratios <10 as well as obese men (who have increased levels of aromatase activity) [54, 55]. These agents are particularly important for utilization in men with KS, in whom it has been shown that normalizing serum T prior to TESE increases rates of successful sperm retrieval [19]. Similar benefits have not been conclusively demonstrated in other men with HG and infertility, but clinicians may prefer to medically optimize T levels before surgical sperm retrieval in all patients.

Conclusions

HG is a prevalent and potentially treatable condition that is associated with male infertility. Scrotal varices have recently been associated with HG in addition to subfertility, and recent evidence supports the use of surgical varicocele repair for improving T levels as well as fertility potential. Patients with primary testicular failure have impaired testicular sperm and T production. Traditional HG treatment with TRT is contraindicated in these patients since it impairs sperm production through negative feedback. There are multiple other medical options that address HG and/or sperm production and should be utilized instead of TRT. Therapies in this category include estrogen receptor modulators, aromatase inhibitors, hCG, hMG, urinary and recombinant FSH, and GnRH. The specific treatment and regimen is tailored to the individual patient and is largely based on the underlying cause of the disorder. Logistical and financial considerations are also relevant and may guide medical decision making.

Although it is desirable to correct T levels in men with HG and infertility, normalization of T levels alone is generally considered ineffective for improving or restoring spermatogenesis in patients with primary testicular failure. Men with infertility related to HH, on the other hand, are relatively responsive to a variety of therapeutic agents that help stimulate testicular sperm production as well as increase T levels. Induced spermatogenesis may be sufficient for natural conception or at least for use with ARTs.

The message that TRT should not be reflexively used to treat men with HG who desire fertility cannot be overemphasized. This concept may be counterintuitive unless the underlying physiology of the hypothalamic-pituitary axis is appreciated. Patients and physicians should be aware of medical options to restore normogonadism that may restore, improve, or, at the very least, fail to impair spermatogenesis.

References

1. Practice Committee of the American Society for Reproductive Medicine. Definitions of infertility and recurrent pregnancy loss. Fertil Steril. 2008;89(6):1603.
2. Simmons FA. Human infertility. NEJM. 1956;255(24):1140.
3. Mosher WD, Pratt WF. Fecundity and infertility in the United States: incidence and trends. Fertil Steril. 1991;56(2):192–3.
4. Thonneau P, Marchand S, Tallec A, Ferial ML, Ducot B, Lansac J, Lopes P, Tabaste JM, Spira A. Incidence and main causes of infertility in a resident population (1,850,000) of three French regions (1988–1989). Hum Reprod. 1991;6(6):811–6.
5. Male Infertility Best Practice Policy Committee of the American Urological Association and the Practice Committee of the American Society for Reproductive Medicine. Report on optimal evaluation of the infertile male. Fertil Steril. 2006;86 Suppl 4:S202–9.
6. Stahl PJ, Stember DS, Goldstein M. Contemporary management of male infertility. Annu Rev Med. 2012;63:525–40.
7. Sigman M, Jarow JP. Endocrine evaluation of infertile men. Urology. 1997;50(5):659–64.
8. Morse HC, Horike N, Rowley MJ, Heller CG. Testosterone concentrations in testes of normal men: effects of testosterone propionate administration. J Clin Endocrinol Metab. 1973;37 (6):882.
9. McLachlan RI, O'Donnell L, Meachem SJ, Stanton PG, de K, Pratis K, Robertson DM. Hormonal regulation of spermatogenesis in primates and man: insights for development of the male hormonal contraceptive. J Androl. 2002;23(2):149.

10. Bagatell CJ, Dahl KD, Bremner WJ. The direct pituitary effect of testosterone to inhibit gonadotropin secretion in men is partially mediated by aromatization to estradiol. J Androl. 1994;15(1):15.
11. Sabanegh E, Agarwal A. Male infertility. In: Wein AJ, Kavoussi LR, Novick AC, Partin AW, Peters CA, editors. Campbells urology. 10th ed. Philadelphia, PA: Saunders Elsevier; 2011.
12. Sokol RZ. Endocrinology of male infertility: evaluation and treatment. Semin Reprod Med. 2009;27(2):149–58.
13. Bhasin S, Cunningham GR, Hayes FJ, Matsumoto AM, Snyder PJ, Swerdloff RS, Montori VM, Task Force, Endocrine Society. Testosterone therapy in men with androgen deficiency syndromes: an Endocrine Society clinical practice guideline. J Clin Endocrinol Metab. 2010;95(6):2536–59.
14. Foresta C, Galeazzi C, Bettella A, et al. Analysis of meiosis in intratesticular germ cells from subjects affected by classic Klinefelter's syndrome. J Clin Endocrinol Metab. 1999;84 (10):3807–10.
15. Verit FF, Verit A. Klinefelter syndrome: an argument for early aggressive hormonal and fertility management. Fertil Steril. 2012;98(5):e25.
16. Houk CP, Rogol A, Lee PA. Fertility in men with Klinefelter syndrome. Pediatr Endocrinol Rev. 2010;8 Suppl 1:182–6.
17. Tournaye H, Staessen C, Liebaers I, Van Assche E, Devroey P, Bonduelle M, et al. Testicular sperm recovery in nine 47 XXY Klinefelter patients. Hum Reprod. 1996;11(8):1644–9.
18. Schiff JD, Palermo GD, Veeck LL, Goldstein M, Rosenwaks Z, Schlegel PN. Success of testicular sperm extraction [corrected] and intracytoplasmic sperm injection in men with Klinefelter syndrome. J Clin Endocrinol Metab. 2005;90(11):6263–7.
19. Ramasamy R, Ricci JA, Palermo GD, Gosden LV, Rosenwaks Z, Schlegel PN. Successful fertility treatment for Klinefelter's syndrome. J Urol. 2009;182(3):1108–13.
20. Zitzmann M, Nieschlag E. Hormone substitution in male hypogonadism. Mol Cell Endocrinol. 2000;161(1–2):73–88.
21. Zitzmann M, Nordhoff V, von Schönfeld V, Nordsiek-Mengede A, Kliesch S, Schüring AN, Luetjens CM, Kamischke A, Cooper T, Simoni M, Nieschlag E. Elevated follicle-stimulating hormone levels and the chances for azoospermic men to become fathers after retrieval of elongated spermatids from cryopreserved testicular tissue. Fertil Steril. 2006;86(2):339–47.
22. Pryor JL, Howards SS. Varicocele. Urol Clin North Am. 1987;14(3):499.
23. Romeo C, Santoro G. Varicocele and infertility: why a prevention? J Endocrinol Invest. 2009;32(6):559.
24. Zini A, Boman JM. Varicocele: red flag or red herring? Semin Reprod Med. 2009;27(2):171–8.
25. Male Infertility Best Practice Policy Committee of the American Urological Association, Practice Committee of the American Society for Reproductive Medicine. Report on varicocele and infertility. Fertil Steril. 2004.
26. Tanrikut C, Goldstein M, Rosoff JS, Lee RK, Nelson CJ, Mulhall JP. Varicocele as a risk factor for androgen deficiency and effect of repair. BJU Int. 2011;108(9):1480–4.
27. Andò S, Giacchetto C, Colpi G, Panno ML, Beraldi E, Lombardi A, Sposato G. Plasma levels of 17-OH-progesterone and testosterone in patients with varicoceles. Acta Endocrinol (Copenh). 1983;102(3):463–9.
28. Hsiao W, Rosoff JS, Pale JR, Powell JL, Goldstein M. Varicocelectomy is associated with increases in serum testosterone independent of clinical grade. Urol. 2013;81(6):1213–8.
29. Jarow JP, Espeland MA, Lipshultz LI. Evaluation of the azoospermic patient. J Urol. 1989;142 (1):62–5.
30. Knuth UA, Maniera H, Nieschlag E. Anabolic steroids and semen parameters in body builders. Fertil Steril. 1989;52(6):1041–7.
31. Foresta C, Bettella A, Garolla A, Ambrosini G, Ferlin A. Treatment of male idiopathic infertility with recombinant human follicle-stimulating hormone: a prospective, controlled, randomized clinical study. Fertil Steril. 2005;84(3):654–61.

32. Petak SM, Nankin HR, Spark RF, Swerdloff RS, Rodriguez-Rigau LJ, American Association of Clinical Endocrinologists. American Association of Clinical Endocrinologists Medical Guidelines for clinical practice for the evaluation and treatment of hypogonadism in adult male patients-2002 update. Endocr Pract. 2002;8(6):440–56.
33. Guo YL, Hu LQ, editors. Nan ke xue. Beijing: People's Medical Publishing House; 2004. p. 1389–99.
34. Pitteloud N, Hayes FJ, Dwyer A, Boepple PA, Lee H, Crowley Jr WF. Predictors of outcome of long-term GnRH therapy in men with idiopathic hypogonadotropic hypogonadism. J Clin Endocrinol Metab. 2002;87(9):4128–36.
35. Happ J, Ditscheid W, Krause U. Pulsatile gonadotropin releasing hormone therapy in male patients with Kallmann's syndrome or constitutional delay of puberty. Fertil Steril. 1985;43 (4):599–608.
36. Liu L, Banks SM, Barnes KM, Sherins RJ. Two-year comparison of testicular responses to pulsatile gonadotropin releasing hormone and exogenous gonadotropins from the inception of therapy in men with isolated hypogonadotropic hypogonadism. J Clin Endocrinol Metab. 1988;67(6):1140–5.
37. Schopohl J. Pulsatile gonadotropin releasing hormone versus gonadotropin treatment of hypothalamic hypogonadism in males. Hum Reprod. 1993;8 Suppl 2:175–9.
38. Buchter D, Behre HM, Kliesch S, Nieschlaq E. Pulsatile GnRH or human chorionic gonadotropin/human menopausal gonadotropin as effective treatment for men with hypogonadotropic hypogonadism, a review of 42 cases. Eur J Endocrinol. 1998;139(3):298–303.
39. Han TS, Bouloux PM. What is the optimal therapy for young males with hypogonadotropic hypogonadism? Clin Endocrinol. 2010;72(6):731–7.
40. Ramasamy R, Stahl PJ, Schlegel PN. Medical therapy for spermatogenic failure. Asian J Androl. 2012;14(1):57–60.
41. Whitten SJ, Nangia AK, Kolettis PN. Select patients with hypogonadotropic hypogonadism may respond to treatment with clomiphene citrate. Fertil Steril. 2006;86(6):1664–8.
42. Ioannidou-Kadis S, Wright PJ, Neely RD, Quinton R. Complete reversal of adult-onset isolated hypogonadotropic hypogonadism with clomiphene citrate. Fertil Steril. 2006;86 (5):1513.
43. Vandekerckhove P, Lilford R, Vail A, Hughes E. Clomiphene or tamoxifen for idiopathic oligo/astheno-spermia. Cochrane Database Syst Rev. 2000;(2).
44. Torok L. Treatment of oligozoospermia with tamoxifen (open and controlled studies). Andrologia. 1985;17(5):497–501.
45. Finkel DM, Phillips JL, Synder PJ. Stimulation of spermatogenesis by gonadotropins in men with hypogonadotropic hypogonadism. N Engl J Med. 1985;313:651–5.
46. Matsumoto AM, Paulsen CA, Bremner WJ. Stimulation of sperm production by human luteinizing hormone in gonadotropin-suppressed normal men. J Clin Endocrinol Metab. 1984;59(5):882.
47. Schaison G, Young J, Pholsena M, Nahoul K, Couzinet B. Failure of combined follicle-stimulating hormone – testosterone administration to initiate and/or maintain spermatogenesis in men with hypogonadotropic hypogonadism. J Clin Endocrinol Metab. 1993;77(6):1545–9.
48. Sokol RZ. Male factor infertility. In: Lobo R, Mishell Jr DR, Paulson RJ, Shoupe D, editors. Infertility, contraception, and reproductive endocrinology. 4th ed. Malden, MA: Blackwell Science; 1997.
49. Di FS, Cui YG, Jia Y. The application of gonadotropin in treatment of male central hypogonadism. Zhonghua Nei Ke Za Zhi. 2005;44(11):836–9.
50. Butcher D, Behre HM, Kliesch S, Nieschlaq E. Pulsatile GnRH or human chorionic gonadotropin/human menopausal gonadotropin as effective treatment for men with hypogonadotropic hypogonadism: a review of 42 cases. Eur Endocrinol. 1998;139(3):298–303.
51. Barrio R, de Luis D, Alonso M, Lamas A, Moreno JC. Induction of puberty with human chorionic gonadotropin and follicle-stimulating hormone in adolescent males with hypogonadotropic hypogonadism. Fertil Steril. 1999;71(2):244–8.

52. Bouloux PM, Nieschlag E, Burger HG, Skakkebaek NE, Wu FC, Handelsman DJ, Baker GH, Ochsenkuehn R, Syska A, McLachlan RI, Giwercman A, Conway AJ, Turner L, van Kuijk JH, Voortman G. Induction of spermatogenesis by recombinant follicle-stimulating hormone (puregon) in hypogonadotropic azoospermic men who failed to respond to human chorionic gonadotropin alone. J Androl. 2003;24(4):604–11.
53. Hopps CV, Mielnik A, Goldstein M, Palermo GD, Rosenwaks Z, Schlegel PN. Detection of sperm in men with Y chromosome microdeletions of the AZFa, AZFb and AZFc regions. Hum Reprod. 2003;18(8):1660–5.
54. Raman JD, Schlegel PN. Aromatase inhibitors for male infertility. J Urol. 2002;167 (2 Pt 1):624–9.
55. Kim ED, Crosnoe L, Bar-Chama N, Khera M, Lipshultz LI. The treatment of hypogonadism in men of reproductive age. Fertil Steril. 2013;99(3):718–24.

Chapter 11
Varicoceles and Hypogonadism

Akanksha Mehta

Introduction

Varicoceles are abnormal dilatations of the internal spermatic veins of the pampiniform plexus of the spermatic cord. First described by the Greek physician Celsus during the first century A.C. [1], varicoceles have classically been associated with testicular pain, decreased testicular volume, impaired semen quality, and decline in Leydig cell function [2]. Clinical varicoceles are present in approximately 15 % of the general male population, and in up to 35 % of men with primary- and 75 % of men with secondary infertility [3]. Since Tulloch's first report on varicocelectomy as a treatment for male subfertility [4], a multitude of studies have investigated the optimal timing, method, and impact of varicocele repair on improvement in testicular function. The vast majority of these studies suffer from methodological flaws; they are largely retrospective and uncontrolled in nature, lack standardized definitions of varicoceles, and fail to account for confounding variables such as female factor infertility. Additionally, pregnancy rates and live birth outcomes are rarely reported as the primary outcome measure [5]. Nevertheless, the repair of clinically palpable varicoceles is indicated and accepted for the treatment of male infertility in the setting of one or more abnormal semen parameters [6, 7].

There is growing interest in the effect of varicoceles and varicocele repair on serum testosterone levels as a marker of Leydig cell function. It is well accepted that testosterone exerts pleiotropic effects on the body, ranging from supporting spermatogenesis and improving sexual function to increasing bone density and muscle mass. The association between varicoceles and hypogonadism, characterized by low serum testosterone and symptoms of androgen deficiency, is long standing [8–11]. It is less clear whether this negative impact of varicoceles on

A. Mehta (✉)
Department of Urology, Emory University School of Medicine, 1365 Clifton Road NE, Clinic B, Suite 1400, Atlanta, GA 30322, USA
e-mail: Akanksha.mehta@emory.edu

J.P. Mulhall and W. Hsiao (eds.), *Men's Sexual Health and Fertility*,
DOI 10.1007/978-1-4939-0425-9_11,

Leydig cell function is discreet or progressive. Emerging evidence indicates that varicocele repair has the potential to improve Leydig cell function, leading to improvement in serum testosterone levels [8]. However, whether the resultant improvement in serum testosterone is sufficient to obviate the need for exogenous testosterone therapy in hypogonadal men remains uncertain.

This chapter discusses the available literature on the relationship between varicoceles and hypogonadism and evaluates the role of varicocele repair in the management of hypogonadal men. Surgical and nonsurgical approaches to varicocele repair are also reviewed.

Etiology and Pathophysiology of Varicoceles

The development of varicoceles is attributed to incompetent valves in the internal spermatic veins, leading to venous stasis and venous enlargement over time [3, 12]. Reversal of blood flow in the internal spermatic veins may also occur as a result of incompetent valves, particularly during maneuvers that increase intra-abdominal pressure. Some authors have proposed that the longer length of the left testicular vein, and its angle of insertion into the left renal vein, predisposes it to elevated hydrostatic pressures compared to its right-sided counterpart, accounting for the higher prevalence of left-sided varicoceles. The so-called nutcracker effect, compression of the left testicular vein between the aorta and the superior mesenteric artery, may be an additional factor contributing to varicocele formation [13].

The exact mechanism by which varicoceles affect testicular function remains unclear. Proposed theories include elevated scrotal and testicular temperatures due to venous stasis and impaired countercurrent heat exchange, reflux of toxic renal and adrenal metabolites via the testicular veins, and increased levels of reactive oxygen species within the testes. The net result is a decrease in the quantity and quality of spermatogenesis, as well as a decline in Leydig cell function. On physical examination, this deterioration in testicular function is reflected in testicular volume and consistency [14], while laboratory testing reveals abnormal semen parameters [15], increased sperm DNA fragmentation rates [16], and declining serum testosterone levels [17].

The hypothesis that varicoceles have a progressive deleterious effect on testicular function derives from the higher incidence of varicoceles noted among men presenting for secondary compared to primary infertility [18, 19], and from a single study demonstrating a decline in sperm counts over time in 13 men with untreated varicoceles [20]. However, this hypothesis has been refuted by Jarow et al. who reported similar rates of varicocele detection in men with primary and secondary infertility [21]. Only one prospective, longitudinal study assessing semen quality in men with untreated varicoceles has been performed to date. This questionnaire-based study included 77 men (39 with varicoceles and 38 men without); all affected men had palpable grade 3 varicoceles. Seventy-six percent of subjects completed the questionnaire and 61 % gave semen samples for analysis after a follow-up period of 8 years. While no patients underwent a varicocele repair, the men with varicocele did not show any significant decline in semen parameters over the 8-year follow-up period [22].

Various confounding factors such as the inclusion of study subjects with subclinical varicoceles diagnosed on ultrasonography, the implicit subjectivity in grading a varicocele on physical examination, and the failure to control for fertility potential of the female partner may account for the discrepant conclusions in the abovementioned studies. Nevertheless, opinion on the long-term impact of varicoceles remains divided.

Clinical and Laboratory Evaluation

Physical examination is the cornerstone of any varicocele evaluation and should be performed with the patient in both the supine and upright positions, with and without use of the Valsalva maneuver. Varicoceles are graded according to the Dubin and Amelar classification as grade I (palpable only during Valsalva), grade II (palpable without Valsalva), or grade III (visible without palpation) [23]. Assessment of testicular consistency and size is also important, as changes in these observations over time may be indicative of a progressive decline in testicular function due to the presence of varicoceles. However, the physical examination is limited by its inherent subjectivity, as well as the experience of the examiner. Additionally, results of the examination may be indeterminate in patients with a small scrotum, history of prior scrotal surgery, or obesity.

As a result, some clinicians have encouraged the use of color Doppler ultrasonography, using venous diameters between 2.5 and 3.5 mm, combined with reversal of venous blood flow during Valsalva, as being indicative of clinically significant varicoceles [24–26]. Although Doppler ultrasonography is more sensitive and specific for the diagnosis of varicoceles than physical examination alone, its use for varicocele evaluation has not been standardized, and its results are subject to operator experience and interpretation [24]. It is well established that the repair of subclinical varicoceles identified by ultrasonography does not improve clinical outcomes. Therefore, while ultrasonography is a valuable adjunctive tool for the evaluation of varicoceles in men with a difficult physical examination, its routine use is not recommended [6].

Indications for Varicocelectomy

Guidelines relating to varicoceles and infertility have been put forth by the American Urological Association (AUA) [6] and the American Society of Reproductive Medicine (ASRM) [7]. Both reports recommend varicocele repair for a clinically palpable varicocele with either documented infertility or one or more abnormal semen parameters, and in the setting of normal or potentially correctable female fertility. Varicocele repair is also recommended in individuals with palpable varicoceles and abnormal semen parameters who are not actively trying to conceive and in adolescents who have reduced ipsilateral testicular size in the setting of a palpable varicocele. In addition to abnormal semen parameters, varicoceles have been associated with abnormal sperm DNA quality, testicular hypotrophy, impaired testosterone production, and testicular pain. Several authors have advocated for varicocelectomy in these settings, especially given the possibility of a progressive effect of varicocele on testicular function.

Surgical Approaches to Varicocelectomy

Surgical options for varicocele repair include the traditional inguinal (Ivanissevich) or high retroperitoneal (Palomo) approaches, laparoscopic repair, and microsurgical repair via an inguinal or subinguinal incision. Complications of varicocelectomy include hydrocele formation, persistence or recurrence of the varicocele, and, rarely, testicular atrophy [3]. Although no specific recommendations exist as to the optimal surgical technique for varicocelectomy, the use of magnification to preserve lymphatics and testicular arteries is recommended. As such, microsurgical varicocelectomy is considered the gold standard technique for varicocelectomy in both adults and adolescents, due to lower postoperative recurrence and complication rates compared to other techniques [27, 28]. A recent meta-analysis also found microsurgical varicocelectomy to be associated with higher postoperative spontaneous pregnancy rates in infertile men with clinically palpable varicoceles [29].

Nonsurgical Approaches to Varicocelectomy

Percutaneous embolization and sclerotherapy is the primary nonsurgical option for varicocele repair. Sclerosants such as ethanol or sodium tetradecyl sulfate foam can permanently occlude the internal spermatic vein, resulting in a minimally invasive procedure, associated with little pain and rapid recovery [30]. As such, this approach has often been used in the pediatric population [31, 32]. Complications of varicocele embolization are uncommon and include pampiniform phlebitis and venous thromboembolism into the renal vein or pulmonary artery. Since this procedure avoids manipulation of lymphatic channels, there is no apparent risk of hydrocele formation. However, between 10 and 15 % of patients develop recurrent varicoceles following embolization, due to collateral vessels, including the external spermatic, gubernacular, and splanchnic veins [30]. Although some studies have reported improvement in one or more semen parameters following varicocele embolization [33, 34], no conclusive reports of a correlation between improvement in semen quality and pregnancy rate have been published to date.

Varicocele Repair and Testosterone Levels

Data from both human and animal studies demonstrates a negative impact of varicoceles on Leydig cell function [8–10, 35]. The available evidence is summarized in Table 11.1. Men with clinical varicoceles have been shown to have lower testosterone levels at every age when compared to a fertility proven control group of vasectomy reversal patients without varicoceles [17]. However, until recently, the impact of varicocele repair on serum testosterone levels was not well appreciated, due to a paucity of adequately sized comparative studies performed using standardized techniques of varicocele repair and standardized serum testosterone assays.

Emerging evidence demonstrates a beneficial effect of varicocelectomy on serum testosterone levels (Table 11.2). In a series of 200 patients who underwent microsurgical varicocelectomy, 70 % of patients experienced an increase in testosterone postoperatively by an average of 100 ng/dL [17]. The improvement in testosterone occurred regardless of patient age, laterality of varicocele, or varicocele grade. Similar results were reported by Hsiao et al. who retrospectively reviewed the records of 272 men who underwent microsurgical varicocelectomy [36]. Study subjects were stratified by age. Men with low baseline testosterone (defined as $T < 400$ ng/dL) experienced a mean increase of over 100 ng/dL following surgery, even in the fifth and sixth decades of life. Interestingly, men with normal baseline testosterone (defined as $T > 400$ ng/dl) showed no statistically significant rise in serum testosterone after varicocelectomy [36].

Subsequently, a prospective study of 200 infertile men with clinical varicoceles who underwent either microsurgical varicocelectomy or assisted reproductive technology (ART) procedures in equal numbers showed that testosterone increased by an average of 80 ng/dL following microsurgical varicocelectomy, resulting in normalization of total testosterone levels in 78 % of treated men versus 16 % of controls [37]. A smaller, but similar study by Zohdy et al. sought to study the impact of varicocele repair on serum testosterone levels and erectile function in men with infertility [38]. The authors compared serum testosterone levels in 103 infertile men who underwent varicocele repair to 38 infertile men who underwent treatment with ART and found that 75 % of hypogonadal men (defined as $T < 300$ ng/dL) in the varicocelectomy group had normalization of serum testosterone levels versus only 20 % in the ART group [38]. Interestingly, erectile function, assessed by the abbreviated International Index of Erectile Function (IIEF-5), was significantly improved in hypogonadal men following varicocelectomy.

Li et al. recently published a meta-analysis including these and other studies investigating the impact of varicocelectomy on serum testosterone levels. This meta-analysis of nine studies, spanning 1995–2011 and involving 814 patients,

Table 11.1 Varicoceles and serum testosterone

Reference	Study design	No. of patients	Summary of observations
Comhaire and Vermeulen [10]	Retrospective cohort	33 Men with varicoceles and 31 men with psychogenic sexual dysfunction	Significant inverse linear correlation between age and serum testosterone in men with varicoceles ($r = -0.56, p < 0.01$) compared to controls
Ando et al. [9]	Prospective cohort	108 Men with palpable varicoceles, 46 controls	Men with varicoceles had significantly lower mean serum testosterone levels than controls, 416 versus 487 ng/dL ($p < 0.01$)
Tanrikut et al. [17]	Nested case control	325 Men with palpable varicoceles, 510 controls	Men with varicoceles had significantly lower mean serum testosterone levels than controls, 416 versus 469 ng/dL ($p < 0.001$)
Luo et al. [35]	Randomized controlled animal study	20 Rats underwent surgery for creation of varicocele, 20 control rats underwent a sham operation	Intratesticular testosterone levels were significantly lower and Leydig cell apoptotic index was significantly higher in the varicocele group compared to controls ($p < 0.01$)

has showed an approximate 100 ng/dL increase in serum testosterone following varicocelectomy [39]. Unfortunately, however, the vast majority of the included studies were retrospective, and the only study to include a control group was not a randomized trial.

Based on the above data, several authors have suggested that varicocelectomy be considered as an option for the prevention and treatment of low serum testosterone, even in men with semen parameters in the normal range. Intuitively, the improvement in serum testosterone following varicocelectomy could obviate the need for exogenous testosterone supplementation in a subset of hypogonadal men. However, given the retrospective nature of the majority of available studies, the level of evidence to support this suggestion is low. Moreover, longitudinal data on the long-term maintenance of higher testosterone levels following varicocelectomy are not available. Further randomized controlled studies are needed to better define the impact of varicocele repair on serum testosterone levels.

Table 11.2 Varicocele repair and serum testosterone

Reference	Study design	Patient population	Type of repair	Outcome
Tanrikut et al. [17]	Retrospective cohort	200 Men with palpable varicoceles	Microsurgical subinguinal varicocelectomy	Mean testosterone levels significantly increased after varicocelectomy from 358 to 454 ng/dL ($p < 0.001$)
Hsiao et al. [36]	Retrospective cohort	106 Men with palpable varicoceles	Microsurgical subinguinal varicocelectomy	Patients with a baseline testosterone $\leq$400 ng/dL ($n = 76$) had a mean increase of $\geq$110 ng/dl after varicocelectomy ($p < 0.001$)
Sathya Srini et al. [37]	Prospective cohort	200 Infertile men with palpable varicoceles who underwent either varicocelectomy ($n = 100$) or assisted reproduction ($n = 100$)	Microsurgical subinguinal varicocelectomy	Mean testosterone levels significantly increased in the varicocelectomy group, 164 versus 246 ng/dL ($p < 0.001$), but not the assisted reproduction group
Zohdy et al. [38]	Prospective cohort	141 Men with palpable varicoceles, who underwent either varicocelectomy ($n = 103$) or assisted reproduction ($n = 38$)	Microsurgical subinguinal varicocelectomy	Mean testosterone levels significantly increased in the varicocelectomy group, 379 versus 450 ng/dL ($p < 0.0001$), but not the assisted reproduction group
Li et al. [39]	Meta-analysis	9 Studies, including 814 patients	Microsurgical and non-microsurgical inguinal and subinguinal varicocelectomy, retroperitoneal varicocelectomy, and sclerotherapy	Mean testosterone levels significantly increased after varicocele repair by an average of 97.5 ng/dL ($p = 0.0004$)

Summary

The relationship between varicoceles and impaired Leydig cell function is long standing. Several studies have investigated differences in serum testosterone levels before and after varicocele repair as a marker of Leydig cell function. Data from these studies suggests that the presence of varicoceles is associated with decreased serum testosterone in a subset of men and that varicocelectomy is associated with variable improvement in serum testosterone in some of these cases. However, the majority of studies on this topic are retrospective in nature. Therefore, randomized controlled studies are certainly needed to better study these associations and definitively demonstrate the impact of varicocele repair on serum testosterone levels.

References

1. Saypol DC, Howards SS, Turner TT, Miller Jr ED. Influence of surgically induced varicocele on testicular blood flow, temperature, and histology in adult rats and dogs. J Clin Invest. 1981;68(1):39–45. Comparative Study Research Support, U.S. Gov't, P.H.S.
2. World Health Organization. The influence of varicocele on parameters of fertility in a large group of men presenting to infertility clinics. Fertil Steril. 1992;57(6):1289–93. Comparative Study Research Support, Non-U.S. Gov't.
3. Goldstein M. Surgical management of male infertility. In: Wein A, Kavoussi LR, Novick AC, Partin AW, Peters CA, editors. Campbell-Walsh urology. Tenthth ed. Philadelphia: Elsevier Saunders; 2012. p. 648–87.
4. Tulloch WS. Varicocele in subfertility; results of treatment. Br Med J. 1955;2(4935):356–8.
5. Kroese AC, de Lange NM, Collins J, Evers JL. Surgery or embolization for varicoceles in subfertile men. Cochrane Database Syst Rev. 2012;10:CD000479. Meta-Analysis Review.
6. AUA. Report on varicocele and infertility: an AUA Best Practice Policy and ASRM Practice Committee Report. 2001.
7. ASRM. Report on varicocele and infertility. Fertil Steril. 2008;90 Suppl 5:S247–9. Review.
8. Schlegel PN, Goldstein M. Alternate indications for varicocele repair: non-obstructive azoospermia, pain, androgen deficiency and progressive testicular dysfunction. Fertil Steril. 2011;96(6):1288–93. Review.
9. Ando S, Giacchetto C, Colpi G, Beraldi E, Panno ML, Lombardi A, et al. Physiopathologic aspects of Leydig cell function in varicocele patients. J Androl. 1984;5(3):163–70.
10. Comhaire F, Vermeulen A. Plasma testosterone in patients with varicocele and sexual inadequacy. J Clin Endocrinol Metab. 1975;40(5):824–9.
11. Pirke KM, Vogt HJ, Sintermann R, Spyra B. Testosterone in peripheral plasma, spermatic vein and in testicular tissue under basal conditions and after HCG-stimulation in patients with varicocele. Andrologia. 1983;15(6):637–41.
12. Barthold JS. Abnormalities of the testes and scrotum and their surgical management. In: Wein A, Kavoussi LR, Növick AC, Partin AW, Peters CA, editors. Campbell-Walsh urology. Tenthth ed. Philadelphia, PA: Saunders Elsevier; 2012.
13. Graif M, Hauser R, Hirshebein A, Botchan A, Kessler A, Yabetz H. Varicocele and the testicular-renal venous route: hemodynamic Doppler sonographic investigation. J Ultrasound Med. 2000;19(9):627–31.

14. Diamond DA, Zurakowski D, Bauer SB, Borer JG, Peters CA, Cilento Jr BG, et al. Relationship of varicocele grade and testicular hypotrophy to semen parameters in adolescents. J Urol. 2007;178(4 Pt 2):1584–8.
15. Jarow JP. Effects of varicocele on male fertility. Hum Reprod Update. 2001;7(1):59–64. Review.
16. Zini A, Dohle G. Are varicoceles associated with increased deoxyribonucleic acid fragmentation? Fertil Steril. 2011;96(6):1283–7. Review.
17. Tanrikut C, Goldstein M, Rosoff JS, Lee RK, Nelson CJ, Mulhall JP. Varicocele as a risk factor for androgen deficiency and effect of repair. BJU Int. 2011;108(9):1480–4. Research Support, Non-U.S. Gov't.
18. Gorelick JI, Goldstein M. Loss of fertility in men with varicocele. Fertil Steril. 1993;59 (3):613–6.
19. Witt MA, Lipshultz LI. Varicocele: a progressive or static lesion? Urology. 1993;42(5):541–3.
20. Chehval MJ, Purcell MH. Deterioration of semen parameters over time in men with untreated varicocele: evidence of progressive testicular damage. Fertil Steril. 1992;57(1):174–7.
21. Jarow JP, Coburn M, Sigman M. Incidence of varicoceles in men with primary and secondary infertility. Urology. 1996;47(1):73–6.
22. Lund L, Larsen SB. A follow-up study of semen quality and fertility in men with varicocele testis and in control subjects. Br J Urol. 1998;82(5):682–6. Clinical Trial Controlled Clinical Trial Research Support, Non-U.S. Gov't.
23. Dubin L, Amelar RD. Varicocele size and results of varicocelectomy in selected subfertile men with varicocele. Fertil Steril. 1970;21(8):606–9.
24. Stahl P, Schlegel PN. Standardization and documentation of varicocele evaluation. Curr Opin Urol. 2011;21(6):500–5. Review.
25. Pilatz A, Altinkilic B, Kohler E, Marconi M, Weidner W. Color Doppler ultrasound imaging in varicoceles: is the venous diameter sufficient for predicting clinical and subclinical varicocele? World J Urol. 2011;29(5):645–50.
26. Hoekstra T, Witt MA. The correlation of internal spermatic vein palpability with ultrasonographic diameter and reversal of venous flow. J Urol. 1995;153(1):82–4.
27. Mirilas P, Mentessidou A. Microsurgical subinguinal varicocelectomy in children, adolescents, and adults: surgical anatomy and anatomically justified technique. J Androl. 2012;33 (3):338–49.
28. Mehta A, Goldstein M. Microsurgical varicocelectomy: a review. Asian J Androl. 2013;15 (1):56–60.
29. Cayan S, Shavakhabov S, Kadioglu A. Treatment of palpable varicocele in infertile men: a meta-analysis to define the best technique. J Androl. 2009;30(1):33–40. Meta-Analysis Review.
30. Lord DJ, Burrows PE. Pediatric varicocele embolization. Tech Vasc Interv Radiol. 2003;6 (4):169–75. Review.
31. Storm DW, Hogan MJ, Jayanthi VR. Initial experience with percutaneous selective embolization: a truly minimally invasive treatment of the adolescent varicocele with no risk of hydrocele development. J Pediatr Urol. 2010;6(6):567–71.
32. Alqahtani A, Yazbeck S, Dubois J, Garel L. Percutaneous embolization of varicocele in children: a Canadian experience. J Pediatr Surg. 2002;37(5):783–5.
33. Ferguson JM, Gillespie IN, Chalmers N, Elton RA, Hargreave TB. Percutaneous varicocele embolization in the treatment of infertility. Br J Radiol. 1995;68(811):700–3.
34. Nabi G, Asterlings S, Greene DR, Marsh RL. Percutaneous embolization of varicoceles: outcomes and correlation of semen improvement with pregnancy. Urology. 2004;63(2):359–63. Comparative Study Evaluation Studies Review.
35. Luo DY, Yang G, Liu JJ, Yang YR, Dong Q. Effects of varicocele on testosterone, apoptosis and expression of StAR mRNA in rat Leydig cells. Asian J Androl. 2011;13(2):287–91.
36. Hsiao W, Rosoff JS, Pale JR, Greenwood EA, Goldstein M. Older age is associated with similar improvements in semen parameters and testosterone after subinguinal microsurgical

varicocelectomy. J Urol. 2011;185(2):620–5. Comparative Study Research Support, Non-U.S. Gov't.

37. Sathya Srini V, Belur Veerachari S. Does varicocelectomy improve gonadal function in men with hypogonadism and infertility? Analysis of a prospective study. Int J Endocrinol. 2011;2011:916380.
38. Zohdy W, Ghazi S, Arafa M. Impact of varicocelectomy on gonadal and erectile functions in men with hypogonadism and infertility. J Sex Med. 2011;8(3):885–93.
39. Li F, Yue H, Yamaguchi K, Okada K, Matsushita K, Ando M, et al. Effect of surgical repair on testosterone production in infertile men with varicocele: a meta-analysis. Int J Urol. 2012;19 (2):149–54.

Chapter 12
Nutraceuticals for Fertility and Erectile Health: A Brief Overview of What Works and What Is Worthless

Mark A. Moyad

Introduction: Lifestyle Changes Matter

Clinicians should not dismiss the importance of lifestyle changes on overall health and male fertility and sexual function. Most heart unhealthy behaviors also negatively impact almost all other areas of men's health [1], including fertility and erectile health [2, 3]. Thus, improving or encouraging heart healthy changes in patients may improve overall mental and physical health [4], which could provide the optimum scenario to enhance any specific conventional medical options.

Heart healthy recommendations are also arguably the most logical and practical suggestions that simultaneously can also improve quality and perhaps quantity of life for patients across a broad spectrum of specialties [5]. It should be remembered and reiterated that cardiovascular disease (CVD) is the number 1 overall cause of mortality in the USA and in other industrialized countries [6, 7]. CVD is currently the number 1 cause of death worldwide, and is the number 1 cause of death in virtually every region of the world. Cancer is the second leading cause of death in the USA and in most developed countries, and is expected to potentially mirror the number of deaths from CVD in the next several years in various regions of the world.

If cancer becomes the primary cause of mortality, the majority of what is known concerning lifestyle and dietary change for CVD prevention directly appears to apply to cancer prevention [2, 5]. Heart healthy changes are tantamount to overall urologic health improvements regardless of the part of the human anatomy that is receiving focus, including the bladder, kidney, penis, testicles, or prostate. Heart healthy changes need to be advocated in urology clinics because it places probability and the research into perspective.

M.A. Moyad (✉)
Department of Urology, University of Michigan, 1500 E. Medical Center Drive, Ann Arbor, MI 48109, USA
e-mail: moyad@med.umich.edu

J.P. Mulhall and W. Hsiao (eds.), *Men's Sexual Health and Fertility*,
DOI 10.1007/978-1-4939-0425-9_12,

If multiple lifestyle changes, or if achieving numerous healthy parameters over time appears to be strongly correlated with some of the largest improvements in health then this theory should have arguably been well tested. And it has been tested over the years and the results are profound and exemplary. For example, data from the National Health and Nutrition Examination Survey (NHANES) was utilized that included 44,959 US adults 20 years of age or older [8]. Mean age was 46–47 years and approximately half of the participants were women. Median follow-up was 14.5 years. A total of only 1–2 % of the participants met all seven of the health parameters. There was a remarkable 51 % reduction in all-cause mortality, 76 % reduction in cardiovascular mortality, and 70 % reduction in ischemic heart disease (IHD) mortality for participants meeting six or more metrics compared to one or fewer. Achieving a higher number of cardiovascular health parameters also appeared to be correlated with a lower risk for all-cancer mortality. These seven basic goals/parameters only achieved by 1–2 % of Americans are listed in Table 12.1.

Reviewing the impact of obesity, high cholesterol, blood pressure and glucose, lack of exercise, improper diet, tobacco use and other potential overall and specific health contributors such as stress and depression, which individually or combined can increase oxidative stress all have some minor or major impact on fertility and erectile health. This is arguably the most holistic approach to changing patient lives and improving overall outcomes [2, 3, 9, 10]. In other words, it is the ultimate two for one beneficial impact on your patients.

Applying comprehensive heart healthy lifestyle data to determine its true objective efficacy in urologic health may not appear to be simple, but in reality it is not difficult. When discussed with patients the observations from this research is quite profound throughout urology. For example, a unique 2-year randomized trial from Italy of vigorous aerobic exercise and diet to improve erectile dysfunction (ED) should have received more clinical attention [11, 12]. It still should change the way health care professionals treat men with ED. A total of 110 obese men (body mass index or BMI of 36–37 = morbidly obese) with ED, waist-to-hip ratio (WHR) of 1.01–1.02, age 43 years, erectile dysfunction score 13–14 out of 25 (IIEF), and without diabetes, high cholesterol, or hypertension were included. A total of 55 men were randomized to an aggressive intervention group that involved caloric restriction and increased physical activity via personalized dietary counseling (Mediterranean-style diet), and regular appointments with a personal trainer. Another group of 55 men were in the control group and were given general educational information about exercise and healthy food choices. After 2 years, the BMI significantly decreased on average from 36.9 to 31.2 in the intervention group, and serum levels of interleukin-6 and C-reactive protein also decreased significantly. The average physical activity level increased significantly from 48 to 195 min per week in the intervention group, and the mean erectile function score increased significantly from 13.9 to 17. A total of 17 men in the intervention group actually reported an erectile score of 22 or higher (normal function). Several changes were independently and significantly correlated with a higher rate of improved erections including a lower BMI or BMI reduction, increased physical

Table 12.1 Seven steps for improved overall, reproductive, and erectile health that only 1–2 % of the US population has been able to achieve

1. Avoiding all tobacco products
2. BMI 25 or less
3. Being physically active almost every day of the week
4. Overall diet that is heart healthy (fruits/veggies/fiber/fish...)
5. Total cholesterol equal to or less than 200 mg/dl[a]
6. Blood pressure equal to or less than 120/80
7. Fasting blood glucose less than 100 mg/dl

[a]An exception is the fact that an unusually high HDL could lead to high total cholesterol, regardless of the fact that an LDL less than 100 mg/dl is another target in these individuals

activity, and a lower C-reactive protein levels. Again, approximately 33 % of the men in this study with E.D. regained normal erectile function after 2 years of following healthy behaviors primarily from exercise, weight reduction, caloric control, and healthy dietary changes. Although a major limitation of this trial was the lack of analysis on psychological factors and social intervention, these lifestyle changes could have improved mood, self-esteem, and reduced depression, and this could have also been a reason for improved erectile function. Still, the combined healthy changes in the intervention group that occurred after 2 years were notable, diverse, and included the following heart healthy and urologic healthy parameters:

- Total caloric reduction of −390 cal per day (2,340–1,950)
- Complex carbohydrate increase and simple sugar reduction
- Fiber consumption increased by 10 g a day (15–25)
- Protein consumption increased significantly (13–16 % of caloric intake)
- No change in the overall percentage of fat in the diet (30 % of calories), but a reduction in saturated fat (14–9 %) and an increased intake in monounsaturated fat (9–14 %)
- Ratios of omega-6 to omega-3 fatty acids was reduced by half (12–6)
- Cholesterol was reduced from dietary sources by 84 mg per day (360–276)
- Exercise time (mainly walking) increased from about 7 min per day to almost 30 min per day
- Average weight loss was 33 lb (226.6–193.6)
- Average BMI decreased by almost 6 points (36.9–31.2)
- WHR decreased by 0.09 (1.02–0.93)
- Erectile function scores increased by 3 points (13.9–17 points)
- Systolic (127–124 mmHg) and diastolic (86–82 mmHg) blood pressure decreased by 3–4 points
- Total cholesterol decreased by 11 mg/dl (213–202), but HDL (good cholesterol) increased by 9 points (39–48 mg/dl)
- Triglycerides decreased by 19 mg/dl (169–150)
- Glucose decreased by 8 mg/dl (103–95) and insulin level also decreased by 7 points (21–14 μU/ml)

- C-reactive protein (CRP) was reduced by1.4 mg/L (3.3–1.9)
- Interleukin 6 was reduced by 1.4 pg/ml (4.5–3.1)
- Interleukin-8 (IL-8, another inflammatory marker) was reduced by 1.2 pg/ml (5.3–4.1)

Additionally, how many more laboratory, cross-sectional, or prospective studies are needed in the area of heart healthy interventions and the potential for improved fertility [13–15], before these recommendations become a part of clinical urologic guidelines? Heart health is tantamount to improved probability of male fertility and erectile health, and this is the theme of this chapter, which includes primarily nutraceutical recommendations.

In addition, clinicians need to keep in mind that lifestyle changes can immediately increase nutrient levels before supplementation with an antioxidant pill is recommended because obesity, substance abuse, insulin resistance, and other heart unhealthy changes accelerate the depletion or dilution of a variety of antioxidants in the serum not only in adults but also in adolescents [2, 16, 17]. For example, there is plenty of discourse of vitamin D supplementation for overall health but there appears to be little discourse on weight loss as a "natural" way to significantly increase serum vitamin D levels without additional supplementation. Lifestyle changes and minimal supplement dosages are more logical, practical, safe, and heart healthy compared to high doses of antioxidants from pills and no lifestyle alterations. In other words, patients that adhere to heart healthy parameters have the highest chance of success in my opinion in combination with conventional medicine as needed. In other words, lifestyle matters!

Nutraceuticals/Dietary Supplements: Fertility

There is a consistent suggestion that up to 80 % of male factor subfertility cases are believed to be the result of "oxidative stress" [18]. Perhaps some of the strongest evidence to espouse the use of dietary supplements for male infertility has been published. A Cochrane Systematic review was arguably one of the most extensive ever published in male fertility and dietary supplements, as it reviewed 34 randomized clinical trials with 2,876 couples in total [19]. Studies used in this analysis were for couples undergoing assisted reproduction technologies (ART), for example in vitro fertilization (IVF), intrauterine insemination (IUI), or intracyclic sperm injection (ICSI). The inclusion criteria were randomized controlled trials that included men as part of a couple with unexplained subfertility or subfertility that were using ART with their own gametes. Trials were excluded in there were non-randomized, included men taking any other fertility-enhancing medications, or men that had used chemotherapy treatment. The primary outcome was the live birth rate per couple randomized. And there were multiple secondary outcomes:

- Pregnancy rate per couple
- Miscarriage rate per couple or spontaneous abortion

- Stillbirth rate per couple
- Level of sperm DNA damage after treatment
- Sperm concentration and sperm motility
- Adverse effects associated with dietary supplements and withdrawals

The overall findings continue to surprise a number of health care professionals and patients, in my opinion, by concluding that antioxidant supplementation in males appears to have a positive role in improving the outcomes of live birth and pregnancy rates in couples participating in ART [19]. In fact, for live births the p-value was 0.0008 and for pregnancy rates it was $p < 0.00001$. Critics of this analysis on "live births" will arguably point toward the small number of such events, 20 live births that occurred from a total of 214 couples in only three studies that was used in this part of the analysis, or the "pregnancy rates," which actually was derived from 96 pregnancies in 15 trials that included 964 couples. However, it is still interesting that this is a viable minimal or moderate option for some men given the low cost of most "antioxidants" utilized in these studies. Additionally, acute side effects were similar to a placebo with no serious adverse events reported in any trial.

The common question that will result from this or any other positive analysis for male fertility and antioxidants is which specific nutraceuticals and at what dosage and frequency? Interestingly, this Cochrane review could not identify one specific antioxidant or combination product from these trials [5], so readers and patients are left with multiple questions. Thus, a summary of antioxidant supplements used in past well-designed placebo-controlled trials is needed with an overall cost, safety, and health perspective to determine which products should be recommended and perhaps avoided by patients. This was a primary weakness of the Cochrane review and other reviews in male fertility [19], which is the overall lack of specific recommendations based on overall safety and efficacy of these agents long-term for overall health and fertility maintenance. This chapter will attempt to provide clarity on this issue of which supplements to recommend or avoid based on heart healthy and overall heath sensitivity and recommendations. And the specific end-points of past studies matter so that clinicians need to constantly ask themselves in which of the following areas does this supplement impact:

- Oxidative stress reduction/markers
- Total Sperm Number
- Sperm concentration
- Sperm morphology
- Sperm motility (% motility and/or forward progression)
- Pregnancy rate
- Live births
- Short and long-term safety
- Miscellaneous (ejaculate volume, pH, viscosity, sperm agglutination, other parameters...)

The impact on pregnancy and live birth rates along with overall safety are the more important variables and are in need of more results in these areas for all of the dietary supplements mentioned in this chapter. And it is also of interest that if some supplements may improve male infertility when dealing with ART then it may impact those with motility issues (asthenospermia) or idiopathic oligoasthenoteratozoospermia (OAT) because of the overlap in those that use ART and men with this condition.

First Do No Harm Specific Supplementation for Infertility

Coenzyme Q10 (CoQ10, Also Known as "Ubiquinone")

CoQ10 appears to be a safe dietary supplement that requires a low and realistic dose for male fertility preservation. CoQ10 (also known as "ubiquinone") supplements have a consistent overall safety profile, and actually have some clinical data to suggest that they may reduce blood pressure, but primarily in those with some form of hypertension, and these supplements might have some role in reducing myalgia from statin therapy [20, 21], but these results have been inconsistent yet still at least proven to be safe at a variety of dosages [22]. The role of CoQ10 in the respiratory pathway as a method to improve energy production and reduce oxidative stress has been well known in basic human physiology. It is for this reason that there is interest in utilizing this dietary supplement for oxidative stress reduction.

Seminal fluid also contains a measurable quantity of CoQ10 that appear to be correlated with sperm count and motility. Patients with idiopathic asthenozoospermia may benefit in terms of spermatozoa motility when consuming 200 mg per day of CoQ10 for 6 months [23]. Another study of 212 infertile men taking 300 mg over 26-weeks found significant improvements in multiple parameters including sperm density, motility, and acrosome reaction [24]. Serum levels of FSH and LH were significantly reduced. However, in a randomized trial of men with oligoasthenoteratozoospermia at a dosage of 200 mg per day compared to placebo, it appeared to reduce markers of oxidative stress but did not demonstrate significant impacts on sperm concentration, motility, and morphology [25].

CoQ10 can be a costly nutraceutical so patients should compare prices from multiple commercial resources to determine the most cost effective product. I have not observed profound differences in clinical effects with low cost compared to high cost CoQ10 products. CoQ10 appears to be a heart healthy or safe supplement [20], except it does have the rare potential to reduce the impact of warfarin because of vitamin K-like properties [26], but ironically its minimal anti-platelet effects may increase bleeding when combined with aspirin or clopidogrel. Regardless, it is a supplement that could be encouraged for fertility improvement in most men at a dosage of 200–300 mg per day for a trial period of 3–6 months.

The biggest reservation about CoQ10 is not adverse effects, or locating a low cost product, but its true efficacy over time. This is due to the initial promise and then slight to moderate disappointment in this product in other areas of medicine. For example, the impact on statin induced myalgia reduction was interesting initially [21], but is not an absolute solution today [22], and this is also true for this product in terms of its antihypertensive [27] and Parkinson's disease research [28]. In other words, the excitement and hype on this supplement was initially tremendous, but more rigorous trials in other areas of medicine have proven adequate consistent safety but efficacy was disappointing. For example, the National Institute of Neurological Disorders and Stroke (NINDS) stopped the QE3 phase 3 study of CoQ10 for the treatment of early stage Parkinson's disease, acting on the recommendation of the study's safety board [28]. An interim analysis showed minimal likelihood of benefit at dosages of 1,200 and 2,400 mg per day for up to 16 months. All subjects also received vitamin E at a dosage of 1,200 IU per day. The study enrolled 600 patients at 67 clinical trial sites and the reason CoQ10 was utilized was due to the close association of oxidative stress and mitochondrial dysfunction as contributors to Parkinson's disease and some past positive data from a Cochrane Database of Systematic Review of four randomized past trials [29], so CoQ10 became a logical treatment choice. This is somewhat similar to the theory and origins of utilizing CoQ10 to improve fertility parameters [30]. Still, the benefit outweighs the risk, so it should be a part of the current dietary supplement discussion for men with subfertility.

L-Carnitine

The story of L-carnitine for male fertility arguably mirrors that for CoQ10 in terms of initial excitement, safety and then some controversy over the lack of impact in other areas of medicine. L-Carnitine is a potential amino acid dietary supplement for male fertility, but large dosages may be needed, and it is not a low cost product. L-Carnitine transports fatty acids from the cytosol to the mitochondria for energy production in each cell of the body [31], which is arguably why there has always been interest in this compound. Humans can produce carnitine de novo in the liver from lysine and methionine (25 %), but dietary intake is the primary source of carnitine (75 %). Foods high in carnitine include dairy and meat and a plant-based diet is in general a poor source of carnitine. Excretion of carnitine occurs from the kidneys, but reabsorption is also efficient so that vegans are still able to maintain close to normal blood levels of this amino acid despite only 10 % or less the consumption of carnitine compared to omnivores.

L-Carnitine had preliminary research that it may slightly reduce fatigue in some cancer patients in higher dosages, but a phase 3 trial demonstrated 2,000 mg per day worked no better than placebo for this specific situation over a 4-week testing period [32]. Even subset analysis revealed that those individuals that had lower blood levels of carnitine at baseline experienced no benefit. The future of L-carnitine in terms of energy production for patients with fatigue is now questionable, but there is still adequate data in other areas of medicine, for example, the ability of this product to increase the body weight or nutritional status of high-risk cachetic patients [33], improve peripheral artery disease [34], and the impact of this supplement on male fertility—primarily motility [31].

It is of interest that vitamin C (ascorbic acid) is needed to synthesize carnitine in the human body [31]. The highest concentration of carnitine apart from supplements occurs in red meat and dairy products so vegetarians that are trying to maintain fertility would potentially be better candidates for this supplement. There are several minimally different forms of L-carnitine available for purchase utilized in clinical trials including L-carnitine, acetyl-L-carnitine (ALC), and propionyl-L-carnitine (PLC). These other types of L-carnitine have been tested because L-carnitine itself tends to be unstable. Yet these other forms of L-carnitine do not necessarily have better fertility data, especially when compared to each other at 3,000 mg per day [35], and are more costly for the patient. Some clinical trials have suggested that the combination of these supplements may improve motility [36], but again this is not my interpretation from these same studies with similar authors [36, 37]. Thus, multiple clinical trials have demonstrated the ability of L-carnitine, or other forms of carnitine to improve primarily sperm motility and potentially pregnancy rates [35–43]. Yet there has been inconsistent or minimal evidence that it can impact sperm concentration and morphology. A small US randomized, double-blind placebo-controlled study in men with idiopathic asthenospermia has challenged the potentially positive results with carnitine [44]. Male patients with sperm motility of 10–50 % were utilized and over 24 weeks 2,000 mg of L-carnitine and 1,000 mg of L-acetyl-carnitine per day were ingested compared to placebo ($n = 12$ vs. $n = 9$). No significant differences in motility or total motile sperm counts occurred at 12 or 24 weeks. These researchers called into question the clinical significance of the effect of L-carnitine for infertile men, but in terms of objectivity their trial was well executed but the small number of participants was a methodological limitation. They also reviewed past studies and suggested several methodology issues such as exclusion of some patients from final analysis as an issue [37], and also found carnitine to cause statistical significance in the past, but the clinical significance of the results are questionable. Another concern is lack of improvement in seminal plasma or sperm carnitine levels following supplementation [37, 44], which could be the result of adequate baseline levels or simply no ability to improve these concentrations with these supplements [44]. After this critical publication a systematic review of nine clinical trials was published by independent researchers on the impact of L-carnitine for male infertility [45], and thus far a significant improvement in pregnancy rates ($p < 0.0001$), total and forward sperm motility ($p = 0.04$), and atypical sperms cell ($p < 0.00001$), but no impact was found for sperm concentration or semen volume. Therefore, again clinicians and patients are left to decide on this controversial supplement. L-Carnitine causes an unpredictable change or minimal to moderate increase in sperm motility without a consistent change in sperm morphology and concentration or increase in seminal plasma carnitine levels, but there is a potential increase in pregnancy without any current consistent safety issues. Is this adequate to endorse the utilization of high doses of carnitine for male infertility? It should not be endorsed for preventive measures to preserve fertility, but its other features (especially safety) make it a controversial option at least.

Adverse events using L-carnitine or serious drug interactions have not been identified. Yet a recent concern over L-carnitine utilization by potentially heart disease producing flora received attention [46], but so did a meta-analysis demonstrating a lower risk of cardiovascular events with L-carnitine from secondary prevention studies [47]. Another recent phase 3 trial in cancer to reduce chemotherapy induced neuropathy actually found an increase in neuropathy with this supplement at 3,000 mg per day [48]. Therefore, the controversy of whether or not this supplement could be beneficial will continue. I am not that concerned about toxicity in healthy patients but similar to CoQ10 the question of whether or not it can improve fertility parameters is open.

Doses of 2–4 g (2,000–4,000 mg per day, divided doses two to three times a day) on average have been used in clinical trials. L-Carnitine or acetyl-L-carnitine or a combination of both was used in these past studies. There was no commentary as to whether L-carnitine was ingested with or without a meal so it seems there is flexibility in regard to this issue.

Omega-3 Fatty Acids

Omega-3 supplements appear to also mirror the previous description with CoQ10 and carnitine due to the initial hype and now the lack of efficacy in other prominent areas of medicine. Additionally, omega-3 supplements simply lack sufficient clinical data in infertility to be recommended at this time. Therefore, recommending dietary sources of omega-3 compounds containing high quantities of EPA and DHA (principal marine sources of omega-3) should be encouraged in most individuals but not individual supplementation. There are numerous marine or fish sources that contain high levels of omega-3 fatty acids, vitamin D, and protein including salmon, tuna, sardines, and a variety of other baked, broiled, raw, but not fried fish are potentially beneficial [49]. Variety should be encouraged to increase compliance and exposure. The benefit of fish consumption to potentially reduce CVD is encouraging from past studies [50] or utilizing fish oil consumption in patients with a history of heart disease has good safety and some positive data [51, 52]. Still, the overall and most up to date clinical trial data with fish oil supplementation on primary endpoints in cardiovascular medicine has been minimal to controversial and more recently discouraging [53], and in otherwise healthy individuals it is not currently espoused [54]. In fact, during the submission of this chapter, arguably the most rigorous primary prevention trial in cardiovascular medicine thus far found no safety issues, but no impact on primary or secondary endpoints with 1,000 mg per day of omega-3 supplementation in a randomized trial of over 12,500 patients and a median follow-up of 5 years [55]. And in arguably the longest and most methodologically rigorous clinical trials of omega-3 supplements to reduce the progression of macular degeneration (AREDS2 trial), no benefit was observed with 1,000 mg per day of fish oil with a median follow-up of 5 years [56]. Thus, fish oils supplements should probably be reserved for patients with high triglycerides [49], where they are FDA approved for this purpose.

The data on fish oil for male subfertility is minimal and controversial because of insufficient data. For example, a randomized trial of DHA at 400 or 800 mg per day compared to placebo over 3 months for 28 asthenozoospermic (50 % or less motility) men appeared to increase serum and potentially seminal plasma DHA levels, but without impacting DHA into the spermatozoa phospholipid, which may have explained why it did not impact sperm motility compared to placebo [57]. A later trial of men with idiopathic oligoasthenoteratospermia (OAT) randomized to 1,840 mg of total omega-3 (EPA and DHA) product compared to placebo over 32 weeks found a significant increase in sperm count, concentration, morphology, and motility, which may have been associated with the reductions in markers of oxidative stress in men with low omega-3 fatty acid levels [58]. Several cases of reflux, itching and diarrhea occurred in the omega-3 group, which are known rare side effects of these supplements [49]. Again, until more research is conducted taking one to two omega-3 supplements that equates to 1,000–1,840 mg of EPA and DHA daily could be of some benefit, but this is speculative based on this one clinical trial.

Regardless, dietary sources of healthy fish can be encouraged. Mercury concentrations in specific fish have been reported by the Food and Drug Administration (FDA) and in the overall medical literature, but the preliminary data is controversial and it is not known at this time what kind of clinical impact these mercury levels may have on the individual [49]. Four types of larger predatory fish have been most concerning because these fish (king mackerel, shark, swordfish, and tilefish) have the ability to retain greater amounts of methyl-mercury. Moderate consumption (two to three times per week) of most fish should have minimal impact on overall human mercury serum levels, but more ongoing research in this area should soon provide better clarity. The positive impact of consuming fish seems to outweigh the negative impact in the majority of individuals with the exception of women considering pregnancy or who are pregnant. Table 12.2 is a summary of a variety of fish that have consistently demonstrated low levels of mercury, and this table should also teach patients that a variety of fish and shellfish are healthy [49]. It should be kept in mind that approximately two servings per week of fatty oily low mercury fish is the equivalent to approximately ingesting one 250–500 mg fish oil pill per day. Clinicians that still desire to recommend high-dosages of fish oil supplements must keep in mind that these supplements could increase the risk of internal bleeding at higher dosages and especially in combination with other blood thinners. Although the risk of bleeding events is extremely rare, it has been observed in some clinical trials of healthy individuals and in combination with statins at a dosage of only 1,800 mg per day [52].

It is interesting that low cost small and short lived fish such as anchovies and sardines are low in mercury, and have some of the highest levels of omega-3 oils,

Table 12.2 Seafood with some omega-3 fatty acids demonstrating minimal levels of mercury

Anchovies
Catfish
Cod
Crab
Flounder/sole
Haddock
Herring
Lobster
Mahi-mahi
Ocean perch
Oysters
Rainbow trout
Salmon (farmed and wild)
Sardines
Scallops
Shrimp
Spiny lobster
Tilapia
Trout (farmed)
White fish (Great Lakes)

and are used primarily more than any other fish in the manufacturing of fish oil pills to be utilized by the public and in many clinical trials [49]. Patients that cannot eat fish or do not want to utilize fish oil because of an allergy or a personal belief could be recommended algae based omega-3 oils or regularly consume the largest plant based source of omega-3 fatty acids which are found in plant oils (canola and soy), flaxseed, and chia seed.

*Tonkat Ali (*Eurycoma longifolia*)*

This is an extract derived from a plant or a common shrub found along the slopes of hilly areas in the Malaysian rainforest. It has preliminary human data that shows it could improve various aspects of male health including sex drive, increase testosterone in men with age-related androgen deficiency, and especially improve sperm quality and quantity at 200–300 mg a day [59–61].

Multiple laboratory studies have shown an ability of this herbal product to potentially improve male fertility status [62–65], and there is a history of using this product in Malaysia and other nearby locations to enhance fertility and male sexual health. An open label study involved 75 men with idiopathic infertility that utilized the supplement at 200 mg daily for at least the first 3 months [61]. Significant improvement in all semen parameters occurred and 11 (14.7 %) spontaneous pregnancies occurred. However, multiple methodological issues still need to be resolved in a placebo-controlled trial. For example, the authors claims that 350 men started the trial and only 75 completed one full cycle of supplementation (3 months) and fulfilled the inclusion criteria, but only 17 men completed all 9 months of supplementation, which is an concerning exclusion and/or non-compliance rate that needs further investigation. The authors also point toward the possibility of a "bioactive peptide" that can increase testosterone levels in animals and humans, and may reduce oxidative stress.

The product that has the most research and only one with real clinical data is the standardized water-soluble extract (Physta) of *Eurycoma longifolia* root from the company Biotropics Malaysia Berhad, Kuala Lumpur, Malaysia. The company has also financially supported most of these studies. Their proprietary standardized water-soluble extract from the root of the plant and other Tongkat Ali studies show that this root has multiple diverse ingredients such as [59–66]:

- Tannins
- High-molecular-weight polysaccharides
- Glycoproteins mucopolysaccharides
- Quassinoid alkaloids
- Amino acid isoleucine
- Calcium, magnesium, and potassium

It is theorized to also benefit in the area of male health via pro-hormone effect or DHEA mimic (yet DHEA supplementation has not been adequately researched for its impact on male fertility), or perhaps it is acting more like a diverse multivitamin for men to increase energy levels and slightly enhancing testosterone production in men and women via SHBG reduction or via some unrecognized pathway [67]. It could be that this product is no better than a really low cost source or another supplement of Tongkat Ali, but the problem is that other brands or just generic Tongkat Ali does not have adequate clinical trials or quality control testing (for lead, arsenic…). Therefore, Tongkat Ali does not have enough clinical evidence to recommend its use in men with idiopathic infertility but few herbal supplements have even received adequate laboratory and clinical testing in this area with quality control and standardization measures. Thus, it could be utilized for a trial period if other less costly products appear not to be efficacious.

Vitamin C

There is enough indirect information and long-term safety of vitamin C that this is a supplement may have a small role in improving male subfertility [19]. Some positive preliminary data exists for improving fertility in men consuming 200–1,000 mg of vitamin C supplements per day in combination with other antioxidants [19]. Whether or not vitamin C alone can perform as well as the combination supplement treatments is not adequately known. Vitamin C utilization for potentially improving male fertility has a history, but a lack of adequate placebo controlled trials [68, 69]. One small placebo controlled trial of vitamin C (1,000 mg) in combination with high-dose vitamin E (800 mg) for 31 patients with asthenospermia showed no difference compared to placebo for 56 days and no pregnancies [70]. Interestingly, prolonged abstinence increased sperm count, concentration, total number of motile spermatozoa, and ejaculate volume. This highlights the difficulty in identifying what is working to improve fertility in some of these antioxidant studies.

Vitamin C supplementation improves seminal plasma vitamin C in nonsmokers and smokers and could be correlated with improved morphology [71–73]. Seminal plasma has concentrations of vitamin C that are several orders of magnitude higher than that found in the bloodstream. Smoking has the ability to profoundly reduce vitamin C concentration [74]. A placebo controlled trial of smokers found improvements in sperm quality at 200 and 1,000 mg per day [75]. Therefore, in smokers, ex-smokers or those that have recently quit or are on smoking cessation regimens and trying to improve subfertility, including vitamin C supplementation up to 1,000 mg per day seems logical. Whether or not it is needed outside of this population is debatable. Perhaps, this is why there was also such early interest in vitamin C years ago as opposed to recently because such a large percentage of the population was smokers. It is also possible that the low cost of this supplement does not lead to much industry support for this product and fertility. Regardless of the reason it still seems appropriate for all patients to be encouraged to eat a healthy diet high in vitamin C.

Some of the best dietary sources of vitamin C are listed in Table 12.3 [49, 76], but keep in one should be careful about getting an excessive amount of calories from them. Regardless, being able to achieve vitamin C concentrations from diet that are similar to the dosage utilized in clinical trials of supplementation is simply unrealistic. Still, a combination of regular vitamin C intake from food and daily dietary supplementation may be one of the best methods of maintaining adequate ascorbic acid and antioxidant blood levels that could improve fertility.

There is some relevant concern about oxalate increases with large dosages of plain vitamin C supplements (1,000 mg and higher) over many years, especially in those with a history of oxalate stones. Recently, this concern has been escalated in a large prospective study of men (COSM or Cohort of Swedish Men) utilizing high dosages (1,000 mg or more) of plain vitamin C over an 11-year follow-up period [77]. There were 436 first incident stone cases, and ascorbic acid was associated with a statistically significant twofold increased risk. This would equate to one new kidney stone per 680 high-dose users per year [78].

If this concern is accurate, low cost buffered vitamin C or calcium ascorbate may be a safer alternative for these specific patients [79], but this also needs more research. The most practical criticism or real concern I hear from colleagues today about vitamin C is also relevant, which is sperm spends minimal time in seminal secretions before ejaculation. Thus, any true DNA injury would occur before entry in the seminal vesicle and ejaculatory ducts. In other words, vitamin C is more of a protective antioxidant after ejaculation and during transit time in the female reproductive tract. Still, overall, the safety of vitamin C at dosages of 200–1,000 mg maximum on general health is adequate [49], and arguably as adequate as any supplement mentioned in this chapter. And the negative effects of tobacco and

Table 12.3 Sources of vitamin C (foods and beverages)

Fruit	*Portion size*	*Vitamin C amount (in mg)*
Guava	1 (medium)	100
Strawberries	1 cup	95
Papaya	1 cup	85
Kiwi	1 (medium)	75
Orange	1 (medium)	70
Cantaloupe	¼ (medium)	60
Mango	1 cup	45
Cantaloupe melon	1 cup	40
Grapefruit	½ fruit	40
Honeydew melon	1/8 (medium)	40
Lemon	1 (medium)	40
Tangerines or tangelos	1 (medium)	25
Watermelon	1 cup	15
Apple	1 (medium)	10
Avocado	1 (medium)	10
Apricot	1 (medium)	10
Banana	1 (medium)	10
Blueberry	1 cup	10
Crabapple	1 (medium)	10
Grape	1 cup	10
Pawpaw	1 (medium)	10
Pineapple	1 cup	10
Plum	1 (medium)	10
Juice	*Portion size*	*Vitamin C amount (in mg)*
Grape juice	½ cup	120
Apple juice	½ cup	50
Orange (fortified) juice	½ cup	50
Cranberry juice	½ cup	45
Grapefruit juice	½ cup	35
Tomato juice	6 oz	35
Vegetables	*Portion size*	*Vitamin c amount (in mg)*
Pepper (raw red or green)	½ cup	65
Broccoli (cooked)	½ cup	60
Kale (cooked)	1 cup	55
Brussels sprouts (cooked)	½ cup	50
Snow peas (fresh cooked)	½ cup	40
Mustard greens (cooked)	1 cup	35
Potato (sweet or regular baked)	1 (medium)	25–30
Cauliflower (raw or cooked)	½ cup	25
Cabbage (red, raw to cooked)	½ cup	20–25
Plantains (sliced and cooked)	1 cup	15
Tomato (raw)	½ cup	15
Cabbage (raw to cooked)	½ cup	10–15
Asparagus (cooked)	½ cup	10

its relationship to vitamin C levels again make this ideal group to at least consider vitamin C supplementation.

Combination Products

Proxeed (Sigma-Tau) is a popular combination dietary supplement for male infertility in some countries, and in my opinion, appears to have no unsafe amounts of any ingredients. It is a combination of L-carnitine (145 mg), acetyl-L-carnitine (64 mg), fructose (250 mg), citric acid (50 mg), selenium (50 μg), coenzyme Q10 (20 mg), zinc (10 mg), vitamin C (90 mg), B12 (1.5 μg), and folic acid (200 μg) given once a day [80]. In an open trial of 114 men with idiopathic asthenoteratozoospermia (96 men completing the trial) for at least 18 months, the mean sperm progressive motility significantly increased from 18.3 to 42.1 and 16 patients "achieved pregnancy." No significant improvement was noted for sperm density and the rate of morphologically normal forms. Whether or not it works the same, better, or worse compared to other less costly supplements mentioned in this chapter is not known. It will be difficult to get clarity from this anytime soon because these comparison trials are not only lacking, but I cannot visualize how the manufacturers of these products will ever be motivated to conduct such head to head studies. Of course they would be welcomed and provide a unique perspective but personally I am not optimistic these will occur. Currently, it would make sense to follow the plethora of the data and I could argue that the lower cost individual or combined supplements for a trial period is completely logical and if not effective then switching to a more commercial combination product would be the next step. I believe the one advantage to these commercial combination products used by health care professionals is quality control, but the downside is cost and lack of impressive research beyond what has already been potentially observed with other antioxidants.

I could further argue that the simplest compounds used in most studies do not have concerning quality control issues overall. Part of the reason for this is that no herbal products (more notorious for quality control because of the need for standardization) are utilized to any extent in past studies and only single ingredient vitamins, minerals and other simplistic compounds. The only recent exception to this list is *Eurycoma longifolia* (Tonkat Ali). Why not just encourage the use of a daily multivitamin, which has good long-term safety data in men and is heart healthy, safe, and may provide caner preventive impacts when only one pill is used per day [81, 82], and also some minimal infertility data [83]. These unanswered, but logical approaches are for clinicians and their patients to decide.

First Do No Harm: Potentially Harmful Supplementation for Infertility

Folic Acid/Vitamin B9 (High Dose)

Folic acid is not an ideal antioxidant for male fertility in my opinion, and should not be used at this time in certain patients, for example those with a personal history or strong family history of cancer, especially prostate cancer. Folate is a water-soluble B-vitamin, which is also known as vitamin "B9," and it occurs naturally in many healthy foods and multiple diverse beverages and foods [84]. Folic acid is the synthetic, human-produced, or manufactured form of folate that is found in dietary supplements and added to a variety of grain products, which are also known as "fortified foods." Folate from foods and folic acid both assist in the production of DNA, RNA, and other items that are critical for the production and maintenance of cells, especially ones involved in rapid cell division and growth such as in pregnancy and infancy [85]. Humans of all ages need folate to produce normal red blood cells and to prevent macrocytic anemia. Folate is also critical for metabolizing an amino acid known as "homocysteine," which may cause cellular damage in abnormally high amounts and is important for the synthesis of methionine. Folate has diverse roles in the development of a human being, which is why this compound is probably best known for preventing neural tube defects (NTDs) [84].

Green leafy vegetables, fruits, legumes and peas are just some of the natural sources of folate. Still, due to the vital role of folate in the prevention of NTDs, the Food and Drug Administration (FDA) required the addition of folic acid to grain products such as breads, cereals, corn, flours, meals, pastas, and rice. In 1998, the USA and Canada officially began fortifying grain products with folic acid [84]. The recommended daily allowance (RDA) is only 400 μg a day [86]. Table 12.4 is a partial listing of food and other sources of folate and folic acid in order of highest to lowest concentrations [86]. It is important to keep in mind that folic acid is generally added to foods that are labeled "enriched" and/or "fortified" in the USA and other countries. It is for this reason it is easy to find recommended daily allowances of folate for example on many breakfast cereals.

Synthetic folic acid was believed to be more bioavailable compared to folate from food, which may have been one of the many reasons to fortify foods around the world, along with the fact that a deficiency of folate in women of reproductive age can have detrimental consequences. Research has now suggested that folate from foods may be only slightly less absorbable (approximately 20 %) compared to what was previously believed [87].

Critical issues with the overall safety and impact of folic acid on male health now exist. A meta-analysis of the randomized trial data on folic acid and other B-vitamin supplementation to reduce the risk of CVD, cancer, or impact all-cause mortality concluded there was minimal to no impact of these supplements in reducing the risk of these conditions [88]. It does not appear to impact the risk of

Table 12.4 A selected list of beverage/food and other sources of folate and folic acid

Food/beverage or other	Micrograms (μg)
100 % Fortified breakfast cereals	400
Multivitamin (on average-1 pill)	400
B-complex vitamin (on average-1 pill)	400–800
Brewer's yeast (1 tablespoon)	250
Beef liver (cooked, 3-oz)	185
Spinach (cooked, ½ cup)	100
Asparagus (4 spears)	85
Rice (white, enriched, ½ cup)	65
Beans (baked, 1 cup)	60
Green peas (boiled, ½ cup)	50
Avocado (½ cup)	45
Broccoli (2 spears)	45
Lettuce (½ cup)	40
Peanuts (dry roasted, 1 oz)	40
Orange or orange juice (6 oz)	30–35
Tomato juice (6 oz)	35
Bread (white, whole wheat, enriched, 1 slice. . .)	25
Egg (whole)	25
Banana (medium)	20
Wheat germ (1 tablespoon)	20
Rice (brown, ½ cup)	5–10

most chronic diseases, despite the fact that it can reduce blood homocysteine levels by at least 25 %.

Folic acid supplements may increase or encourage the growth of a variety of common tumors and precancerous lesions or polyps in high-risk individuals with adequate or high baseline folate status [89], but it may reduce adenoma risk in those with baseline deficiency of folic acid [90], especially in countries that do not require mandatory fortification. The cancer receiving the most attention in terms of concern is the potential increased risk in prostate cancer [91, 92]. Serum levels of folic acid also appear to be increasing in the elderly such that unmetabolized folic acid (UMFA) has become a concern in men [93].

The controversy over the clinical significance of a potential increased risk of prostate cancer will and should continue without any resolution in the near future. A meta-analysis of randomized trials found a significant increased risk of prostate cancer [94]. Arguably, another larger meta-analysis of randomized trials in cancer suggested that there was no risk and that past meta-analyses were influenced by a higher rate of cancer from one clinical trial [91, 95], where prostate cancer incidence in the folic acid arm was probably increased due to chance [95]. Although these researchers make a compelling argument, the problem with this theory is that most of the major trials looking at prostate cancer incidence still found at least non-significant increases in risk that cannot be disregarded due to chance, and this is confirmed by other recent meta-analysis [96], including recent population studies [97]. The sum of the data is not demonstrating a neutral or reduced effect, but only an increased risk overall, and the argument is whether or not it is statistically or clinically significant [98].

Clinicians should not encourage supplemental folic acid use especially in men with a history of cancer concerned about fertility, despite some minimal positive or just non-impressive data in the area of fertility itself [99, 100], because other supplements are safer, just as effective and do not appear to require mega-dosage (like folic acid) for a clinical impact. Some of the early and only clinical trials that involved folic acid were utilizing dosages such as 5 mg per day (along with zinc), which is 12.5 times the recommended daily intake [99]. Only sperm concentration, but not motility or morphology, was improved. Food sources of folate can be recommended, because these have not been concerning overall, but the concentrated nutraceuticals do not follow the mantra right now of benefit exceeding risk.

Selenium and Vitamin E

Selenium or vitamin E supplements should not be recommended to improve fertility in subfertile men strictly based entirely on their overall safety issues and not on efficacy. For example, the initiation and even the final results of the SELECT trial of selenium and/or vitamin E to prevent prostate cancer were concerning for a multitude of reasons [101, 102]. Both agents failed to prevent prostate cancer, and there were multiple past and current safety issues with these nutritional supplement agents. Selenium had a history of potentially increasing the risk of skin cancer recurrence [103], and there were concerns over an increased risk of type-2 diabetes [104]. Interestingly, SELECT observed a non-significant increased risk of type 2 diabetes when the trial was terminated [101]. And there was a non-significant increase in the risk of aggressive (Gleason 7–10) prostate cancer with vitamin E and/or selenium [102].

Vitamin E supplements were also replete with some similar but even more concerning issues compared to selenium during the SELECT trial. Past meta-analysis of other clinical trials found a potential increased risk of all-cause mortality with higher doses of vitamin E supplements [105]. Other large clinical trials found a significant increased risk of heart failure in those with vascular disease or diabetes [106]. A significant increased risk of hemorrhagic stroke was found for vitamin E supplements in another major chemoprevention trial of healthy male physicians (Physicians' Health Study II) that was concurrently being conducted during the time of SELECT [107]. And again SELECT found a non-significant ($p = 0.06$) increased risk of prostate cancer in the vitamin E arm when the study was terminated, and a significantly higher risk with greater follow-up after termination [101, 102]. Thus, both of these supplements have no impressive overall or heart health research unless there is a deficiency in these compounds [108–112], and multiple past and ongoing concerns abound [113, 114], as also outlined earlier. There needs to be more clinician and patient awareness over the multiple serious safety issues with vitamin E and selenium, and these supplements should not be encouraged for any healthy individual attempting to improve fertility despite past trials in infertility demonstrating some benefit [115–117]. It is also interesting that all of the past trial of vitamin E and/or selenium that have suggested benefit in male subfertility have also been at dosages equivalent or actually larger than past clinical trials in other areas of health that found large concerns [101, 102, 105–107]. Since these supplements have not been found to have profound benefits beyond what has been observed with other supplements discussed in this chapter [19], then it would be prudent again to not recommend this particular compounds with such as negative and nebulous history.

Zinc

The excitement for the use of zinc with or without other supplements is supported by some older clinical trials. For example, over 100 subfertile and fertile men experienced a large improvement in sperm counts (74 % significant increase) over 24 weeks, which was not observed in the placebo group [99]. This older study was published in 2002, and 66 mg of zinc sulfate (six times the recommend daily dietary intake) was used alone or combined with 5 mg of folic acid (over 12 times the recommend dietary intake). Additionally, there was no difference in the serum or seminal plasma level of zinc between the subfertile and fertile men in this study, and zinc supplements did not increase those levels, and the study did not include pregnancy as a clinical endpoint.

Another older clinical trial of 100 men with asthenozoospermia was randomized to 250 mg twice daily (over 45 times the recommended dietary intake) of zinc for 3 months compared to no treatment [118]. Significant improvement in sperm quality, sperm count, motility, fertilizing capacity, and the incidence of anti-sperm antibodies was observed in the zinc group. After 12 months of follow-up, there were 11 pregnancies (22.5 %) in the zinc group and 2 (4.3 %) in the control group ($p < 0.03$). There were no hormonal differences found between the groups. Other studies have methodology issues including a lack of controls or short treatment periods [119].

The issue with zinc currently is that the recommended dietary intake is only 11 mg [120], and mega-doses of zinc supplements are replete with issues especially in urology [121]. One of the largest prospective studies to look at high-dose zinc supplement intake found an increased risk of advanced prostate cancer [122]. And arguably the largest dietary supplement study to use high-dose zinc (macular degeneration) found an increased risk of hospital admissions from this exact same trial (Age Related Eye Disease Study or AREDS) in regard to genitourinary complications (BPH, stones, and UTI) in the 80 mg zinc arm [123, 124]. Thus, whether or not this will be further confirmed is not the issue because at this time zinc supplements in high doses like the ones needed in the fertility trials are too concerning, short and long-term. In fact, some countries such as Canada now discourages the sale of high-dose zinc supplements (40 mg or more) unless research suggests a specific benefit otherwise and proven safety simply because of these issues [125, 126]. Some major clinical trials (AREDS 2) tested lower zinc dosages compared to the older effective higher dosage based on this history of adverse events [127].

First Do No Harm Specific Supplementation for Improved Erectile Function

L-Arginine or L-Arginine Aspartate + Pycnogenol

Nitric oxide (NO) is produced from L-arginine by nitric oxide synthase (NOS) [22], thus the idea of utilizing L-arginine supplements to enhance the treatment of ED appears logical and is an option for some patients. In fact, L-arginine with its ability to increase NO and lower blood pressure makes it a potential preventive or treatment option in other areas of medicine such as hypertension and preeclampsia [128–130].

However, three serious problems with L-arginine supplementation in terms of metabolism include:

- The potential for extensive first pass liver metabolism (arginase enzyme) that occurs when ingesting this compound [131–133].
- The additional intestinal enzymes (gut arginases) that also exist in the GI tract to further potentially deactivate this agent [131–133].
- The presence of an endogenous inhibitor of NOS, which is known as ADMA (asymmetrical dimethylarginine) [134, 135].

Thus, large dosages of L-arginine will usually needed to achieve some success in general medicine and in the area of ED and FSD, and this can be daunting for the patient. For example, 3–6 g of L-arginine would require 6–12 large pills or capsules per day.

Perhaps, this is one reason large intakes of dietary arginine or supplemental arginine have not been proven beneficial in other areas of medicine such as athletic performance [136, 137]. And this is also the case with erectile function where moderate dosages of L-arginine alone (1,500 mg per day) do not appear to work better compared to placebo [138] for ED. Other studies of high-dosages of L-arginine (5 g per day, $n = 50$) over 6 weeks appear to work mildly to moderately better than placebo in terms of subjective (not objective) outcomes, especially for those that with organic ED that may produce or secrete low amounts of nitrite and nitrate (metabolites of nitric oxide that are fairly stable) from urinary measurements [139]. Urinary nitric oxide metabolites appear to double when taking 5 g per day. One area that needed better research was whether L-arginine efficacy could be enhanced when combining it with other agents.

An impressive amount of clinical data has been garnered for the use of L-arginine aspartate at a lower dosage (2,800–3,000 mg) when used with pycnogenol (80 mg) [140–142]. The most commonly tested supplement in this form is Prelox (Horphag Research Ltd, London, UK). Perhaps, this solves part of the metabolism problem when utilizing L-arginine alone.

A randomized, double-blind, placebo-controlled crossover study of 50 participants with moderate ED (IIEF score of 11–17) and a mean age of 37 years was conducted [141]. The total daily dose of Prelox was 3,000 mg of L-arginine aspartate and 80 mg of pycnogenol. This total dosage was divided into four tablets, two taken between 7 and 9 a.m. and two between 7 and 9 p.m. with 200 ml of water. IIEF scores from 11 to 17 at baseline approximately doubled to 26–30 ($p > 0.001$) after 1 month. The earliest improvement was 1 day and the latest response was after 9 days (mean 4.9 days). IIEF domains including orgasmic function, sexual desire, intercourse satisfaction, overall satisfaction and percent sexual response also approximately doubled ($p > 0.001$). Systolic and diastolic blood pressure also dropped significantly ($p < 0.001$), and side effects were similar to placebo. It should be kept in mind that men with severe CVD or hypertension were excluded from this study.

The clinical trial that has established Prelox as a definite nutraceutical option for men with mild to moderate ED in my opinion and arguably one of the better nutraceutical options for ED was based on a 6-month randomized, double blind trial, placebo-controlled parallel-arm study ($n = 124$, mean age 44 years) [142]. Men in this trial had IIEF scores at baseline of 11–17, and diabetics and those with severe hypertension were excluded. Again, two tablets were utilized in the morning and evening and each table contained 700 mg L-arginine aspartate and 20 mg of pycnogenol (total daily dose was 2,800 mg L-arginine aspartate and 80 mg pycnogenol). The erectile domain of the IIEF (questions 1–5 and 15) improved from a baseline of 15–25 after 3 months and 27 after 6 months compared to placebo where an increase of 15–19 was observed ($p < 0.05$). These results are in the same range of prescription PDE-5 inhibitors. There was an insignificant drop in blood pressure in the Prelox group from a systolic of 139–131 and a diastolic from 86 to 82 (6 point drop in the placebo arm). Total testosterone also increased significantly ($p < 0.05$) from 15.9 to 18.9 nmol/l in the Prelox group (16.9–17.3 nmol/l with placebo). It is plausible that testosterone increased from increased sexual activity and/or another mechanism, and this should be followed in patients to answer this question because it would be an ancillary benefit for some men if this was the case. Increases in the domain of orgasmic function, sexual desire, intercourse satisfaction, and overall satisfaction were all significantly improved over placebo ($p < 0.05$) with Prelox. A total of 13 men were lost to follow-up in this trial, so 111 men completed the trial. The question is whether or not the data was analyzed based on intention to treat principle, which is important because all significant values reached the minimum of $p < 0.05$? Regardless, there is adequate efficacy with Prelox and it should be offered as an option for healthy men with mild to moderate ED and no significant co-morbidity and no hepatic or renal abnormalities. The number of pills needed per day (four) could be problematic long-term along with cost, and whether or not those with CVD should utilize it are questionable. Two clinical trials demonstrated potential adverse events or worse outcomes in those with a previous myocardial event or existing peripheral artery disease (PAD) [143, 144], but other clinical studies have challenged the merit of these findings [145, 146]. Still, the overall efficacy is still notable and again makes it one of the best over the counter options available based on the scientific evidence for men with mild to moderate ED.

L-Citrulline

The major source of L-arginine within the endothelial cell is from L-citrulline, and both L-arginine and L-citrulline raise vascular NO levels [147]. In some individuals L-citrulline may be at least twice as efficient at increasing nitric oxide levels compared to L-arginine, which could solve some of the dosage and other issues mentioned with L-arginine. In a double-blind, randomized, placebo-controlled crossover study, 20 (mean age 57 years) healthy volunteers received six different dosing regimens of placebo, citrulline, and arginine. L-Citrulline was significantly more effective at increasing L-arginine plasma levels compared to L-arginine itself ($p < 0.01$). At a dosage of only 1.5 g per day of oral L-citrulline, L-arginine blood levels were raised to a similar degree as 3.2 g per day of oral L-arginine. L-Citrulline raised the ratio of L-arginine to ADMA, and the arginine/ADMA ratio is again thought to determine substrate availability of arginine to the endothelium. The correlation observed in this study between increases in the arginine/ADMA ratio and forearm flow-mediated vasodilatation indicated a dose–response relationship with NO production. The highest dose of L-citrulline (3 g twice a day or 6 g total) was the most effective at raising nitric oxide levels compared to L-arginine ($p < 0.01$). Urinary nitrate (a marker of NO) and cGMP (another potential indicator of systemic NO production and bioactivity) were significantly ($p = 0.01$, $p = 0.04$) increased over arginine. Neither blood urea nitrogen (BUN) nor serum creatinine was changed, and there were no safety issues over placebo.

It is of interest that the 1.5 g of L-citrulline used as one dosage in the previously mentioned study was the same daily dosage found to be effective in 1-month crossover trial of men with mild to moderate ED [148]. A total of 24 men (mean age is 56.5 ± 9.8 years) took 1.5 g of L-citrulline a day or placebo for 1 month. An improvement in erection hardness score (validated ED instrument) was found after 1 month in the L-citrulline group compared to placebo ($p < 0.01$). No adverse events occurred over placebo, and 37.5 % of participants had hypertension, 21 % high cholesterol, 12.5 % BPH, and 12.5 % had diabetes. This is preliminary but potentially exciting research suggesting that L-citrulline could be one of the better nutraceutical options for ED and should also be researched as ancillary supplementation to conventional ED options.

The question of short and long-term safety with L-citrulline needs to be addressed. High dosages of L-citrulline have been utilized in some short-term clinical trials with good safety [149, 150]. Citrulline can be used to increase arginine availability without affecting urea excretion and may enhance nitrogen balance. It does appear that adequate renal function is needed for maximum citrulline conversion into arginine and this should be considered.

Citrulline from synthetic or watermelon extract supplements have not been known to cause acute side effects and is another source of citrulline and arginine, but blood pressure reductions could occur, especially in prehypertensive and hypertensive patients and this has to be noted to anyone before starting citrulline supplementation [151]. Citrulline from dietary sources only are difficult if not impossible to obtain, since watermelon is the only source and the rind contains the majority of this compound, but excessive quantities would need to be consumed to equate to several hundred milligrams of this amino acid. Thus, nutraceutical sources of citrulline are the only realistic option for patients recommended more citrulline for erectile health.

Since nitric oxide (NO) production inhibits platelet aggregation as demonstrated from L-arginine infusion studies [152], it should be expected that L-citrulline can do the same but needs more research. And more short and long-term studies are needed in the area of ED to determine the best potential use of this interesting amino acid from watermelon. Since citrulline has the potential to be heart healthy this also makes it a potential ideal candidate in the area of ED in the future [153].

Panax ginseng ***and Ginsenosides (Korean Red Ginseng and Others)***

Ginseng actually refers to the root of several species in the genus *Panax*, of which *Panax ginseng* is one of the most widely utilized species and is native to Asian countries such as China and Korea [154–157]. Ginsenosides, which are also known as ginseng saponins or glycosylated steroidal saponins, are unique to the *Panax* species, and are the primary active ingredients in ginseng. More than 30 different ginsenosides have been isolated from the root of *Panax ginseng*, and although ginseng contains other diverse compounds, the individual and collective ginsenosides appear to be the generally agreed upon active ingredients from basic science and clinical trials.

Ginsenosides have multiple mechanisms of action, and each ginsenoside may have tissue-specific impacts [158–161]. The backbone of each ginsenoside is similar and consists of a common four-ring steroid-like structure that includes multiple carbon atoms with attached sugar moieties. Each ginsenoside has a different type, position, and number of sugar moieties attached by a glycosidic bond at C-3 and C-6. Each type of ginsenoside also has at least three side chains at the C-3, C-6, or C-20 position. These side chains are free or are attached to monomers, dimers, or trimers of sugars. It is these sugar compounds that may provide the cellular-specific or receptor effects of each ginsenoside. The ginseng species, age, part of the plant, harvest season, preservation, and extraction method can all impact the compounds found in ginseng and even alter somewhat the ginsenoside content.

Over several decades, the content of ginsenoside standardized extracts utilized in clinical trials has varied, from approximately 4 % ginsenosides in the 1990s to 4–7 % ginsenosides in the mid-2000s, and higher standardized extracts are offered today (>8 % for example) [162, 163]. The ginsenoside content should be considered when comparing different efficacy doses from clinical trials. When the ginsenoside concentration is isolated, it appears to elicit the same or better results than the sum of the total ginseng components [163], which again supports the accepted general philosophy that ginsenosides are the active medical components of *Panax ginseng*.

One of the more influential evidence based endorsements for ginseng and male sexual function was a clinical evidence guideline of conventional and alternative medicines [164]. The authors used *Panax ginseng* data from six randomized trials conducted over a period of approximately 15 years that included a total of 349 men. The investigators found that ginseng significantly ($p < 0.00001$) improved erectile function compared with placebo over 4–12 weeks. Approximately 58 % of men experienced an improvement in some aspect of sexual function compared with 20 % of men who received the placebo. No other dietary or truly CAM supplement was recommended. Ginseng was found to have "moderate-quality evidence" and the investigators concluded that ginseng is "likely to be beneficial" in men with erectile dysfunction of any etiology (organic and psychogenic causes). The final clinical evidence-based guideline provided in this review stated "Ginseng is a traditional Asian remedy with rare adverse effects in the recommended dose of 0.5–2.0 g daily." What was not mentioned in this review and any other to date to my knowledge is that these dosages recommended were for older less concentrated form of ginseng (4–7 % ginsenosides). And, in this same systematic review [164], the authors mentioned that they still needed to evaluate a more concentrated ginsenoside randomized trial by Park and colleagues that was published in Korean in the Korean Journal of Urology [165], but that the article was being translated. Interestingly, the author of this chapter had this study by Park and colleagues translated into English, and it arguably provides some of the best preliminary clinical data to date for a dietary supplement compared with placebo over 8 weeks for men with ED. This was a multicenter, randomized, double-blind, placebo-controlled study of 69 participants that used a highly concentrated ginsenoside product (800 mg per day) [165]. The primary endpoint was the response to the erectile function domain of the International Index of Erectile Function (IIEF) questionnaire at baseline and 8 weeks. The other domains of the IIEF were secondary endpoints, and safety was monitored. Every single sexual health domain from the IIEF-15 was significantly improved by Korean ginseng compared with placebo: erectile function (primary endpoint), sexual desire, orgasmic function, intercourse satisfaction, and overall satisfaction. Additionally, every question on the IIEF (15 out of 15) was improved significantly in this specific clinical trial. The sexual desire domain, frequency, and degree of sexual desire were all also significantly increased ($p < 0.001$). In other words, both the primary and the secondary endpoints significantly favored ginseng over placebo. No significant differences in adverse events have been reported for ginseng compared with placebo. The results of this trial will strengthen the clinical evidence for *Panax ginseng* and the evidence that highly concentrated ginsenosides are the active or effective ingredients in ginseng [165]. The product used was from a Korean Ginseng Company (BT Gin). Still, the current and future cost of this and other products need to be discussed because again they can be quite high depending on the source and time of year.

The onset of action or efficacy of ginseng could arguably occur within days to months [164–166]. The time period is variable and requires further elucidation, but at least 4–8 weeks should be attempted on a *Panax ginseng* supplement before deciding upon efficacy. The onset of action will not be as rapid on average as PDE-5 inhibitors, but the impact on libido, lower cost in some cases, and safety affords ginseng its own set of advantages for certain patients. In addition, the potential for combining ginseng with conventional ED treatments should be explored since PDE-5 inhibitors have no significant effect on libido.

In terms of *Panax ginseng* the laboratory data for ginsenosides suggest multiple mechanisms of action. In cultured bovine endothelial cells, ginsenosides were shown to stimulate the conversion of [14C]L-arginine to [14C]L-citrulline and to promote vasorelaxation [167]. More specific studies in rabbit corpus cavernosum tissue continue to support the potential of increasing endogenous nitric oxide (NO) concentrations via the addition of ginsenosides [168]. Other basic laboratory investigations and reviews support this thought and mechanism whereby the stimulation of nitric oxide synthase may produce higher quantities of NO and peripheral neurophysiologic enhancement may also occur [169–172].

Ginsenosides also compete with agonists for binding to GABA-A and GABA-B receptors [173, 174], which could also explain a central mechanism of action impacting desire or arousal. Anxiolytic effects have also been demonstrated in mice and maze models. Ginseng and ginsenosides have been shown to positively impact striatal dopaminergic activity and dopamine receptors [175], which could translate to a minimal apomorphine like effect. Ginseng may exert a direct effect on the hypothalamus or pituitary to also suppress prolactin secretion, but these hormonal changes I believe are minor at best because past clinical trials measuring hormonal changes in men did not find significant or consistent increases in prolactin or testosterone [176].

A rare but still surprising issue with some herbal preparations in my opinion is the chance for them to be inappropriately and falsely tagged with an acute safety issue on the basis of isolated case reports or uncontrolled investigation without an examination of the totality of the objective laboratory and clinical evidence. One perpetuated example is a 1979 observational series in a notable medical journal that associated the self-reported utilization of ginseng products with hypertension in 14 individuals after 3 months of use [177]. Yet despite no control group, and other basic methodology quality-control issues, which included a lack of correction for other confounders (such as high intake of caffeine and potentially other stimulants) the investigation was used by some as proof of cause and effect [178–180]. These hypertensive effects have not been replicated since 1979 in a controlled setting. Randomized trials of hypertensive and non-hypertensive individuals have demonstrated no impact or a partial reduction in blood pressure with *Panax* or American ginseng and isolated ginsenosides, regardless of dose utilized and time period (up to 3 months) [181–186].

Regardless, long-term studies (several years) are needed to confirm this consistent finding in the acute setting. In my experience, other compounds found with ginseng commercial products such as caffeine or caffeine mimics I believe have the ability to exacerbate the stimulant effects of ginseng itself, or be the sole cause of blood pressure or heart rate increases in rare patients. It is for this reason that a patient with controlled or uncontrolled hypertension should receive some objective education on the past history of ginseng in combination with adulterants that could theoretically change blood pressure values. Ginseng (*Panax quinquefolius*—somewhat similar to *Panax ginseng*) alone has been shown to increase energy levels in cancer patients with fatigue, but again the safety was similar to a placebo in a large phase 3 like randomized trial ($n = 290$) [187]. This again speaks to the safety and another potential mechanism of action of ginseng (reduced fatigue).

Potential interactions with warfarin or hemostatic issues have also been suggested on the basis of case reports [188], but controlled studies have not been able to substantiate any consistent impact of ginseng on warfarin anticoagulation or hemostasis in general (prothrombin time, partial thromboplastin time, and international normalized ratio [INR]) [189]. Still, this needs to be further elucidated based on studies of other types of ginseng that could have some impact on platelet activity and this could explain some cardiovascular benefits. And since ginseng may improve nitric oxide levels (NO), and NO is known, as mentioned earlier in the chapter, to inhibit platelet aggregation, it is plausible that there could be a blood thinning type effect.

Past human studies of ginseng and sexual health have reported gastrointestinal side effects [164, 166], for example, stomach upset, but these were not reported at a rate significantly higher than the rate for placebo. Ingesting ginseng with a meal seems more appropriate because of potential gastrointestinal issues with most dietary supplement interventions or placebo, and there are no reports that ginseng is less or more efficacious in this scenario. More rigorous monitoring of ginseng safety in clinical trials should be conducted to provide some clarity on adverse events. The dose of ginseng and ginsenoside concentration should always be noted in clinical trials and again reviews on this topic have been lacking. Ginsenoside concentrations should be required for publication in any clinical trial of ginseng.

Panax ginseng has arguably the longest and perhaps one of the most impressive nutraceutical records to date for use in men with mild to moderate ED. Approximately ten randomized trials have suggested that *Panax ginseng* and its ginsenosides have potential efficacy in diverse areas of male sexual health [164, 165, 190, 191]. Still, this is not meant to suggest that it is the most effective ED nutraceutical option because others (arginine combinations and citrulline) have their own advantages and disadvantages, and methodological quality of future clinical trials needs to be improved. The isolation of the more active ginsenosides also needs more research and in my experience quality control is a real problem with many ginseng products. Also, price issues need to be resolved because at the time of this writing Korean Red ginseng and Chinese ginseng with more concentrated ginsenosides were no longer of low cost.

SAM-e for SSRI-Induced Sexual Dysfunction

S-Adenosyl methionine (SAMe) is a naturally occurring compound that functions as a methyl donor in human metabolism may have a individual treatment role for major depressive disorder (MDD), or an ancillary role to enhance conventional treatment [153, 192–196]. A clinical study of 73 serotonin reuptake inhibitor non-responders with MDD over 6 weeks found a benefit in those receiving 800 mg twice daily of SAM-e compared to placebo [193]. A significantly higher response and remission rate occurred with SAM-e over placebo. Side effects were similar to placebo. Gastrointestinal side effects and headaches have occurred in other studies [194], and SAM-e is not a low cost CAM in general.

Preliminary research also suggests that in those with MDD this dietary supplement may have a positive effect on male arousal and ED, such that scores improved in these areas compared to placebo [197]. SSRIs and other antidepressant medications could have a profound impact on male and female sexual function [198]. I am hopeful that research on SAM-e to support its minimal or even positive effect on sexual function (ED or FSD) in those with MDD continues. It is also of interest that SAM-e has been used as a prescription drug, given as an IV or an injectable in numerous European countries since the 1970s and its ability to reduce osteoarthritic pain is also notable, well published, and on par with NSAIDs but with less toxicity at dosages of up to 600 mg per day [199, 200].

First Do No Harm: Potentially Harmful or Ineffective Nutraceuticals for Erectile Function

Androstenedione and/or DHEA

On January 20, 2005 it became illegal to sell androstenedione dietary supplements in the USA [201, 202]. Androstenedione was considered a "prohormone" supplement that some men used in an attempt to build muscle. It was utilized by some notable US professional athletes before being banned, and it created enormous controversy. It was a potentially dangerous supplement because it had been associated with a reduction in "good cholesterol" or HDL and it had potentially other health consequences such as significantly increasing estrogen (estrone and estradiol) in healthy young men (ages 26–32 years) taking 100 or 300 mg per day for 7 days, and significantly increasing testosterone levels at 300 mg per day (from 526 to 872 ng/dl on average in one study) [203]. Other studies of young men demonstrated just increases in estrogen with these dosages [204], which is why it would not been surprising that some individual reports of ED from these supplements can also occur because of arguable the suppression of the pituitary and gonadal axis [205]. The individual variability in the response is also what is striking about androstenedione (or DHEA) in men and women, except for the estrogen increases in young and older primarily eugonadal men. Men ages 35–65 years taking 200 mg of androstenedione had significant increases in estrogen but not testosterone over 12 weeks [206]. In postmenopausal women a significant increase in estrone occurred but the individual variability in the response was always notable, which is again part of the problem [207]. Regardless of the population studied the variability or unpredictability of the physiologic response should be mentioned to patients. This has also been my experience that men (and women) without overt hormone deficiencies have variable results and men experience dramatic increases in estrogen and potentially a small increase in testosterone the more testosterone deficient the male [153].

Therefore, there were so many concerns with these supplements that eventually the FDA and the US government decided to remove almost all of them, including androstenedione, from the market [201]. Other so-called prohormone supplements like DHEA were not banned, but are still being allowed for sale. Now, if DHEA is similar to androstenedione in that it has similar effects, then why is this supplement still allowed for sale over the counter? This is part of the strange circumstances surrounding some dietary supplements and the inconsistency in the policies that are applied. DHEA supplements enjoy a unique exemption under federal law, because of a bill approved by Congress in late 2004. How did DHEA survive when other similar to identical supplements did not? Sports officials were in favor of an overall ban on steroids and related products, including DHEA. DHEA has been banned by the Olympics, the World Anti-Doping Agency, the National Collegiate Athletic Association, the National Football League, the National Basketball Association, and minor league baseball. The 2005 law that impacts prohormone supplements, passed without objection, also gave the Drug Enforcement Administration more authority to ban new or novel steroids, with one exemption, DHEA. The term "anabolic steroid" is defined now as any drug or hormonal substance, chemically and pharmacologically related to testosterone (other than estrogens, progestins, corticosteroids, and DHEA). In my opinion, since such a large percentage of Congressional officials use dietary supplements and some perceived DHEA as unique, the proposal to ban all over the counter pro-hormone supplements in the USA would have not passed Congress if DHEA were included in the proposal. Now, with this pertinent history, what about any new data to support DHEA for men's health or sexual health?

Population studies such as the Massachusetts Male Aging Study have suggested a higher risk of ED with lower blood levels of DHEA-S [208]. Yet what gets missed in referencing these studies is that there were also inverse associations of HDL with ED and a higher risk of ED in those with heart disease, hypertension, smoking and diabetes for example, which is a more tangible and productive conversation. It should be kept in mind that DHEA levels decrease substantially with aging, and this has been utilized in deceptive advertising in my opinion to encourage men and women to purchase this supplement. Other studies suggest that a lower level of DHEA and an increase risk of ED is only an anemic association [209]. DHEA is produced primarily by the adrenal cortex and in smaller amounts by the testes and the ovaries, and then it is quickly sulfated by sulfotransferases into DHEA-S, which is more stable with a longer half-life and its concentrations stay stable most of the day [210]. DHEA is arguably the most abundant steroid in the human body (more than testosterone), thus for this and many other reasons there will always be sufficient physiologic facts to give it some advertising attraction. It does not appear to have a role for androgen deficient or insufficient men because it is not predictable.

Small studies of men utilizing 50 mg for 6 months (DHEAS level <1.5 μmol/l) showed some improvements in function in those with hypertension and ED or those without organic etiology, but not in those with diabetes or neurologic issues [211, 212]. These men were all generally tested with prostaglandin E1 first to ensure that they were capable of having a full erection with pharmacologic intervention. The problem with DHEA is a lack of large studies with good methodology and no really novel findings with DHEA and ED or in the area of male sexual health. DHEA-S levels are also not easy to acutely or chronically predict with lifestyle interventions; for example, in some studies there is minimal or large changes in this hormonal marker for men and women after large reduction in weight [213–215]. Perhaps this is due to the fact that DHEA levels need to be monitored over many years. Obesity appears to attenuate the association or correlation between higher DHEA and lower morbidity [216].

*Fenugreek (***Trigonella foenum-graecum***)*

Fenugreek has been promoted by numerous commercial entities as an option for testosterone replacement, or a testosterone-enhancing supplement via an aromatase inhibitor mechanism of action (blocks the conversion of testosterone to estrogen) [153]. Human studies have failed to demonstrate that this herb/spice supplement increases testosterone consistently, especially in hypogonadal men. In fact, fenugreek has been used as a spice and is utilized in Indian Ayurvedic and in Chinese Medicine as a stimulus for lactation for breastfeeding women [153, 217]. This supplement has a partial notorious history for being touted as a breast enhancement supplement for women without human research to support this claim. Yet allergic reactions to the powder and mild gastrointestinal upset are not uncommon side effects and increased bleeding can occur beyond what is expected in those on aspirin or anti-inflammatory drugs [217].

In terms of fenugreek as a TRT supplement, in one clinical study, fenugreek (standardized to 70 % trigimannose) actually significantly reduced levels of free testosterone [218]. Men had a 40 ng/ml free testosterone at baseline, reduced to 33 ng/ml at 4 weeks, and then to 36 ng/ml at 8 weeks ($p = 0.02$) when taking 500 mg per day. DHT levels were reduced in the fenugreek group. Other studies demonstrate that fenugreek either causes no change or slightly increases testosterone in men have been for those with an already normal testosterone at baseline [219, 220]. In other words, it is an unpredictable supplement in the area of TRT. One clinical trial of fenugreek of 500 mg per day (standardized for Grecunin) over 8 weeks showed an average increases of 6.6 and 12.3 % for total testosterone and bioavailable testosterone [219]. Even if fenugreek operates as an aromatase inhibitor, as explained earlier in this chapter, I do not recognize this as a positive mechanism of action because it could cause bone loss in healthy men based on some past clinical trials of prescription drugs that have this same mechanism of action.

One ancillary health advantage of fenugreek is that the natural seeds can be purchased at health food stores and used in most diet plans (soups, yogurt, oatmeal...) and they may slightly lower blood sugar and cholesterol because they are a good source of fiber (1 tablespoon = 3 g of fiber) [153, 221].

Tribulus terrestris

This is an herbal product that has been suggested by some commercial entities to have a DHEA or pro-hormone type effects (for ED and TRT), and it had been around for decades but there is simply no positive or adequate evidence to support its use for ED. Human studies have failed to demonstrate that this herb acts like "DHEA" to increase testosterone, or just increases testosterone by an independent mechanism, which is what it is advertised to do in many places [153]. For example, a small clinical trial of elite male rugby players ($n = 22$) were placed on Tribulus or placebo for 5 weeks and no alterations in testosterone or muscle mass occurred [222]. Another small trial of healthy men ages 20–36 years of age with body weights ranging from 60 to 125 kg ($n = 14$) was published [223]. Participants consumed 10 or 20 mg/kg body weight of Tribulus (divided into three daily intakes) for 4 weeks. No significant changes in any parameter occurred in the Tribulus group and this included testosterone, androstenedione, or LH. The authors concluded that this supplement does not contain any indirect or direct testosterone-enhancing properties. In fact, the only adequate clinical trials where a dose of Tribulus (750 mg or more) appears to increase testosterone is when it is combined with 150 mg of DHEA and 300 mg of androstenedione [224–227]. And drops of 5.0 mg/dl in HDL or "good cholesterol" were observed which have to be somewhat concerning [225], but again was probably due to the DHEA and androstenedione components. Preliminary clinical trials have failed to demonstrate an impact of Tribulus on body composition or exercise performance and no impact on hormone levels.

Yohimbine Hydrochloride (Not Really a Dietary Supplement or CAM)

Yohimbine comes from the West African Yohimbe tree and can be found as a supplement and a prescription drug (Yocon® etc.) [153, 228]. Whether or not it even works is controversial, but what is not controversial is that it is a "alpha-2-adrenoreceptor antagonist," and some of the side effects include headache, sweating, nausea, dizziness, nervousness/agitation, tremors, sleeplessness, antidiuresis, and elevated blood pressure and heart rate [229]. And it cannot be used by individuals with kidney disease, those on anti-depressants, or other mood-altering drugs, and in some individuals with specific cardiovascular, neurological, and psychological issues.

Many media and other credible sources appear to suggest yohimbine is as an alternative medicine or over the counter dietary supplement, but this is really not the case based on its clinical trial efficacy. It is usually characterized as an "alternative medicine" by some individuals and reviews [220], some may assume this is a dietary supplement, and there are many companies that sell "yohimbe" or tout that they sell "yohimbine HCL." The positive data with the drug or compound derived from this tree, yohimbine hydrochloride, came from European and other studies at a total of 5–10 mg per day (divided doses) [230]. Yohimbine HCL is a prescription drug, but many dietary supplements that mimic this drug have quality serious control problems and are dangerous [228, 229]. Again, yohimbine HCL is the active ingredient found in the bark of a West African tree, but many dietary supplements really sell "yohimbe" which in many cases has little to no or variable quantities of the active ingredient "yohimbine HCL" in it. Again, if there is an interest in yohimbine HCL in the area of ED I believe the prescription drug should be utilized because of quality control issues and because the successful clinical trials utilized this version.

Conclusion

Other supplements in the area of fertility and erectile health simply have shown no benefit, such as magnesium [231], or should not be recommended because of the need for more efficacy and/or safety data (for example L-carnitine for ED) [153]. Tongkat ali (*Eurycoma longifolia*) has some initial positive data for fertility and sexual enhancement [60, 61], but the mechanism of action and tangible effects

Table 12.5 Summary of some of the nutraceutical products discussed in this chapter for fertility and erectile function that could be recommended or discouraged

Fertility nutraceuticals	*Commentary/recommendations*
CoQ10	200–300 mg per day has excellent safety but efficacy is mixed
Folic acid	Not recommended beyond the dose found in a multivitamin (200–400 μg). Has controversial ability to potentially increase the growth of colon polyps and prostate cancer in individuals with already high baseline levels of folate
L-Carnitine	2,000–4,000 mg per day has mixed data but overall safety has been adequate
Multivitamin	Minimal clinical data to improve fertility and could be utilized based on the safety of one pill a day
Omega-3 fatty acid (EPA and DHA)	Increasing dietary intake of marine sources of omega-3 fatty acids is recommended over supplementation
Proxeed (commercial product)	Combination nutraceutical product with minimal clinical data but a long history of physician use and can be utilized. Cost could be the only issue
Selenium and/or vitamin E	Not recommended based on the overall safety concerns in men's health with increasing dosages of selenium (type 2 diabetes or skin cancer recurrence) and vitamin E (prostate cancer)
Tongkat Ali (*Eurycoma longifolia*)	One company (Biotropics Malaysia Berhad, Kuala Lumpur, Malaysia) has a standardized extract at 200 mg per day and could be of benefit
Vitamin C	Up to 1,000 mg per day is recommended and generally safe short-term but can increase oxalate levels significantly. Non-buffered or pH neutral vitamin C (also known as "calcium ascorbate") could cause minimal changes in oxalate and appears to be as effective. Smokers, ex-smokers or those that have recently quit or are on smoking cessation regimens and trying to improve subfertility are the best candidates
Zinc	Not recommended based on the potential for urologic toxicity when used in large dosages (80 mg+) over long periods of time
Erectile function/health nutraceuticals	*Commentary/recommendations*
DHEA/androstenedione	Not recommended, can reduce HDL cholesterol, unpredictable testosterone changes and can increase estrogen levels in men
Fenugreek (*Trigonella foenum-graecum*)	Touted to increase testosterone but has not consistently demonstrated a benefit and could potentially reduce free testosterone
L-Arginine	Not generally recommended alone because of the large dosages needed to overcome first pass metabolism and deactivating enzymes (arginases). Blood pressure reductions with this supplement can occur
L-Arginine aspartate + pycnogenol	One of the most clinically researched and efficacious nutraceuticals for men with mild to moderate ED. Dosages of 2,800–3,000 mg of L-arginine aspartate + 80 mg daily of pycnogenol (Prelox is the most commercialized researched product) has demonstrated adequate efficacy. Cost and pill count may be an issue for some individuals and blood pressure reductions are not uncommon

(continued)

Table 12.5 (continued)

L-Citrulline	Dosages as low as 1,500 mg per day can be recommended for ED based on moderate clinical data and an ability to be as efficacious as L-arginine in producing nitric oxide (NO) at lower dosages. Still requires more clinical research for ED, especially whether or not blood pressure reduction occurs rarely or commonly with higher dosages
MACA (*Lepidium meyenii*)	Not enough research but preliminary data in fertility or ED is promising and should continue
Panax ginseng (Korean Red ginseng and others)	Dosages of 800–3,000 mg (lower dosages with more concentrated ginsenoside products) have been used in multiple randomized trials to benefit men with mild to moderate ED. A consistent impact on libido could make this an option with conventional prescription agents. Cost may become an issue with concentrated ginsenoside products
SAM-e (*S*-adenosyl methionine)	May be used for the treatment of major depressive disorder (MDD) with and without SSRIs medication and has not been shown to reduce sexual function and may even provide a benefit, which is unusual for an anti-depressant. Dosages as high as 800 mg bid have been used but cost is an issue with this supplement
Tribulus terrestris	Not recommended. Suppose to act as a DHEA mimic but in general has not demonstrated any impressive testosterone-enhancing properties
Yohimbine hydrochloride	Not a true nutraceutical because all of the positive and adequate clinical trials used a prescription form of this compound. Yohimbe supplements claim to contain adequate amounts of the active compound (yohimbine HCL) but this has not been proven and in fact quality control and safety has been shown to be an issue with these over the counter products

on erectile health need more clinical research. The testosterone increases are statistically significant but arguably not clinically significant as of yet. Horny Goat Weed (Epimedium species) contains a compound(s) known as "icariin" that may have a PDE-5 like effect [232–234], but clinical research is needed because the majority of the impressive research was derived from basic science studies, but still it is also one clinicians should monitor. MACA (*Lepidium meyenii*) has some preliminary positive clinical data in fertility and ED, but needs more consistent research on standardization of active ingredients and efficacy, but is commonly used in other countries such as Peru [235, 236]. An overview of most nutraceutical products that are discussed in this chapter is provided in Table 12.5.

It is time to view fertility and erectile function nutraceuticals with a wider perspective because a plethora of research has been performed on numerous compounds. Large and authoritative meta-analyses actually endorsed the utilization of multiple products for men attempting to maintain or improve fertility and erectile function [19, 164]. However, before endorsement of a specific supplement becomes logical it would seem imperative to teach clinicians and patients about the overall safety and efficacy of these interventions outside of fertility and ED.

Current conventional options are not perfect and have a host of their own issues from side effects, efficacy and especially price as exemplified by the current cost of PDE-5 inhibitors for example or assisted reproductive technology. Thus, if a nutraceutical that is safe and heart healthy and cost effective can be utilized with or without a conventional agent then it should be embraced. This has arguably already occurred in the area of fertility but in the area of ED nutraceuticals the unctuous history of these products, including the highest rate of recall of any supplement category in FDA history [237], makes it difficult for some clinicians to appreciate the few truly efficacious products amongst a sea of ineffective and tainted products. It is my hope this chapter provided more objectivity to this issue and for clinicians and patients to appreciate a better sense of nutraceuticals that are worthwhile and others that are worthless. This is critical in my opinion, because it could be argued that clinicians are one of the last bastions of objectivity for those that require real answers to the questions that currently abound over nutraceuticals.

References

1. Moyad MA, Lowe FC. Educating patients about lifestyle modifications for prostate health. Am J Med. 2008;121(8 Suppl 2):S34–42.
2. Moyad MA. Heart health = urologic health and heart unhealthy = urologic unhealthy: rapid review of lifestyle changes and dietary supplements. Urol Clin North Am. 2011;38:359–67.
3. Cabler S, Agarwal A, Flint M, du Plessis SS. Obesity: modern man's fertility nemesis. Asian J Androl. 2010;12:480–9.
4. Yusuf S, Hawken S, Ounpuu S, et al. Effect of potentially modifiable risk factors associated with myocardial infarction in 52 countries (the INTERHEART study): case–control study. Lancet. 2004;364:937–52.
5. Eyre H, Kahn R, Robertson RM, et al for the ACS/ADA/AHA Collaborative Writing Committee. Preventing cancer, cardiovascular disease, and diabetes: a common agenda for the American Cancer Society, the American Diabetes Association, and the American Heart Association. CA Cancer J Clin. 2004;54:190–207.
6. Lloyd-Jones D, Adams RJ, Brown TM, Carnethon M, Dai S, de Simone G, et al for the American Heart Association Statistics Committee and Stroke Statistics Subcommittee. Heart disease and stroke statistics-2010 update: a report from the American Heart Association. Circulation. 2010;121:e46–215.
7. World Heart Federation web site. Available at: http://www.world-heart-federation.org. Accessed 20 Mar 2013.
8. Yang Q, Cogswell ME, Flanders WD, Hong Y, Zhang Z, Loustalot F, et al. Trends in cardiovascular health metrics and associations with all-cause and CVD mortality among US adults. JAMA. 2012;307:1273–83.
9. Kasturi SS, Tannir J, Brannigan RE. The metabolic syndrome and male infertility. J Androl. 2008;29:251–9.
10. Campagne DM. Should fertilization treatment start with reducing stress? Hum Reprod. 2006;21:1651–8.
11. Esposito K, Giugliano F, Di Palo C, Giugliano G, Marfella R, D'Andrea F, et al. Effect of lifestyle changes on erectile dysfunction in obese men. JAMA. 2004;291(24):2978–84.
12. Giugliano D, Giugliano F, Esposito K. Sexual dysfunction and the Mediterranean diet. Public Health Nutr. 2006;9:1118–20.

13. Jensen TK, Heitmann BL, Jensen MB, Halldorsson TI, Andersson AM, Skakkebaek NE, et al. High dietary intake of saturated fat is associated with reduced semen quality among 701 young Danish men from the general population. Am J Clin Nutr. 2013;97:411–8.
14. Gaskins AJ, Colaci DS, Mendiola J, Swan SH, Chavarro JE. Dietary patterns and semen quality in young men. Hum Reprod. 2012;27:2899–907.
15. Saez Lancellotti TE, Boarelli PV, Romero AA, Funes AK, Cid-Barria M, et al. Semen quality and sperm function loss by hypercholesterolemic diet was recovered by addition of olive oil to diet in rabbit. PLoS One. 2013;8:e52386.
16. Oliveira RM, Novaes JF, Azeredo LM, Candido AP, Leite IC. Association of vitamin D insufficiency with adiposity and metabolic disorders in Brazilian adolescents. Public Health Nutr. 2013;9:1–8.
17. Di Martino G, Matera MG, De Martino B, Vacca C, Di Martino S, Rossi F. Relationship between zinc and obesity. J Med. 1993;24:177–83.
18. Tremellen K. Oxidative stress and male infertility—a clinical perspective. Hum Reprod Update. 2008;14:243–58.
19. Showell MG, Brown J, Yazdani A, Stankiewicz MT, Hart RJ. Antioxidants for male subfertility. Cochrane Database Syst Rev. 2011;1, CD007411.
20. Littarru GP, Tiano L. Clinical aspects of coenzyme Q10: an update. Nutrition. 2010;26:250–4.
21. Wyman M, Leonard M, Morledge T. Coenzyme Q10: a therapy for hypertension and statin-induced myalgia? Cleve Clin J Med. 2010;77:435–42.
22. Bogsrud MP, Langslet G, Ose L, Arnesen KE, Sm Stuen MC, Malt UF, et al. No effect of combined coenzyme Q10 and selenium supplementation on atorvastatin-induced myopathy. Scand Cardiovasc J. 2013;47(2):80–7.
23. Balercia G, Buldreghini E, Vignini A, Tiano L, Paggi F, Amoroso S, et al. Coenzyme Q10 treatment in infertile men with idiopathic asthenozoospermia: a placebo-controlled randomized trial. Fertil Steril. 2009;91:1785–92.
24. Safarinejad ME. Efficacy of coenzyme Q10 on semen parameters, sperm function and reproductive hormones in infertile men. J Urol. 2009;182:237–48.
25. Nadjarzadeh A, Sadeghi MR, Amirjannati N, Vafa MR, Motevalian SA, Gohari MR, et al. Coenzyme Q10 improves seminal oxidative defense but does not affect on semen parameters in idiopathic oligoasthenoteratozoospermia: a randomized double-blind, placebo-controlled trial. J Endocrinol Invest. 2011;34:e224–8.
26. Mousa SA. Antithrombotic effects of naturally derived products on coagulation and platelet function. Methods Mol Biol. 2010;663:229–40.
27. Young JM, Florkowski CM, Molyneux SL, McEwan RG, Frampton CM, Nicholis MG, et al. A randomized, double-blind, placebo-controlled crossover study of coenzyme Q10 therapy in hypertensive patients with the metabolic syndrome. Am J Hypertens. 2012;25:261–70.
28. National Institute of Neurological Disorders and Stroke. Statement on the termination of QE3 Study. www.ninds.nih.gov/disorders/clinical_trials/CoQ10-Trial-Update.htm. Accessed 15 Feb 2013.
29. Liu J, Wang L, Zhan SY, Xia Y. Coenzyme Q10 for Parkinson's disease. Cochrane Database Syst Rev. 2011;12, CD008150.
30. Mancini A, De Marinis L, Littarru GP, Balercia G. An update of Coenzyme Q10 implications in male infertility: biochemical and therapeutic aspects. Biofactors. 2005;25:165–74.
31. Acetyl-L-carnitine. Monograph. Altern Med Rev. 2010;15:76–83.
32. Cruciani RA, Zhang JJ, Manola J, Cella D, Ansari B, Fisch MJ. L-Carnitine supplementation for the management of fatigue in patients with cancer: an eastern cooperative oncology group phase III, randomized, double-blind, placebo-controlled trial. J Clin Oncol. 2012;30:3864–9.
33. Kraft M, Kraft K, Gartner S, Mayerle J, Simon P, Weber E, et al. L-Carnitine-supplementation in advanced pancreatic cancer (CARPAN)—a randomized multicenter trial. Nutr J. 2012;11:52.

34. Goldenberg NA, Krantz MJ, Hiatt WR. L-Carnitine plus cilostazol versus cilostazol alone for the treatment of claudication in patients with peripheral artery disease: a multicenter, randomized, double-blind, placebo-controlled trial. Vasc Med. 2012;17:145–54.
35. Balercia G, Regoli F, Armeni T, Koverech A, Mantero F, Boscaro M. Placebo-controlled double-blind randomized trial on the use of L-carnitine, L-acetylcarnitine, or combined L-carnitine and L-acetylcarnitine in men with idiopathic asthenozoospermia. Fertil Steril. 2005;84:662–71.
36. Lenzi A, Sgro P, Salacone P, Paoli D, Gillio B, Lombardo F, et al. A placebo-controlled double-blind randomized trial of the use of combination l-carnitine and l-acetyl-carnitine treatment in men with asthenozoospermia. Fertil Steril. 2004;81:1578–84.
37. Lenzi A, Lombardo F, Sgro P, Salacone P, Caponecchia L, Dondero F, et al. Use of carnitine therapy in selected cases of male factor infertility: a double-blind crossover trial. Fertil Steril. 2003;79:292–300.
38. Li Z, Chen GW, Shang XJ, Bal WJ, Han YF, et al. A controlled randomized trial of the use of combined L-carnitine and acetyl-L-carnitine treatment in men with oligoasthenozoospermia. Zhonghua Nan Ke Xue. 2005;11:761–4.
39. Cavallini G, Ferraretti AP, Gianaroli L, Biagiotti G, Vitali G. Cinnoxicam and L-carnitine/acetyl-L-carnitine treatment for idiopathic and varicocele-associated oligoasthenospermia. J Androl. 2004;25:761–70.
40. Moncada ML, Vivari E, Cimino C, Calogero AE, Monglol A, D'Agata R. Effect of acetylcarnitine treatment in oligoasthenospermic patients. Acta Eur Fertil. 1992;23:221–4.
41. Costa M, Canale D, Filicori M, D'lddio S, Lenzi A. L-Carnitine in idiopathic asthenozoospermia: a multicenter study. Italian Study Group on carnitine and male infertility. Andrologia. 1994;26:155–9.
42. Vitali G, Parente R, Melotti C. Carnitine supplementation in human idiopathic asthenospermia: clinical results. Drugs Exp Clin Res. 1995;21:157–9.
43. Vicari E, Calogero AE. Effects of treatment with carnitines in infertile patients with prostato-vesciculo-epididymitis. Hum Reprod. 2001;16:2338–42.
44. Sigman M, Glass S, Campagnone J, Pryor JL. Carnitine for the treatment of idiopathic asthenospermia: a randomized, double-blind, placebo-controlled trial. Fertil Steril. 2006;85:1409–14.
45. Zhou X, Liu F, Zhai S. Effect of L-carnitine and/or L-acetyl-carnitine in nutrition treatment for male infertility: a systematic review. Asia Pac J Clin Nutr. 2007;16 Suppl 1:383–90.
46. Koeth RA, Wang Z, Levison BS, Buffa JA, Org E, Sheehy BT, et al. Intestinal microbiota metabolism of L-carnitine, a nutrient in red meat, promotes atherosclerosis. Nat Med. 2013;19:576–85.
47. Dinicolantonio JJ, Lavie CJ, Fares H, Menezes AR, O'Keefe JH. L-Carnitine in the secondary prevention of cardiovascular disease: systematic review and meta-analysis. Mayo Clin Proc. 2013;88:544–51.
48. Hershman DL, Unger JM, Crew KD, Minasian LM, Awad D, Moinpour CM, et al. Randomized double-blind placebo-controlled trial of acetyl-l-carnitine for the prevention of taxane-induced neuropathy in women undergoing adjuvant breast cancer therapy. J Clin Oncol. 2013;31(20):2627–33.
49. Moyad MA. Dr. Moyad's no bogus science health advice. Ann Arbor, MI: Ann Arbor Editions Publishing; 2009.
50. Burr ML, Fehlly AM, Gilbert JF, Rogers S, Holliday RM, Sweetnam PM, et al. Effects of changes in fat, fish, and fibre intakes on death and myocardial reinfarction: diet and reinfarction trial (DART). Lancet. 1989;2:757–61.
51. Marchioli R, Barzi F, Bomba E, Chieffo C, Di Mascio R, Franzosi MG, et al. Early protection against sudden cardiac death by n-3 polyunsaturated fatty acids after myocardial infarction: time-course analysis of the results of the Gruppo Italiano per lo Studio della Sopravvivenza nell'Infarto Miocardico (GISSI)-Prevenzione. Circulation. 2002;105:1897–903.

52. Matsuzaki M, Yokoyama M, Saito Y, Origasa H, IshikawaY, Oikawa S, et al for the JELIS investigators. Incremental effects of eicosapentaenoic acid on cardiovascular events in statin-treated patients with coronary artery disease. Circ J. 2009;73:1283–90.
53. Mozaffarian D, Marchioli R, Macchia A, Silleta MG, Ferrazzi P, Gardner TJ, et al for the OPERA Investigators. Fish oil and postoperative atrial fibrillation: the omega-3 fatty acids for prevention of post-operative atrial fibrillation (OPERA) randomized trial. JAMA. 2012;308:2001–11.
54. Rizos EC, Ntzani EE, Bika E, Kostapanos MS, Elisaf MS. Association between omega-3 fatty acid supplementation and risk of major cardiovascular disease events: a systematic review and meta-analysis. JAMA. 2012;308:1024–33.
55. Risk and Prevention Study Collaborative Group. N-3 fatty acids in patients with multiple cardiovascular risk factors. N Engl J Med. 2013;368:1800–8.
56. Age-Related Eye Disease Study 2 Research Group. Lutein + zeaxanthin and omega-3 fatty acids for age-related macular degeneration: the age-related eye disease study 2 (AREDS2) randomized clinical trial. JAMA. 2013;309:2005–15.
57. Conquer JA, Martin JB, Tummon I, Watson L, Tekpetey F. Effect of DHA supplementation on DHA status and sperm motility in asthenozoospermic males. Lipids. 2000;35:149–54.
58. Safarinejad MR. Effect of omega-3 polyunsaturated fatty acid supplementation on semen profile and enzymatic anti-oxidant capacity of seminal plasma in infertile men with idiopathic oligoasthenoteratospermia: a double-blind, placebo-controlled, randomized study. Andrologia. 2011;43:38–47.
59. Tambi MI, Imran MK, Henkel RR. Standardized water-soluble extract of Eurycoma longifolia, Tongkat ali, as testosterone booster for managing men with late-onset hypogonadism. Andrologia. 2012;44 Suppl 1:226–30.
60. Ismall SB, Wan Mohammad WM, George A, Nik Hussain NH, Musthapa Kamal ZM, Liske E. Randomized clinical trial on the use of PHYSTA freeze-dried water extract on Eurycoma longifolia for the improvement of quality of life and sexual well-being in men. Evid Based Complement Alternat Med. 2012;2012:429268.
61. Tambi MI, Imran MK. Eurycoma longifolia Jack in managing idiopathic male infertility. Asian J Androl. 2010;12:376–80.
62. Low BS, Das PK, Chan KL. Standardized quassinoid-rich Eurycoma longifolia extract improved spermatogenesis and fertility in male rats via the hypothalamic-pituitary-gonadal axis. J Ethnopharmacol. 2013;13(145):706–14.
63. Erasmus N, Solomon MC, Fortuin KA, Henkel RR. Effect of Eurycoma longifolia Jack (Tongkat ali) extract on human spermatozoa in vitro. Andrologia. 2012;44:308–14.
64. Wahab NA, Mokhtar NM, Halim WN, Das S. The effect of Eurycoma longifolia Jack on spermatogenesis in estrogen-treated rats. Clinics (Sao Paulo). 2010;65:93–8.
65. Chan KL, Low BS, The CH, Das PK. The effect of Eurycoma longifolia on sperm quality of male rats. Nat Prod Commun. 2009;4:1331–6.
66. Chua LS, Abdul-Rahman N, Rosidi B, Lee CT. Plant proteins, minerals and trace elements of Eurycoma longifolia (Tongkat Ali). Nat Prod Res. 2013;27(4–5):314–8.
67. Henkel RR, Wang R, Bassett SH, Chen T, Liu N, Zhu Y, Tambi MI. Tongkat Ali as a potential herbal supplement for physically active male and female seniors—a pilot study. Phytother Res. 2013; epub ahead of print.
68. Abel BJ, Carswell G, Elton R, Hargreave TB, Kyle K, Orr S, et al. Randomised trial of clomiphene citrate treatment and vitamin C for male infertility. Br J Urol. 1982;54:780–4.
69. Hargreave TB, Kyle KF, Baxby K, Rogers AC, Scott R, Tolley DA, et al. Randomised trial of mesterolone versus vitamin C for male infertility. Scottish Infertility Group. Br J Urol. 1984;56:740–4.
70. Rolf C, Cooper TG, Yeung CH, Nieschlag E. Antioxidant treatment of patients with asthenozoospermia or moderate oligoasthenozoospermia with high dose vitamin C and vitamin E: a randomized, placebo-controlled, double-blind study. Hum Reprod. 1999;14:1028–33.

71. Colagar AH, Marzony ET. Ascorbic acid in human seminal plasma: determination and its relationship to sperm quality. J Clin Biochem Nutr. 2009;45:144–9.
72. Fraga CG, Motchnik PA, Shigenaga MK, Helbock HJ, Jacob RA, Ames BN. Ascorbic acid protects against endogenous oxidative DNA damage in human sperm. Proc Natl Acad Sci U S A. 1991;88:11003–6.
73. Dawson EB, Harris WA, Powell LC. Relationship between ascorbic acid and male fertility. World Rev Nutr Diet. 1990;62:1–26.
74. Mostafa T, Tawadrous G, Roala MM, Amer MK, Kader RA, Aziz A. Effect of smoking on seminal plasma ascorbic acid in infertile and fertile males. Andrologia. 2006;38:221–4.
75. Dawson EB, Harris WA, Teter MC, Powell LC. Effect of ascorbic acid supplementation on the sperm quality of smokers. Fertil Steril. 1992;58:1034–9.
76. Vitamin C content in foods. http://www.vitamincfoundation.org/usda.html. Accessed 10 Feb 2013.
77. Thomas LD, Ellinder CG, Tiselius HG, Wolk A, Akesson A. Ascorbic acid supplements and kidney stone incidence among men: a prospective study. JAMA Intern Med. 2013;173:386–8.
78. Fletcher RH. The risk of taking ascorbic acid. JAMA Intern Med. 2013;173:388–9.
79. Moyad MA, Combs MA, Baisley JE, Evans M. Vitamin C with metabolites: additional analysis suggests favorable changes in oxalate. Urol Nurs. 2009;29:383–5.
80. Busetto GM, Koverech A, Messano M, Antonini G, De Berardinis E, Gentile V. Prospective open-label study on the efficacy and tolerability of a combination of nutritional supplements in primary infertile patients with idiopathic asthenoteratozoospermia. Arch Ital Urol Androl. 2012;84:137–40.
81. Gaziano JM, Sesso HD, Christen WG, Bubes V, Smith JP, MacFadyen J, et al. Multivitamins in the prevention of cancer in men: the Physicians' Health Study II randomized controlled trial. JAMA. 2012;308:1871–80.
82. Sesso HD, Christen WG, Bubes V, Smith JP, MacFadyen J, Schvartz M, et al. Multivitamins in the prevention of cardiovascular disease in men: the Physicians' Health Study II randomized controlled trial. JAMA. 2012;308:1751–60.
83. Singh AK, Tiwari AK, Singh PB, Dwivedi US, Trivedi S, Singh SK, et al. Multivitamin and micronutrient treatment improves semen parameters of azoospermic patients with maturation arrest. Indian J Physiol Pharmacol. 2010;54:157–63.
84. Obican SG, Finnell RH, Mills JL, Shaw GM, Scialli AR. Folic acid in early pregnancy: a public health success story. FASEB J. 2010;24:4167–74.
85. Zeisel SH. Importance of methyl donors during reproduction. Am J Clin Nutr. 2009;89:673S–7.
86. Institute of Medicine. Food and Nutrition Board. Folate, Dietary reference intakes for thiamin, riboflavin, niacin, vitamin B6, folate, vitamin B12, pantothenic acid, biotin, and choline. Washington, DC: National Academy Press; 2000. p. 196–305.
87. Winkels RM, Brouwer IA, Siebelink E, Katan MB, Verhoef P. Bioavailability of food folates is 80% of that of folic acid. Am J Clin Nutr. 2007;85:465–73.
88. Clarke R, Halsey J, Lewington S, Lonn E, Armitage J, Manson JE, et al for the B-vitamin Treatment Trialists' Collaboration. Effects of lowering homocysteine levels with B vitamins on cardiovascular disease, cancer, and cause-specific mortality. Meta-analysis of 8 randomized trials involving 37,485 individuals. Arch Intern Med. 2010;170:1622–31.
89. Cole BF, Baron JA, Sandler RS, Halle RW, Ahnen DJ, Bresaller RS, et al for Polyp Prevention Study Group. Folic acid for the prevention of colorectal adenomas: a randomized clinical trial. JAMA. 2007;297:2351–359.
90. Gao QY, Chen HM, Chen YX, Wang YC, Wang ZH, Tang JT, et al. Folic acid prevents the initial occurrence of sporadic colorectal adenoma in Chinese older than 50 years of age: a randomized clinical trial. Cancer Prev Res (Phila). 2013;6(7):744–52.
91. Figueriredo JC, Grau MV, Haile RW, Sandler RS, Summers RW, Bresalier RS, et al. Folic acid and risk of prostate cancer: results from a randomized clinical trial. J Natl Cancer Inst. 2009;101:432–5.

92. Collin SM, Metcalfe C, Refsum H, Lewis SJ, Zuccolo L, Smith GD, et al. Circulating folate, vitamin B12, homocysteine, vitamin B12 transport proteins, and risk of prostate cancer: a case-control study, systematic review, and meta-analysis. Cancer Epidemiol Biomarkers Prev. 2010;19:1632–42.
93. Balley RL, Millis JL, Yetley EA, Gahche JJ, Pfeiffer CM, Dwyer JT, et al. Unmetabolized serum folic acid and its relation to folic acid intake from diet and supplements in a nationally representative sample of adults aged > or =60 y in the United States. Am J Clin Nutr. 2010;92:383–9.
94. Wien TN, Pike E, Wisloff T, Staff A, Smeland S, Klemp M. Cancer risk with folic acid supplements: a systematic review and meta-analysis. BMJ Open. 2012;2(1):e000653.
95. Vollset SE, Clarke R, Lewington S, Ebbing M, Halsey J, Lonn E, et al. Effects of folic acid supplementation on overall and site-specific cancer incidence during the randomized trials: meta-analyses of data on 50,000 individuals. Lancet. 2013;381:1029–36.
96. Qin X, Cui Y, Shen L, Sun N, Zhang Y, Li J, et al. Folic acid supplementation and cancer risk: a meta-analysis of randomized controlled trials. Int J Cancer. 2013;133(5):1033–41.
97. Bassett JK, Severi G, Hodge AM, Baglietto L, Hopper JL, English DR, et al. Dietary intake of B vitamins and methionine and prostate cancer incidence and mortality. Cancer Causes Control. 2012;23:855–63.
98. Miller JW, Ulrich CM. Folic acid and cancer—where are we today? Lancet. 2013;381:974–6.
99. Wong WY, Merkus HM, Thomas CM, Menkveld R, Zielhuis GA, Steegers-Theunissen RP. Effects of folic acid and zinc sulfate on male factor subfertility: a double-blind, randomized, placebo-controlled trial. Fertil Steril. 2002;77:491–8.
100. Murphy LE, Mills JL, Molloy AM, Qian C, Carter TC, Strevens H, et al. Folate and vitamin B12 in idiopathic male infertility. Asian J Androl. 2011;13:856–61.
101. Lippman SM, Klein EA, Goodman PJ, Lucia MS, Thompson IM, Ford LG, et al. Effect of selenium and vitamin E on risk of prostate cancer and other cancers: the selenium and vitamin E cancer prevention trial (SELECT). JAMA. 2009;301:39–51.
102. Klein EA, Thompson Jr IM, Tangen CM, Crowley JJ, Lucia MS, Goodman PJ, et al. Vitamin E and the risk of prostate cancer: the selenium and vitamin E cancer prevention trial (SELECT). JAMA. 2011;306:1549–56.
103. Duffield-Lillico AJ, Slate EH, Reid ME, Turnbull BW, Wilkins PA, Combs GF Jr, et al for the Nutritional Prevention of Cancer Study Group. Selenium supplementation and secondary prevention of nonmelanoma skin cancer in a randomized trial. J Natl Cancer Inst. 2003;95:1477–81.
104. Stranges S, Marshall JR, Natarajan R, Donahue RP, Trevisan M, Combs GF, et al. Effects of long-term selenium supplementation on the incidence of type 2 diabetes: a randomized trial. Ann Intern Med. 2007;147:217–23.
105. Miller III ER, Pastor-Barriuso R, Dalal D, Riemersma RA, Appel LJ, Guallar E. Meta-analysis: high-dosage vitamin E supplementation may increase all-cause mortality. Ann Intern Med. 2005;142:37–46.
106. Lonn E, Bosch J, Yusuf S, Sheridan P, Pogue J, Arnold JM, et al for the HOPE and HOPE TOO Trial Investigators. Effects of long-term vitamin E supplementation on cardiovascular events and cancer: a randomized controlled trial. JAMA. 2005;293:1338–47.
107. Sesso HD, Buring JE, Christen WG, Kurth T, Belanger C, MacFadyen J, et al. Vitamins E and C in the prevention of cardiovascular disease in men: the Physicians' Health Study II randomized controlled trial. JAMA. 2008;300:2123–33.
108. Stranges S, Marshall JR, Trevisan M, Natarajan R, Donahue RP, Combs GF, et al. Effects of selenium supplementation on cardiovascular disease incidence and mortality: secondary analyses in a randomized clinical trial. Am J Epidemiol. 2006;163:694–9.
109. Neve J. Selenium as a risk factor for cardiovascular diseases. J Cardiovasc Risk. 1996;3:42–7.
110. Moyad MA. Selenium and vitamin E supplements for prostate cancer: evidence or embellishment? Urology. 2002;59(4 Suppl 1):9–19.

111. Pearson P, Lewis SA, Britton J, Young IS, Fogarty A. The pro-oxidant activity of high-dose vitamin E supplements in vivo. BioDrugs. 2006;20:271–3.
112. Rayman MP. Selenium and human health. Lancet. 2012;379:1256–68.
113. MacFarquhar JK, Broussard DL, Melstrom P, Hutchinson R, Wolkin A, Martin C, et al. Acute selenium toxicity associated with a dietary supplement. Arch Intern Med. 2010;170(3):256–61.
114. Diskin CJ, Tomasso CL, Alper JC, Glaser ML, Fliegel SE. Long-term selenium exposure. Arch Intern Med. 1979;139:824–6.
115. Keskes-Ammar L, Feki-Chakroun N, Rebai T, Sahnoun Z, Ghozzi H, Hammami S, et al. Sperm oxidative stress and the effect of an oral vitamin E and selenium supplement on semen quality in infertile men. Arch Androl. 2003;49:83–94.
116. Kessopoulou E, Powers HJ, Sharma KK, Pearson MJ, Russell JM, Cooke ID, et al. A double-blind randomized placebo cross-over controlled trial using the antioxidant vitamin E to treat reactive oxygen species associated with male infertility. Fertil Steril. 1995;64:825–31.
117. Safarinejad MR, Safarinejad S. Efficacy of selenium and/or N-acetyl-cysteine for improving semen parameters in infertile men: a double-blind, placebo controlled, randomized study. J Urol. 2009;181:741–51.
118. Omu AE, Dashti H, Al-Othman S. Treatment of asthenozoospermia with zinc sulphate: andrological, immunological and obstetric outcome. Eur J Obstet Gynecol Reprod Biol. 1998;79:179–84.
119. Netter A, Hartoma R, Nahoul K. Effect of zinc administration on plasma testosterone, dihydrotestosterone, and sperm count. Arch Androl. 1981;7:69–73.
120. Food and Nutrition Board, National Academy of Sciences. Dietary reference intakes for vitamin A, vitamin K, arsenic, boron, chromium, copper, iodine, iron, manganese, molybdenum, nickel, silicon, vanadium, and zinc. Washington DC: National Academy Press; 2001. p. 177–204. 351–98.
121. Moyad MA. Zinc for prostate disease and other conditions: a little evidence, a lot of hype, and a significant potential problem. Urol Nurs. 2004;24:49–52.
122. Leitzmann MF, Stampfer MJ, Wu K, Colditz GA, Willett WC, Giovannucci EL. Zinc supplement use and risk of prostate cancer. J Natl Cancer Inst. 2003;96:1004–7.
123. Age-Related Eye Disease Study Research Group. A randomized, placebo-controlled, clinical trial of high-dose supplementation with vitamins C and E, beta-carotene, and zinc for age-related macular degeneration and vision loss: AREDS Report Number 8. Arch Ophthalmol. 2001;119:1417–36.
124. Johnson AR, Munoz A, Gottlieb JL, Jarrard DF. High dose zinc increases hospital admissions due to genitourinary complications. J Urol. 2007;177:639–43.
125. Health Canada Website. Multi-vitamin/Mineral Supplements. http://www.hc-sc.gc.ca/dhp-mps/prodnatur/applications/licen-prod/monograph/multi_vitmin_suppl-eng.php. Accessed 10 Nov 2012.
126. Science M, Johnstone J, Roth DE, Guyatt G, Loeb M. Zinc for the treatment of the common cold: a systematic review and meta-analysis of randomized controlled trials. CMAJ. 2012;184:551–61.
127. AREDS2 Research Group, Chew EY, Clemons T, SanGiovanni JP, Danis R, Domalpally A, McBee W, et al. The age-related eye disease study 2 (AREDS2): study design and baseline characteristics (AREDS2 report number 1). Ophthalmology. 2012;119:2282–9.
128. Dong J-Y, Qin L-Q, Zhang Z, Zhao Y, Wang J, Arigoni F, et al. Effect of oral L-arginine supplementation on blood pressure: a meta-analysis of randomized, double-blind, placebo-controlled trials. Am Heart J. 2011;162:959–65.
129. Vadillo-Ortega F, Perichart-Perera O, Espino S, Avila-Vergara MA, Ibarra I, Ahued R, et al. Effect of supplementation during pregnancy with L-arginine and antioxidant vitamins in medical food on pre-eclampsia in high risk population: randomized controlled trial. BMJ. 2011;342:d2901.

130. Gui S, Jia J, Niu X, Bai Y, Zou H, Deng J, et al. Arginine supplementation for improving maternal and neonatal outcomes in hypertensive disorder of pregnancy: a systematic review. J Renin Angiotensin Aldosterone Syst. 2013; epub ahead of print.
131. Morris Jr SM. Enzymes of arginine metabolism. J Nutr. 2004;134(10 Suppl):2743S–7.
132. Morris Jr SM. Arginases and arginine deficiency syndromes. Curr Opin Clin Nutr Metab Care. 2012;15:64–70.
133. Castillo L, de Rojas TC, Chapman TE, Vogt J, Burke JF, Tannenbaum SR, et al. Splanchnic metabolism of dietary arginine in relation to nitric oxide synthesis in normal adult man. Proc Natl Acad Sci U S A. 1993;90:193–7.
134. Boger RH. Asymmetric dimethylarginine, an endogenous inhibitor of nitric oxide synthase, explains the L-arginine paradox and acts as novel cardiovascular risk factor. J Nutr. 2004;134:2842S–7.
135. Paroni R, Barassi A, Ciociola F, Dozio E, Finati E, Fermo I, et al. Asymmetric dimethylarginine (ADMA), symmetric dimethylarginine (SDMA) and arginine in patients with arteriogenic and non-arteriogenic erectile dysfunction. Int J Androl. 2012;35:660–7.
136. Bescos R, Gonzalez-Haro C, Pujol P, Drobnic F, Alonso E, Santolaria ML, et al. Effects of dietary L-arginine intake on cardiorespiratory and metabolic adaptation in athletes. Int J Sport Nutr Exerc Metab. 2009;19:355–65.
137. Bescos R, Sureda A, Tur JA, Pons A. The effect of nitric-oxide-related supplements on human performance. Sports Med. 2012;42:99–117.
138. Klotz T, Mathers MJ, Braun M, Bloch W, Engelmann U. Effectiveness of oral L-arginine in first-line treatment of erectile dysfunction in a controlled crossover study. Urol Int. 1999;63:220–3.
139. Chen J, Wollman Y, Chernichovsky T, Iaina A, Sofer M, Matzkin H. Effect of oral administration of high-dose nitric oxide donor L-arginine in men with organic erectile dysfunction: results of a double-blind, randomized, placebo-controlled study. BJU Int. 1999;83(3):269–73.
140. Stanislavov R, Nikolova V. Treatment of erectile dysfunction with Pycnogenol and L-arginine. J Sex Marital Ther. 2003;29:207–13.
141. Stanislavov R, Nikolova V, Rohdewald P. Improvement of erectile function with Prelox: a randomized, double-blind, placebo-controlled, crossover trial. Int J Impot Res. 2008;20:173–80.
142. Ledda A, Belcaro G, Cesarone MR, Dugall M, Schonlau F. Investigation of a complex plant extract for mild to moderate erectile dysfunction in a randomized, double-blind, placebo-controlled parallel-arm study. BJU Int. 2010;106:1030–3.
143. Schulman SP, Becker LC, Kass DA, Champion HC, Terrin ML, Forman S, et al. L-Arginine therapy in acute myocardial infarction: the vascular interaction with age in myocardial infarction (VINTAGE MI) randomized clinical trial. JAMA. 2006;295:58–64.
144. Wilson AM, Harada R, Nair N, Balasubramanlan N, Cooke JP. L-Arginine supplementation in peripheral arterial disease: no benefit and possible harm. Circulation. 2007;116:188–95.
145. Bednarz B, Jaxa-Chamiec T, Maciewjewski P, Szpajer M, Janik K, Gniot J, et al. Efficacy and safety of oral L-arginine in acute myocardial infarction. Results of multicenter, randomized, placebo-controlled ARAMI pilot trial. Kardiol Pol. 2005;62:421–6.
146. Oka RK, Szuba A, Giacomini JC, Cooke JP. A pilot study of L-arginine supplementation on functional capacity in peripheral artery disease. Vasc Med. 2005;10:265–74.
147. Schwedhelm E, Maas R, Freese R, Jung D, Lukacs Z, Jambrecina A, et al. Pharmacokinetic and pharmacodynamic properties of oral L-citrulline and L-arginine: impact on nitric oxide metabolism. Br J Clin Pharmacol. 2008;65:51–9.
148. Cormio L, De Siati M, Lorusso F, Selvaggio O, Mirabella L, Sanguedolce F, et al. Oral L-citrulline supplementation improves erection hardness in men with mild erectile dysfunction. Urology. 2011;77:119–22.

149. Rouge C, Des Robert C, Robins A, Le Bacquer O, Volteau C, De La Cochetiere MF, et al. Manipulation of citrulline availability in humans. Am J Physiol Gastrointest Liver Physiol. 2007;293:G1061–7.
150. Moinard C, Nicolis I, Neveux N, Darquy S, Benazeth S, Cynober L. Dose-ranging effects of citrulline administration on plasma amino acids and hormonal patterns in healthy subjects: the Citrudose pharmacokinetic study. Br J Nutr. 2008;99:855–62.
151. Figueroa A, Sanchez-Gonzalez MA, Wong A, Arjmandi BH. Watermelon extract supplementation reduces ankle blood pressure and carotid augmentation index in obese adults with prehypertension or hypertension. Am J Hypertens. 2012;25:640–3.
152. Marietta M, Facchinetti F, Neri I, Piccinini F, Volpe A, Torelli G. L-Arginine infusion decreases platelet aggregation through an intraplatelet nitric oxide release. Thromb Res. 1997;88:229–35.
153. Moyad MA. Dr Moyad's guide to male sexual health: what works and what's worthless? Ann Arbor, MI: Spry publishing; 2012.
154. Choi KT. Botanical characteristics, pharmacological effects and medicinal components of Korean Panax ginseng C A Meyer. Acta Pharmacol Sin. 2008;29:1109–18.
155. Yue PY, Mak NK, Cheng YK, Leung KW, Ng TB, Fan DT, et al. Pharmacogenomics and the Yin/Yang actions of ginseng: anti-tumor, angiomodulating and steroid-like activities of ginsenosides. Chin Med. 2007;2:6.
156. Lee DC, Lau AS. Effects of Panax ginseng on tumor necrosis factor-alpha-mediated inflammation: a mini-review. Molecules. 2011;16:2802–16.
157. Chu SF, Zhang JT. New achievements in ginseng research and its future prospects. Chin J Integr Med. 2009;15:403–8.
158. Kiefer D, Pantuso T. Panax ginseng. Am Fam Physician. 2003;68:1539–42.
159. Christensen LP. Ginsenosides chemistry, biosynthesis, analysis, and potential health effects. Adv Food Nutr Res. 2009;55:1–99.
160. Attele AS, Wu JA, Yuan CS. Ginseng pharmacology: multiple constituents and multiple actions. Biochem Pharmacol. 1999;58:1685–93.
161. Jia L, Zhao Y. Current evaluation of the millennium phytomedicine-ginseng (I): etymology, pharmacognosy, phytochemistry, market and regulations. Curr Med Chem. 2009;16:2475–84.
162. Bucci LR. Selected herbals and human exercise performance. Am J Clin Nutr. 2000;72 (Suppl):624S–34.
163. Jovanovski E, Jenkins A, Dias AG, Peeva V, Sievenpiper J, Arnason JT, et al. Effects of Korean red ginseng (Panax ginseng C.A. Mayer) and its isolated ginsenosides and polysaccharides on arterial stiffness in healthy individuals. Am J Hypertens. 2010;23:469–72.
164. Khera M, Goldstein I. Erectile dysfunction. Clin Evid (online), released June 29, 2011.
165. Ham WS, Kim WT, Lee JS, Ju HJ, Kang SJ, Oh JH, et al. Efficacy and safety of red ginseng extract powder in patients with erectile dysfunction: multicenter, randomized, double-blind, placebo-controlled study. Korean J Urol. 2009;50(2):159–64.
166. Jang DJ, Soo Lee M, Shin B-C, Lee Y-C, Ernst E. Red ginseng for treating erectile dysfunction: a systematic review. Br J Clin Pharmacol. 2008;66:444–50.
167. Kim H, Chen X, Gillis CN. Ginsenosides protect pulmonary vascular endothelium against free radical-induced injury. Biochem Biophys Res Commun. 1992;189:670–6.
168. Chen X, Lee TJ. Ginsenosides-induced nitric oxide-mediated relaxation of the rabbit corpus cavernosum. Br J Pharmacol. 1995;115:15–8.
169. Chen X. Cardiovascular protection by ginsenosides and their nitric oxide releasing action. Clin Exp Pharmacol Physiol. 1996;23:728–32.
170. Choi YD, Xin ZC, Choi HK. Effect of Korean red ginseng on the rabbit corpus cavernosal smooth muscle. Int J Impot Res. 1998;10:37–43.
171. Choi YD, Rha KH, Choi HK. In vitro and in vivo experimental effect of Korean red ginseng on erection. J Urol. 1999;162:1508–11.

172. Kim HJ, Woo DS, Lee G, Kim JJ. The relaxation effects of ginseng saponin in rabbit corporal smooth muscle: is it a nitric oxide donor? Br J Urol. 1998;82:744–8.
173. Kimura T, Saunders PA, Kim HS, Rheu HM, Oh KW, Ho IK. Interactions of ginsenosides with ligand-bindings of GABA(A) and GABA(B) receptors. Gen Pharmacol. 1994;25:193–9.
174. Park JH, Cha HY, Seo JJ, Hong JT, Han K, Oh KW. Anxiolytic-like effects of ginseng in the elevated plus-maze model: comparison of red ginseng and sun ginseng. Prog Neuropsychopharmacol Biol Psychiatry. 2005;29:895–900.
175. Watanabe H, Ohta H, Imamura L, Asakura W, Matoba Y, Matsumoto K. Effect of Panax ginseng on age-related changes in the spontaneous motor activity and dopaminergic nervous system in the rat. Jpn J Pharmacol. 1991;55:51–6.
176. de Andrade E, de Mesquita AA, Claro Jde A, de Andrade PM, Ortiz V, Paranhos M, et al. Study of the efficacy of Korean red ginseng in the treatment of erectile dysfunction. Asian J Androl. 2007;9:241–4.
177. Siegel RK. Ginseng abuse syndrome. Problems with the panacea. JAMA. 1979;241:1614–5.
178. Baldwin CA, Anderson LA, Phillipson JA. What pharmacists should know about ginseng. Pharm J. 1986;237:583–6.
179. Miller LG. Herbal medicinals: selected clinical considerations focusing on known or potential drug-herb interactions. Arch Intern Med. 1998;158:2200–11.
180. Klepser TB, Klepser ME. Unsafe and potentially safe herbal therapies. Am J Health Syst Pharm. 1999;56:125–41.
181. Stavro PM, Woo M, Heim TF, Leiter LA, Vuksan V. North American ginseng exerts a neutral effect on blood pressure in individuals with hypertension. Hypertension. 2005;46:406–11.
182. Stavro PM, Woo M, Leiter LA, Heim TF, Sievenpiper JL, Vuksan V. Long-term intake of North American ginseng has no effect on 24-hour blood pressure and renal function. Hypertension. 2006;47:791–6.
183. Caron MF, Hotsko AL, Robertson S, Mandybur L, Kluger J, White CM. Electrocardiographic and hemodynamic effects of Panax ginseng. Ann Pharmacother. 2002;36:758–63.
184. Han JH, Choe SC, Kim HS, Sohn DW, Nam KY, Oh BH, et al. Effect of red ginseng on blood pressure in patients with essential hypertension and white coat hypertension. Am J Chin Med. 1998;26:199–209.
185. Rhee MY, Kim YS, Bae JH, Nah DY, Kim YK, Lee MM, et al. Effect of Korean ginseng on arterial stiffness in subjects with hypertension. J Altern Complement Med. 2011;17:45–9.
186. Vuksan V, Sung MK, Sievenpiper JL, Stavro PM, Jenkins AL, Di Buono M, et al. Korean red ginseng (Panax ginseng) improves glucose and insulin regulation in well-controlled, type 2 diabetes: results of a randomized, double-blind, placebo-controlled study of efficacy and safety. Nutr Metab Cardiovasc Dis. 2008;18:46–56.
187. Barton DL, Soori GS, Bauer BA, Sloan JA, Johnson PA, Figueras C, et al. Pilot study of Panax quinquefolius (American ginseng) to improve cancer-related fatigue: a randomized, double-blind, dose-finding evaluation: NCCTG trial N03CA. Support Care Cancer. 2010;18:179–87.
188. Ang-Lee MK, Moss J, Yuan CS. Herbal medicines and perioperative care. JAMA. 2001;286:208–16.
189. Jiang X, Williams KM, Liauw WS, Ammit AJ, Roufogalis BD, Duke CC, et al. Effect of St John's wort and ginseng on the pharmacokinetics and pharmacodynamics of warfarin in healthy subjects. Br J Clin Pharmacol. 2004;57:592–9.
190. Kim TH, Jeon SH, Hahn E-J, Paek K-Y, Park JK, Youn NY, et al. Effects of tissue-cultured mountain ginseng (Panax ginseng CA Meyer) extract on male patients with erectile dysfunction. Asian J Androl. 2009;11:356–61.
191. Kim HS, Woo SH, Jo S, Hahn E-J, Youn NY, Lee HL. Double-blind, placebo-controlled, multi-center study for therapeutic effects of Mountain Panax Ginseng C.A. Meyer extract in men with erectile dysfunction: a preliminary report. Korean J Androl. 2006;24(2):84–8.
192. Papakostas GI. Evidence for S-adenosyl-L-methionine (SAM-e) for the treatment of major depressive disorder. J Clin Psychiatry. 2009;70 Suppl 5:18–22.

193. Papakostas GI, Mischoulon D, Shyu I, Alpert JE, Fava M. S-Adenosyl methionine (SAMe) augmentation of serotonin reuptake inhibitors for antidepressant nonresponders with major depressive disorder: a double-blind, randomized clinical trial. Am J Psychiatry. 2010;167:942–8.
194. Alpert JE, Papakostas G, Mischoulon D, Worthington III JJ, Petersen T, Mahal Y, et al. S-Adenosyl-L-methionine (SAMe) as an adjunct for resistant major depressive disorder: an open trial following partial or nonresponse to selective serotonin reuptake inhibitors or venlafaxine. J Clin Psychopharmacol. 2004;24:661–4.
195. Levkovitz Y, Alpert JE, Brintz CE, Mischoulon D, Papakostas GI. Effects of S-adenosyl methionine augmentation of serotonin-reuptake inhibitor antidepressants on cognitive symptoms of major depressive disorder. Eur Psychiatry. 2012;27:518–21.
196. Shippy RA, Mendez D, Jones K, Cergnul I, Karpiak SE. S-Adenosyl methionine (SAM-e) for the treatment of depression in people living with HIV/AIDS. BMC Psychiatry. 2004;4:38.
197. Dording CM, Mischoulon D, Shyu I, Alpert JE, Papakostas GI. SAMe and sexual functioning. Eur Psychiatry. 2011;27:451–4.
198. Kennedy SH, Rizvi S. Sexual dysfunction, depression, and the impact of antidepressants. J Clin Psychopharmacol. 2009;29:157–64.
199. Ringdahl E, Pandit S. Treatment of knee osteoarthritis. Am Fam Physician. 2011;83:1287–92.
200. Soeken KL, Lee WL, Bausell RB, Agelli M, Berman BM. Safety and efficacy of S-adenosyl methionine (SAM-e) for osteoarthritis. J Fam Pract. 2002;51:425–30.
201. Kornblut Anne E, Wilson D. How one pill escaped place on steroid list. The New York Times, Sunday, April 17, 2005, page 1 and page 20.
202. Brown GA, Vukovich M, King DS. Testosterone prohormone supplements. Med Sci Sports Exerc. 2006;38:1451–61.
203. Leder BZ, Longcope C, Catlin DH, Ahrens B, Schoenfeld DA, Finkelstein JS. Oral androstenedione administration and serum testosterone concentrations in young men. JAMA. 2000;283:779–82.
204. King DS, Sharp RL, Vukovich MD, Brown GA, Reifenrath TA, Uhl NL, et al. Effect of oral androstenedione on serum testosterone and adaptations to resistance training in young men: a randomized controlled trial. JAMA. 1999;281:2020–8.
205. Ritter RH, Cryar AK, Hermans MR. Oral androstenedione-induced impotence and severe oligospermia. Fertil Steril. 2005;84:217.
206. Broeder CE, Quindry J, Brittingham K, Panton L, Thomson J, Appakondu S, et al. The Andro Project: physiological and hormonal influences of androstenedione in men 35 to 65 years old participating in a high-intensity resistance training program. Arch Intern Med. 2000;160:3093–104.
207. Leder BZ, Leblanc KM, Longcope C, Lee H, Catlin DH, Finkelstein JS. Effects of oral androstenedione administration on serum testosterone and estradiol levels in postmenopausal women. J Clin Endocrinol Metab. 2002;87:5449–54.
208. Feldman HA, Goldstein I, Hatzichristou DG, Krane RJ, McKinlay JB. Impotence and its medical and psychological correlates results of the Massachusetts Male Aging Study. J Urol. 1994;151:54–61.
209. Reiter WJ, Pycha A, Schatzi G, Klingler HC, Mark I, Auterith A, et al. Serum dehydroepiandrosterone sulfate concentrations in men with erectile dysfunction. Urology. 2000;55:755–8.
210. Traish AM, Kang P, Saad F, Guay AT. Dehydroepiandrosterone (DHEA)—a precursor steroid or an active hormone in human physiology. J Sex Med. 2011;8:2960–82.
211. Reiter WJ, Schatzi G, Mark I, Zeiner A, Pycha A, Marberger M. Dehydroepiandrosterone in the treatment of erectile dysfunction in patients with different organic etiologies. Urol Res. 2001;29:278–81.

212. Reiter WJ, Pycha A, Schatzi G, Pokorny A, Gruber DM, Huber JC, et al. DHEA in the treatment of erectile dysfunction: a prospective, double-blind, randomized, placebo-controlled study. Urology. 1999;53:590–4.
213. Hellbronn LK, de Jonge L, Frisard MI, DeLany JP, Larson-Meyer DE, Rood J, et al for the Pennington CALERIE Team. Effect of 6-month calorie restriction on biomarkers of longevity, metabolic adaptation, and oxidative stress in overweight individuals: a randomized controlled trial. JAMA 2006;295:1539–48.
214. Niskanen L, Laaksonen DE, Punnonen K, Mustajoki P, Kaukua J, Rissanen A. Changes in sex hormone-binding globulin and testosterone during weight loss and weight maintenance in abdominally obese men with the metabolic syndrome. Diabetes Obes Metab. 2004;6:208–15.
215. Ernst B, Wilms B, Thurnheer M, Schultes B. Reduced circulating androgen levels after gastric bypass surgery in severely obese women. Obes Surg. 2013;23:602–7.
216. Voznesensky M, Walsh S, Dauser D, Brindisi J, Kenny AM. The association between dehydroepiandosterone and frailty in older men and women. Age Ageing. 2009;38:401–6.
217. Tiran D. The use of fenugreek for breast feeding women. Complement Ther Nurs Midwifery. 2003;9:155–6.
218. Poole C, Bushey B, Foster C, Campbell B, Willoughby D, Kreider R, et al. The effects of a commercially available botanical supplement on strength, body composition, power output, and hormonal profiles in resistance-trained males. J Int Soc Sports Nutr. 2010;7:34.
219. Steels E, Rao A, Vietta L. Physiological aspects of male libido enhanced by standardized Trigonella foenum-graecum extract and mineral formulation. Phytother Res. 2011;25:1294–300.
220. Wilborn C, Taylor L, Poole C, Foster C, Willoughby D, Kreider R. Effects of a purported aromatase and 5alpha-reductase inhibitor on hormone profiles in college-age men. Int J Sport Nutr Exerc Metab. 2010;20:457–65.
221. Hannan JM, All L, Rokeya B, Khaleque J, Akhter M, Flatt PR, Abdel-Wahab YH. Soluble dietary fibre fraction of Trigonella foenum-graecum (fenugreek) seed improves glucose homeostasis in animal models of type 1 and type 2 diabetes by delaying carbohydrate digestion and absorption, and enhancing insulin action. Br J Nutr. 2007;97:514–21.
222. Rogerson S, Riches CJ, Jennings C, Weatherby RP, Meir RA, Marshall-Gradisnik SM. The effect of five weeks of Tribulus terrestris supplementation on muscle strength and body composition during preseason training in elite rugby league players. J Strength Cond Res. 2007;21:348–53.
223. Neychev VK, Mitev VI. The aphrodisiac herb Tribulus terrestris does not influence the androgen production in young men. J Ethnopharmacol. 2005;101:319–23.
224. Kohut ML, Thompson JR, Campbell J, Brown GA, Vukovich MD, Jackson DA, et al. Ingestion of a dietary supplement containing dehydroepiandrosterone (DHEA) and androstenedione has minimal effect on immune function in middle-aged men. J Am Coll Nutr. 2003;22:363–71.
225. Brown GA, Vukovich MD, Martini ER, Kohut ML, Franke WD, Jackson DA, et al. Effects of androstenedione-herbal supplementation on serum sex hormone concentrations in 30- to 59-year-old men. Int J Vitam Nutr Res. 2001;71:293–301.
226. Brown GA, Vukovich MD, Reifenrath TA, Uhl NL, Parsons KA, Sharp RL, et al. Effects of anabolic precursors on serum testosterone concentrations and adaptations to resistance training in young men. Int J Sport Nutr Exerc Metab. 2000;10:340–59.
227. Antonio J, Uelmen J, Rodriguez R, Earnest C. The effects of Tribulus terrestris on body composition and exercise performance in resistance-trained males. Int J Sport Nutr Exerc Metab. 2000;10:208–15.
228. Moyad MA, Barada JH, Lue TF, Mulhall JP, Goldstein I, Fawzy A, for the Sexual Medicine Society (SMS) Nutraceutical Committee. Prevention and treatment of erectile dysfunction using lifestyle changes and dietary supplements: what works and what is worthless, part II. Urol Clin North Am. 2004;31:259–73.
229. Yohimbe. www.nlm.nih.gov/medlineplus/druginfo/natural/759.html. Accessed 23 Apr 2013

230. Ernst E, Pittler MH. Yohimbine for erectile dysfunction: a systematic review and meta-analysis of randomized clinical trials. J Urol. 1998;159:433–6.
231. Zavaczki Z, Szollosi J, Kiss S, et al. Magnesium-orotate supplementation for idiopathic infertile male patients: a randomized, placebo-controlled clinical pilot study. Magnes Res. 2003;16:131–6.
232. Dell'Agli M, Galli GV, Dal Cero E, Belluti F, Matera R, Zironi E, et al. Potent inhibition of human phosphodiesterase-5 by icariin derivatives. J Nat Prod. 2008;71:1513–7.
233. Shindel AW, Xin ZC, Lin G, Fandel TM, Huang YC, Banie L, et al. Erectogenic and neurotrophic effects of icariin, a purified extract of horny goat weed (Epimedium spp.) in vitro and in vivo. J Sex Med. 2010;7(4 Pt 1):1518–28.
234. Liu WJ, Xin ZC, Xin H, Yuan YM, Tian L, Guo YL. Effects of icariin on erectile function and expression of nitric oxide synthase isoforms in castrated rats. Asian J Androl. 2005;7:381–8.
235. Shin BC, Lee MS, Yang EJ, Lim HS, Ernst E. Maca (L. meyenii) for improving sexual function: a systematic review. BMC Complement Altern Med. 2010;10:44.
236. Gonzales GF, Cordova A, Gonzales C, Chung A, Vega K, Villena A. Lepidium meyenii (Maca) improved semen parameters in adult men. Asian J Androl. 2001;3:301–3.
237. Harel Z, Harel S, Wald R, Mamdani M, Bell CM. The frequency and characteristics of dietary supplement recalls in the United States. JAMA Intern Med. 2013;15:1–3.

Chapter 13
Effects of Phosphodiesterase-5 Inhibitors on Testicular and Sperm Function

Nathaly François, Raunak D. Patel, and Tobias S. Köhler

Introduction

Phosphodiesterase-5 inhibitors (PDE-5i) have been proposed as a possible therapeutic option for male infertility. Given the ubiquitous nature of phosphodiesterase (PDE) isoforms throughout the body, several mechanisms of positive PDE-5i effects on male fertility have been purported. Male patients under pressure to ejaculate either for a semen sample or during timed intercourse can often have problems with erections. The majority of published research relating PDE-5i to fertility focuses upon sperm function and spermatogenesis for which results are mixed, but most favor either a benefit or no effect. The process of sperm capacitation and the acrosomal reaction may also be affected by PDE-5i. Contractile cells surrounding seminiferous tubules, efferent ducts, and epididymal ducts play an important role in spermatozoa transport and can be influenced by PDE-5i. PDE-5i use may also affect male fertility via effects on the vas deferens, seminal vesicles (SV), and prostate. Figure 13.1 summarizes current knowledge on the effect of PDE-5i on male fertility. Additional research is required to definitively assess the effects of PDE-5i in these areas, especially in regard to real world clinical application. At the very least, the preponderance of data shows that PDE-5i do not exert a negative effect on fertility.

T.S. Köhler (✉)
Division of Urology, Department of Surgery, Southern Illinois University School of Medicine, 301 N. Eighth Street, 4B, Springfield, IL 62702, USA
e-mail: tkohler@siumed.edu

J.P. Mulhall and W. Hsiao (eds.), *Men's Sexual Health and Fertility*,
DOI 10.1007/978-1-4939-0425-9_13,

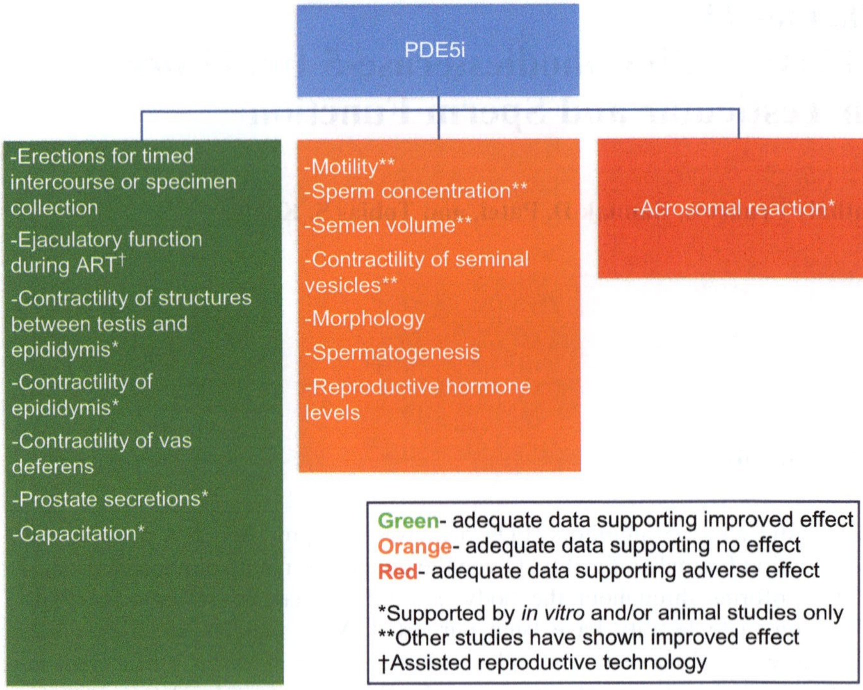

Fig. 13.1 Effects of PDE-5i on testicular and sperm function

Ejaculatory Effects

Involuntary childlessness is a powerful stressor for infertile couples and can result in a high frequency of erectile dysfunction (ED), ejaculatory dysfunction, loss of libido, and decreased frequency of intercourse. These problems are particularly problematic in the context of timed intercourse and multiple specimen collections for assisted reproductive technologies (ART). The use of PDE-5i has been purported to aid in ART compliance [1]. Temporary ED during attempts at ART has been successfully treated with sildenafil [2, 3]. In a study of 20 healthy volunteers not under the stress of ART, 100 mg of sildenafil resulted only in a marked reduction of post-ejaculatory refractory time, but did not affect already normal erectile function or semen characteristics [4]. Ejaculatory dysfunction during infertility treatment has also been successfully treated with PDE-5i [5]. Some investigators have added a 50 mg sertraline dose to PDE-5i to help alleviate temporary ejaculation failure for ART in those who failed PDE-5i doses alone. The utilization of SSRIs in this study is thought to have worked by mitigating associated stresses and anxiety [6].

A Korean study revealed a 43 % ED and 6 % ejaculatory dysfunction rate in 439 men utilizing timed intercourse [7]. Men affected had significantly lower levels of luteinizing hormone, testosterone, and estradiol. In addition, men who required high doses of tadalafil in this cohort had not only higher levels of anxiety, but more self-reported aggression. Use of PDE-5i has also been noted to aid in both erectile and ejaculatory dysfunction for artificial intrauterine insemination (IUI) by improving both the patients' ability to have a full erection and their confidence in obtaining and maintaining an erection. This improvement has been effective for transient sexual dysfunction and ultimately helped result in clinical pregnancies [8].

Effects of PDE-5i on Testicular and Sperm Function

There have been multiple clinical trials conducted to establish the role of PDE-5i in testicular and sperm function. Sildenafil (100 mg) has been shown to reach concentrations of 0.1–0.3 μmol/L in the ejaculate [9], with a presumed inhibitory effect on PDE isoforms. Tadalafil, a strong PDE-5 and -11 inhibitor, has been purported to have an effect as well, given the strong expression of PDE-11 in prostate gland, Leydig cells, and developing germ cells in the testes [10–12]. Nonetheless, many studies have been conflicting, some demonstrating improvements in spermatogenesis and sperm function, others showing no unfavorable effect, and few demonstrating reduced function [13]. Table 13.1 summarizes human studies of PDE-5i on testicular and sperm function.

Improved Function

One prospective, randomized, double-blind, crossover study, in which the investigators sought to assess the acute effect of sildenafil (50 mg) and tadalafil (20 mg) on seminal parameters in young, infertile men, demonstrated an increase in sperm progressive motility in these subjects with sildenafil, and a decrease with tadalafil 20 mg [14]. Eighteen subjects were randomized to the individual drugs, and then instructed to collect semen samples 1 h after sildenafil and 2 h after tadalafil administration. Following a 2-week wash-out period, each subject was switched to the other drug. On microscopic evaluation of each semen sample, concentration, motility, agglutination of spermatozoa, and the presence of other cellular elements were assessed; motility was classified as rapid-progressive, slow-progressive, non-progressive, and immotility. A statistically significant increase was demonstrated in the rapid and total progressive motility with sildenafil, compared to baseline [18.5 % vs. 10.5 %, $p = 0.0006$ and 37.0 % vs. 28.5 % $p = 0.009$, respectively]. Tadalafil showed a significant decrease in these motility parameters [6.0 % vs. 10.5 %, $p = 0.006$ and 21.5 % vs. 28.5 %, $p = 0.015$, respectively]. There were no significant differences noted for the other seminal parameters.

Lefievre et al. have shown that sildenafil enhances human sperm motility and capacitation [15]. Semen samples from healthy volunteers were collected after 3 days of abstinence and centrifuged. Samples with at least 70 % motility were

Table 13.1 Human studies of PDE-5i effects on testicular and sperm function

Author and year	Methods	Findings
Improved function		
Pomara (2007) [14]	Prospective, randomized, double-blind, crossover study. $N = 18$	Increased sperm progressive motility in subjects with sildenafil (50 mg); decreased progressive motility with tadalafil (20 mg)
	Assessed acute effect of sildenafil and tadalafil in young, infertile men	Effect appears to be in sperm, the vas ampulla, or seminal components
	Intervention: sildenafil 50 mg or tadalafil 20 mg	
Lefièvre (2000) [15]	PDE activity, motility, sperm capacitation, and the acrosome reaction were measured in the presence of cAMP and cGMP	Dose-dependent increase in sperm cAMP levels, which triggered sperm motility and capacitation
Rago (2012) [16]	Randomized, open-label, parallel group study. $N = 205$	Increased sperm motility after a single dose of vardenafil (10 mg), and after treatment on alternating days
	Intervention: no treatment, 10 mg vardenafil × 1, 10 mg vardenafil qod × 15 days	
Glenn (2007) [17]	Laboratory analysis of sperm motility after exposure to sildenafil using computer-assisted semen analysis; acrosome reaction assessed by fluorescein isothiocyanate-labeled peanut agglutinin staining. $N = 57$	Sildenafil found to significantly increase the number and velocity of progressively motile sperm in the best- and poor-quality sperm of infertile men Premature acrosome reaction noted with sildenafil
Ali and Rakkah (2007) [18]	Investigated the role of sildenafil on seminal parameters in diabetics Intervention: sildenafil 100 mg given to insulin-dependent and non-insulin-dependent diabetics, and to age-matched controls. $N = 100$	Significant increase in sperm motility and semen volume with sildenafil (100 mg), in diabetic neuropathics
No change		
du Plessis (2004) [19]	Prospective, double-blind, placebo-controlled, crossover, 2-period clinical study. $N = 20$	In vivo study revealed enhanced sperm binding to the oocyte with a single dose of sildenafil (50 mg); no effect on sperm kinematics
	Intervention: sildenafil 50 mg or placebo; 20 μM 8-Bromo-cGMP added in vitro to semen samples	In vitro study showed no effect of sildenafil or exogenous cGMP on semen parameters; no effect of cGMP on the acrosome reaction
Burger (2000) [21]	Sperm incubated in 125, 250, and 750 ng/mL, as well as pentoxifylline as a positive control and Ham's F10 as a reagent control. $N = 12$	No significant effect of sildenafil on motility, viability, or membrane integrity of normal or infertile sperm at 0, 1, or 3 h incubation
Andrade (2000) [20]	10 μL sildenafil added directly to 90 μL semen sample; computer-assisted assessment of sperm parameters at high	No effect of sildenafil on sperm motility at a concentration of 200 μg/mL

(continued)

Table 13.1 (continued)

Author and year	Methods	Findings
	(2,000 μg/mL) and low (200 μg/mL) sildenafil concentrations	
Aversa (2000) [4]	Double-blind, randomized, placebo-controlled, crossover 2-period study. $N = 20$	No changes in sperm number, percent sperm abnormalities, or motility with sildenafil (100 mg); there was a reduction of post-ejaculatory refractory times
	Intervention: sildenafil 100 mg × 1	
Jarvi (2008) [22]	Randomized, double-blind, placebo-controlled, parallel group, multicenter study. $N = 200$	No effect of vardenafil (20 mg) or sildenafil (100 mg), versus placebo, on sperm concentration or other semen characteristics, when given daily for 6 months
	Intervention: vardenafil 20 mg, sildenafil 100 mg, placebo	Vardenafil daily for 6 months does not impact sperm quality in men with normal baseline semen and reproductive hormone parameters
Purvis (2002) [23]	Double-blind, randomized, 4-period, 2-way crossover study. $N = 17$ Intervention: sildenafil 100 mg × 1	No effect of a single sildenafil (100 mg) dose on sperm motility, count, ejaculate volume, or ejaculate quality in healthy males
Hellstrom (2003) [24]	Parallel studies Intervention: 6 months placebo versus tadalafil 10 mg; 6 months placebo versus tadalafil 20 mg. $N = 421$	No significant adverse effect of tadalafil (10 mg or 20 mg) on spermatogenesis or reproductive hormones in men 45 years or older after 6 months of treatment
Hellstrom (2008) [25]	Double-blind, placebo-controlled study. $N = 253$ Intervention: tadalafil 20 mg versus placebo	No significant adverse effect of tadalafil (20 mg) on sperm production or reproductive hormones in men 45 years or older, after 9 months of treatment
Reduced function		
Andrade (2000) [20]	10 μL sildenafil added directly to 90 μL semen sample, computer-assisted assessment of sperm parameters at high (2,000 μg/mL) and low (200 μg/mL) sildenafil concentrations	50 % reduction in sperm motility at a high sildenafil concentration of 2,000 μg/mL
Ali and Rakkah (2007) [18]	Investigated the role of sildenafil on seminal parameters in diabetics. $N = 100$ Intervention: sildenafil 100 mg given to IDDM, NIDDM, and age-matched controls	Significant decrease in total sperm output and concentration with sildenafil (100 mg), in diabetic neuropathics

used in the investigation. PDE activity in the presence of cAMP and cGMP was measured, as were motility, sperm capacitation, and the acrosome reaction (AR). Sildenafil was found to cause a dose-dependent increase in sperm cAMP levels, which triggered sperm motility and capacitation. The mechanism responsible is unclear, but it is hypothesized that sildenafil can also act on PDE types other than type 5 to yield this effect.

In a randomized, open-label, parallel group study Rago et al. also showed an increase in sperm motility after a single dose of vardenafil (10 mg) [16]. Two hundred and five male subjects were randomized to no treatment (group A), one dose of vardenafil (group B), and vardenafil every other day for 15 days (group C). Semen analyses were done 1 h after treatment in group B, and at day 15 after treatment in groups A and C. The IIEF-5 questionnaire was also administered to subjects with erectile dysfunction before and after each treatment period. The two groups taking either a single dose or single dose on alternating days for 15 days demonstrated a significant increase in the percentage of spermatozoa with forward motility [$p < 0.001$]. Subjects taking single doses every other day also experienced a significant increase in the mean semen volume and mean total sperm concentration [$p < 0.001$], the former believed possibly due to stimulation of prostatic secretory function by vardenafil. Furthermore, erectile function as subjectively reported on the IIEF-5 questionnaire was improved in groups taking either single dose of vardenafil or single dose of vardenafil on alternating days.

Glenn et al. also showed a significant increase in the number and velocity of progressively motile sperm in good- and poor-quality sperm [17]. Fifty-seven infertile male subjects, who had presented for fertility evaluation, produced semen samples 2–5 days after abstaining. The sperm samples were divided into populations of sperm with the best-fertilizing potential as would be used in assisted reproduction treatments (90 % fraction) and poor-fertilizing (45 % fraction) potential as similar to sperm of men with infertility. These were then incubated in the presence or absence of sildenafil and assessed. Sildenafil was found to significantly increase the number and velocity of progressively motile sperm in the best- and poor-quality sperm. More specifically, the PDE-5i demonstrated a sustained enhancement of motility, as well as a premature activation of the AR.

Jannini et al. also studied the effect of sildenafil in infertile men, notably its effect on sexual function and reproductive outcome given the known reduction in sexual function in men undergoing investigation and treatment for infertility [8]. A group of healthy men were evaluated after treatment with 50 mg sildenafil before IUI or planned intercourse for a postcoital test. This group found that sildenafil reduced stress levels, reversing the stress-induced transient ED experienced in some of these men, with more complete ejaculation and more good-quality sperm. Sildenafil also improved the percentage of spermatozoa with linear progressive motility, and the number of spermatozoa that successfully penetrated the cervical mucus. They demonstrated two successful pregnancies after sildenafil treatment.

Ali and Rakkah examined the role of sildenafil on seminal parameters in diabetic males [18]. In this study, 50 insulin-dependent and 50 non-insulin-dependent diabetic males with and without evidence of neuropathy, as well as 50 healthy age-matched males were selected for treatment with sildenafil 100 mg daily for 12 months. Semen was obtained 1 h after intake, and a semen analysis completed. Sildenafil was found to significantly increase sperm motility and semen volume in the diabetic neuropathics by about 40 % [$p < 0.005$] and 48 % [$p < 0.001$], respectively; there was no significant difference in the non-neuropathics.

No Change

Studies by Hellstrom et al. showed no significant adverse effect of tadalafil after either 6 or 9 months of treatment [24, 25] in men 45 years or older. In the earlier study, tadalafil 10 or 20 mg versus placebo was given daily for 6 months. Semen analyses and reproductive hormones were assessed at baseline and at the end of treatment, following 2–5 days of abstinence. 76–85 % of patients completed this study. Tadalafil was found to be non-inferior to placebo, with no statistically significant difference between placebo and either the 10 or 20 mg dose of tadalafil in subjects that experienced a 50 % or greater decrease in sperm concentration; there was no significant adverse change in sperm morphology or motility.

In the later study, 253 men used either tadalafil 20 mg ($n = 125$) versus placebo ($n = 128$) which was given for 9 months, followed by 6 months of no treatment. Semen analyses and reproductive hormones were evaluated at baseline and every 10–12 weeks, following 2–5 days of abstinence. Seventy-five percent of subjects completed the treatment phase. Tadalafil was again found to be non-inferior to placebo, with no statistically significant difference between placebo and the 20 mg dose of drug among the subjects with a 50 % or greater decrease in sperm concentration. Overall, tadalafil demonstrated no significant adverse effect on sperm production or reproductive hormones in men 45 years or older. Analysis of secondary endpoints in both studies showed no differences in sperm concentration, sperm number per ejaculate, motility and morphology, or serum concentrations of testosterone, luteinizing hormone (LH), and follicle-stimulating hormone (FSH).

In a prospective double-blind, placebo-controlled, crossover study, du Plessis et al. demonstrated an enhancement in sperm binding to the oocyte, but no effect on sperm kinetics [19]. The investigators did an in vivo study in which subjects randomly received a single dose of sildenafil (50 mg) or placebo, after having abstained for 3 days prior to treatment. Following a 7-day wash-out period, each patient crossed over to receive the placebo. They also conducted an in vitro study in parallel to explore the effects of increased levels of exogenous cyclic guanosine monophosphate (cGMP) on sperm motility, AR, and sperm–oocyte binding. 8-Bromo-cGMP (8-Br-cGMP), a cGMP analogue, was added to the specimens treated with sildenafil or placebo. Neither sildenafil nor 8-Br-cGMP showed any significant effect on semen parameters, including percentage sperm motility, sperm count, concentration, and morphology. 8-Br-cGMP also did not affect the AR when added to the sildenafil or placebo-treated sperm, although cGMP is known as a signal transducer that mediates the AR. Sildenafil and 8-Br-cGMP did, however, increase sperm–zona pellucida binding. Overall, this study suggests that sildenafil by itself cannot initiate the AR, nor does it produce significant effects on semen parameters.

Andrade et al. reported no effect of sildenafil on sperm motility [20]. In this in vitro study, the investigators mixed semen or washed sperm in various doses of sildenafil (or phentolamine), then analyzed the specimens for motility during a 30-min period. Sildenafil demonstrated no effect on sperm motility at a concentration of 200 μg/mL. (Phentolamine demonstrated a dose-related inhibition.)

Burger et al. also showed no effects on motility, viability, or membrane integrity at a range of sildenafil concentrations (125–750 ng/mL) during a 3-h period [21]. After 2 days of abstinence, sperm from six normal, healthy donors and that from six infertile donors was incubated in the presence of sildenafil, as well as pentoxifylline as a positive control and a reagent control. There was no significant change in motility of normal or infertile sperm at 0, 1, and 3 h of incubation with sildenafil. Pentoxifylline, known to improve sperm motion and capacitation, did demonstrate increased percent motility from normal and infertile sperm donors.

Also, in a double-blind, randomized, placebo-controlled, crossover 2-period study, Aversa et al. found no changes in seminal parameters when a group of 20 men were given sildenafil 100 mg orally, with their semen parameters determined 1 h after treatment [4]. They did demonstrate, however, a reduction in the post-ejaculatory refractory times.

The study by Jarvi et al. revealed no clinically significant effect of vardenafil on sperm concentration, compared with sildenafil and placebo, when given daily for 6 months [22]. These investigators obtained semen analyses and levels of reproductive hormones after 2 and 6 months of treatment with vardenafil 20 mg, sildenafil 100 mg, and placebo. The primary variable was the percentage of vardenafil-treated subjects with a $\geq$50 % decrease in mean sperm concentration from baseline compared to placebo-treated subjects. The secondary variables were semen parameters. Neither vardenafil nor sildenafil was found to have any effect versus placebo.

Purvis et al. demonstrated no effect on sperm motility, count, or ejaculate volume, among other semen parameters [23]. Seventeen healthy male volunteers received a single dose of sildenafil 100 mg for two periods and a single dose of placebo for two periods, each period separated by 5–7 days. The study concluded that sildenafil had not adverse effect on sperm function or ejaculate quality.

Reduced Function

In the aforementioned studies, Andrade et al. revealed a 50 % reduction in sperm motility at high sildenafil concentrations, i.e., 2,000 μg/mL [20] and Ali and Rakkah demonstrated a significant decrease in the total sperm output (63 %) and sperm concentration (45 %) [$p < 0.001$] with chronic sildenafil treatment [18].

In addition, of interest is a study conducted by Khalaf et al., in which they demonstrated overall poor effects of tadalafil on the structure and function of rat testes [26]. The investigators studied the effects of chronic tadalafil administered in 60 old albino rats, divided into three groups: (1) saline orally for 90 days, (2) tadalafil 1.8 mg/kg (equivalent to the 20 mg/day human dose) for 3 months, and (3) tadalafil 1.8 mg/kg for 6 months. The animals were closely monitored daily, with their body weight and food consumption recorded weekly. They were then sacrificed at the end of the treatment period. The testes were examined grossly in situ; the epididymis was processed for assessment of sperm parameters. The animals in group 3 were found to have a significantly lower average testicular weight. Sperm count was found to exhibit a significant dose-dependent decrease. Sperm motility also decreased significantly in groups 2 and 3, with a worse effect in group 3. Furthermore, there were increased abnormal forms in groups 2 and 3.

Effects of PDE-5i on Spermatogenesis

Along with the numerous effects that PDE-5i may have on sperm characteristics, studies have also reported the effects of these medications on parameters of spermatogenesis including Leydig cell secretory function (LCSF), Sertoli cell secretory function (SCSF), and reproductive hormones including FSH, LH, and testosterone. In the therapeutic use for erectile dysfunction, PDE-5i have had both positive and non-detrimental effects in regard to SCSF, LCSF, spermatogenesis, and reproductive hormone levels.

Among the various roles of the Leydig cells is maintaining an optimal biochemical environment in seminiferous tubules for sperm growth and development. In one study by Dimitriadis et al., LCSF improvement was seen in males with oligoasthenospermia using vardenafil or sildenafil for 12 weeks [27]. The investigators used insulin-like-3 protein (INSL3) as a marker for increased LCSF and found that INSL3 levels were significantly elevated in patients that used vardenafil 10 mg daily or sildenafil 50 mg for 12 weeks compared to patients with no treatment. Testosterone was also elevated in patients using PDE-5i, though the difference was not statistically significant. The mechanism of this increased LCSF in response to PDE-5i is unclear, but it may be related to the presence of PDE-5 receptors on peritubular cells that regulate testosterone synthesis.

This group also used androgen-binding protein (ABP) as a marker for SCSF in a study of 87 males with azoospermia using vardenafil for 14 weeks. They assessed ABP levels, fertilization rates, and the maintenance of foci of advanced spermatogenesis. Again ABP, which is normally secreted by Sertoli cells to concentrate androgens in the seminiferous tubules, was used as a marker for SCSF. Decreased levels of ABP have been shown to represent decreased SCSF. This study assessed the response to vardenafil treatment in 19 patients with obstructive azoospermia, and 68 men with non-obstructive azoospermia. After ABP levels were initially assessed in the whole sample, biopsy was done to detect the presence of spermatozoa. Intracytoplasmic sperm injection cycles (ICSI) were done on these samples, and those unable to achieve pregnancy were extracted into a subset. Treatment with vardenafil was then begun on patients in this subset. At the end of the 14-week trial, increased levels of ABP in these azoospermic males was noted, though fertilization rate via ICSI was not affected. This study also found that in both obstructive and non-obstructive azoospermic patients, no detrimental effects were observed in small foci of advanced spermatogenesis.

Tadalafil has been tested in men over the age of 45 years with moderate ED to determine whether or not unfavorable adverse effects would arise [24]. A trial of tadalafil in a parallel study which compared 101 patients receiving placebo versus 103 receiving 10 mg daily and 106 patients receiving placebo versus 111 patients receiving 20 mg daily provided similar results. Parameters monitored during the study included semen analysis, testosterone, FSH, and LH at baseline before treatment, 3 months into treatment, and at the end of the 6-month treatment period. Results from the study showed that spermatogenesis and reproductive hormone levels were statistically non-inferior in men receiving treatment compared to those receiving placebo.

Thus, patients using PDE-5i for reasons such as ED may be reassured by these studies that use will, at the very least, not have a detrimental effect on spermatogenesis and reproductive hormone levels.

Capacitation and Acrosomal Reaction

Capacitation

Sperm's ability to prepare for and achieve oocyte penetration via capacitation and the AR may also be affected by PDE-5i. Capacitation involves a modification of proteins and cholesterol derivatives on the exterior sperm membrane after ejaculation in the female genital tract. This allows the sperm to attach to the zona pellucida and begin the AR and dispensing of paternal DNA. Second messenger systems involving cGMP synthesis and cAMP/Protein kinase A interactions have been implicated in capacitation and the AR.

Phosphodiesterase is a universal protein involved in the breakdown of cyclic nucleotides, with various subtypes in different locations. Baxendale et al. used PCR analysis and antibodies to isolate PDE subtypes 1, 4, 6, 8, 10, and 11 from sperm [28]. In regard to specific locations, PDE-1A was found in the flagellum and PDE-4D and PDE-10A both were isolated in the acrosomal region and the flagellum. Inhibition of PDE-4 with rolipram led to increased capacitation and in-vitro fertilization ability. Fournier et al. performed a study on bovine sperm testing the role of PDE inhibition [29]. Since subtypes 1 and 4 have been linked to sperm function and capacitation, this study attempted to assess the effect of PDE-1 and PDE-4 inhibition on capacitation. Sperm were incubated along with either 15 μg/mL heparin as the control group, or the PDE-1 inhibitor vinpocetine and PDE-3 inhibitor rolipram. Capacitation and motility were assessed at 0, 3, and 5 h. Initially at 3 h, increased sperm parameters including capacitation were higher in the vinpocetine group compared to control, though by 5 h there was no difference between the vinpocetine group and control group. Rolipram was ineffective.

Other effects included the fact that vinpocetine reduced sperm mortality more than control. Unfortunately, vinpocetine did not aid in oocyte penetration.

In 2000, Lefievre et al. showed that sildenafil led to a dose-dependent increase in sperm cAMP via inhibition of PDE, which may trigger sperm capacitation [30]. Doses used for treatment included 30, 100, and 200 μmol/L. Sildenafil's ability to improve the AR in this study will be described in the following section. Importantly, this study alludes to the fact that PDE-5i may have a role in influencing PDE subtypes other than 5.

Acrosome Reaction

The process of the AR involves the release of sperm products such as hyaluronidase and acrosin to penetrate the oocyte. In a review done by Biel et al., tricyclic nucleotide cGMP synthesis was implicated in the sperm AR [31]. Sildenafil itself leads to a decrease in cGMP degradation.

Sildenafil's effect on the acrosome reaction was evaluated by Cuadra et al. in 2000 [32]. In this study, sperm were isolated, washed, and incubated with concentrations of Sildenafil ranging from 0 to 40 nmol/L. Fractions of sperm were removed at 0, 4, 24, and 48 h and both sperm motility and the AR were analyzed. A dose-dependent relationship was not found between sildenafil and the AR, though an increase of 50 % over control was found in the percentage of sperm that had undergone the AR. Sperm motility had increased by hour 4, but decreased in the ensuing hours. Conversely, the study done by Lefievre previously mentioned, with improvement in capacitation, found that there was no improvement in the AR in sperm that did and did not undergo acrosomal activity.

Glen et al. studied the effects of sildenafil on premature acrosome activation in 57 males via fluorescein isothiocyanate-labeled peanut agglutinin staining [16]. The sample population was divided into a study group of sperm with the best fertilizing potential and a control group of a poorer population, with 90 and 45 % fractions respectively. Both groups were incubated at 37 °C for 180 min. Sildenafil caused a significant increase in the proportion of acrosome-reacted sperm in both groups. Thus, it was concluded that the use of sildenafil might lead to an increase in premature acrosome activation and a harmful effect on male fertility.

Contractility

Contractile cells surrounding seminiferous tubules, efferent ducts, and epididymal ducts play an important role in spermatozoa transport from the testis to the epididymis [33]. The ability of PDE inhibitors such as sildenafil and tadalafil to have an impact on contractility might depend on their ability to affect the various subtypes of PDE gene families that have been studied in regard to location and function in the reproductive tract. Specifically, PDE-3 has been shown to contribute to epididymal contractility [34], as well as have PDE-5 in myoid cells of rats [33]. PDE-11 is an important subtype, as it is used as a target for drug therapy by tadalafil. One study in mice showed reduced sperm count in a PDE-11 gene knockout [35, 36].

Middendorff et al. showed on electron microscopy and immunohistochemistry that smooth muscle cells and myofibroblasts were present in the tunica albuginea [37]. Other findings in their study suggested an importance of cGMP regulation in contraction and relaxation in this tissue allowing sperm transport through the tunica albuginea. The contractile tissue is highly regulated by cGMP-generating enzymes and showed significant response to agonists such as atrial natriuretic peptide (ANP) on guanylate cyclase A (GCa) and sodium nitroprusside (SNP) on soluble guanylate cyclase (sGC). Along with this, nitric oxide (NO) synthase was identified in the inner zone of the tunica albuginea where contractile cells are located. Increases in spontaneous contractions of these cells near the rete testis had also been revealed physiologically. These responses were opposed by the addition of cGMP, SNP, and ANP. SNP reduced the amplitude of these spontaneous contractions, while ANP reduced both contraction amplitude and frequency of contractions. This was also seen in noradrenaline-induced contractions, where SNP was able to inhibit contractions throughout the testicular capsule [38]. Thus, with evidence revealing an important responsibility of cGMP in regulating contractions in the tunica albuginea, PDE-5i may play an important role in improving fertility in patients with pathology involving decreased sperm transport.

In addition to decreasing cGMP breakdown, one study by Sundkvist et al. also showed that inhibition of PDE resulted in improvements in concentrating cGMP intracellularly [39]. After isolating inside-out vesicles from fresh blood, they were incubated with [3H]-cGMP with or without cGMP efflux inhibitors for 120 min at 37 °C. One inhibitor, sildenafil, showed a high affinity for the efflux pump responsible for actively transporting cGMP extracellularly. Thus, PDE-5i may be useful not only in decreasing breakdown of cGMP, but also in prohibiting cellular efflux of cGMP.

Epididymis

A study by Mewe et al. showed that cGMP regulates contractility in the epididymis by causing smooth muscle relaxation [40]. In this study, evaluation of the role of cGMP was conducted by using cGMP analogs and subsequently performing muscle tension recordings, immunological techniques, and autoradiographic techniques. Protein kinase G (PKG), GCs, and endothelial nitric oxide synthase (eNOS) were localized to epididymal muscle cells. Contractions were found to be dependent on cGMP and inhibition of eNOS and PKG led to increased frequencies of smooth muscle contractions. These data emphasize the importance of cGMP signaling in the control of epididymal peristalsis and aiding in sperm transport and maturation. Translation of these findings to medical therapy, however, has been lacking.

Vas Deferens

PDE-5i may have a more promising role in contractility of the vas deferens. PDE-5i have been studied in regard to their effects on premature ejaculation. Chen et al. showed an improvement in rates of premature ejaculation in patients using sildenafil with paroxetine as opposed to paroxetine alone [41]. This study involved 138 men with moderate primary premature ejaculation as determined by frequency of premature ejaculation on a scale of 0–8 and intravaginal ejaculatory latency time on a scale of 0–3. These scales were also used to measure improvement throughout the study. Treatment was done in a stepwise manner. Initial treatment included topical 5 % lidocaine ointment. Dissatisfied patients took one tablet of paroxetine 20 mg for 30 days as well as one tablet 7 h before intercourse. Those that were dissatisfied with that treatment began sildenafil. The end result showed that 56 of the 58 patients taking sildenafil reported significant improvement in frequency of premature ejaculation and intravaginal ejaculatory latency time.

In a study by Bilge et al., the role of PDE inhibition was examined in relation to contractility [42]. Epididymal and prostatic portions of isolated vas deferens were exposed to noradrenaline, adenosine triphosphate (ATP), alpha, beta-methylene ATP and electrical field stimulation (EFS). Contractions were measured after sildenafil was added, and it was found that contractions caused by ATP and EFS were inhibited, while those caused by noradrenaline and alpha, beta-methylene ATP were unaffected.

Medina et al. studied the effects of sildenafil on the activation of prejunctional potassium channels in tissue from the vas deferens [43]. They found that sildenafil was able to inhibit electrically induced contractions of ring segments of human vas deferens tissue from 34 vasectomies. An inhibitor of guanylate cyclase did not affect this result, but its inhibitory effect was stopped by a potassium channel blocker. This means that sildenafil also works in a manner independent of the cGMP second messenger system and attenuates adrenergic neurotransmission in human vas deferens. This is more likely due to the activation of prejunctional potassium channels.

Seminal Vesicle Effects

Previous studies of the secretory function of the SV utilizing fructose concentrations in seminal plasma have revealed no differences in men treated with PDE-5i [9]. However, several studies have noted functional features in the SV that may be affected by PDE-5i [44–47]. In a study evaluating infertile men determined to have infection induced hypertrophic congestive SV on ultrasound, daily 5 mg tadalafil resulted in improved ultrasound appearance and improvement in total sperm count progressive motility, seminal levels of fructose, and ejaculate volume [48].

Prostate

PDE-5i have been shown to upregulate several prostatic secretions that enhance sperm quality including citrate, zinc, spermine, and semen cholesterol [49]. Citrate helps maintain the osmotic equilibrium of prostate. Zinc stabilizes the sperm nucleus and has antibiotic properties. Spermine correlates with sperm motility. Semen cholesterol stabilizes sperm against environmental stressors and temperature.

Conclusion

PDE-5i are well known for their therapeutic role in the treatment of ED. They are also understood to affect male infertility in varying capacities, including an overall non-detrimental effect on sperm and testicular function as demonstrated in multiple studies. Notably in infertile patients, there are no clear negative effects of the PDE-5i on spermatogenesis or reproductive hormone levels, which is altogether encouraging as these medications are often utilized, as male patients prepare for their role in IUI and in vitro fertilization cycles. In therapeutic doses, PDE-5i have indeed been shown to ultimately improve both the erectile and ejaculatory dysfunction during infertility treatments, and to sometimes improve progressive sperm motility, semen volume, total sperm concentration, capacitation, and contractility. The AR has not been shown to improve with PDE-5i, rather PDE-5i may contribute to a premature AR, although not significantly. These agents have primarily positive or no effect on the vas deferens, SV, and prostate tissues.

Overall, there is a demand for additional research to more definitively identify a consistent role for PDE-5i in testicular and sperm function, given the few studies that refute, and the multiple that collectively demonstrate a positive effect.

References

1. Lenzi A, Lombardo F, Salacone P, Gandini L, Jannini EA. Stress, sexual dysfunctions, and male infertility. J Endocrinol Invest. 2003;26:72–6.
2. Tur-Kaspa I, Segal S, Moffa F, Massobrio M, Meltzer S. Viagra for temporary erectile dysfunction during treatments with assisted reproductive technologies. Hum Reprod. 1999;14:1783–4.

3. Kalsi JS, Bahadur G, Muneer A, Ozturk O, Christopher N, Ralph DJ, et al. Novel PDE5 inhibitors for the treatment of male erectile dysfunction. Reprod Biomed Online. 2003;7:456–61.
4. Aversa A, Mazzilli F, Rossi T, Delfino M, Isidori AM, Fabbri A. Effect of sildenafil (Viagra) administration on seminal parameters and post-ejaculatory refractory time in normal males. Hum Reprod. 2000;15:131–4.
5. Kaplan B, Ben-Rafael Z, Peled Y, Bar-Hava I, Bar J, Orvieto R. Oral sildenafil may reverse secondary ejaculatory dysfunction during infertility treatment. Fertil Steril. 1999;72:1144–5.
6. Lu S, Zhao Y, Hu J, Li X, Zhang H, You L, Chen ZJ. Combined use of phosphodiesterase-5 inhibitors and selective serotonin reuptake inhibitors for temporary ejaculation failure in couple undergoing assisted reproductive technologies. Fertil Steril. 2009;91(5):1806–8.
7. Byun JS, Lyu SW, Seok HH, Kim WJ, Shim SH, Bak CW. Sexual dysfunctions induced by stress of timed intercourse and medical treatment. BJU Int. 2013;111(4 Pt B):227–34.
8. Jannini EA, Lombardo F, Salacone P, Gandini L, Lenzi A. Treatment of sexual dysfunctions secondary to male infertility with sildenafil citrate. Fertil Steril. 2004;81(3):705–7.
9. Dimitriadis F, Giannakis D, Pardalidis N, Zikopoulos K, Paraskevaidis E, Giotitsas N, et al. Effects of phosphodiesterase-5 inhibitors on sperm parameters and fertilizing capacity. Asian J Androl. 2008;10:115–33.
10. First international consultation on erectile dysfunction: sponsored by World Health Organization (WHO), International Consultation on Urological Disease (ICUD), and Société Internationale d'Urologie (SIU). Paris, 1–3 July 1999.
11. Fawcett L, Baxendale R, Stacey P, McGrouther C, Harrow I, Soderling S, et al. Molecular cloning and characterization of a distinct human phosphodiesterase gene family: PDE11A. Proc Natl Acad Sci U S A. 2000;97:3702–7.
12. Baxendale RW Burslem F Phillips SC. Phosphodiesterase type 11 (PDE11) cellular localization: progress towards defining a physiological role in testis and/or reproduction. J Urol Suppl. 2001;165:[abstract]1395.
13. Mostafa T. Oral phosphodiesterase-5 inhibitors and sperm functions. Int J Impot Res. 2008;20(6):530–6.
14. Pomara G, Morelli G, Canale D, Turchi P, Caglieresi C, Moschini C, Liguori G, Selli C, Macchia E, Martino E, Francesca F. Alterations in sperm motility after acute oral administration of sildenafil or tadalafil in young, infertile men. Fertil Steril. 2007;8(4):860–5.
15. De Lefièvre L, Lamirande E, Gagnon C. The cyclic GMP-specific phosphodiesterase inhibitor, sildenafil, stimulates human sperm motility and capacitation but not acrosome reaction. J Androl. 2000;21:929–37.
16. Rago R, Salacone P, Caponecchia L, Marcucci I, Flori C, Sebastianelli A. Effect of vardenafil on semen parameters in infertile men: a pilot study evaluating short-term treatment. J Endocrinol Invest. 2012;35(10):897–900.
17. Glenn DR, McVicar CM, McClure N, Lewis SE. Sildenafil citrate improves sperm motility but causes a premature acrosome reaction in vitro. Fertil Steril. 2007;87(5):1064–70.
18. Ali ST, Rakkah NI. Neurophysiological role of sildenafil citrate (Viagra) on seminal parameters in diabetic males with and without neuropathy. Pak J Pharm Sci. 2007;20(1):35–42.
19. du Plessis SS, de Jongh PS, Franken DR. Effect of acute in vivo sildenafil and in vitro 8-bromo-cGMP treatments on semen parameters and sperm function. Fertil Steril. 2004;81:1026–33.
20. Andrade JR, Traboulsi A, Hussain A, Dubin NH. In vitro effects of SC and phentolamine, drugs used for erectile dysfunction, on human sperm motility. Am J Obstet Gynecol. 2000;182:1093–5.
21. Burger M, Sikka SC, Bivalacqua TJ, Lamb DJ, Hellstrom WJ. The effect of sildenafil on human sperm motion and function from normal and infertile men. Int J Impot Res. 2000;12(4):229–34.
22. Jarvi K, Dula E, Drehobl M, Pryor J, Shapiro J, Seger M. Daily vardenafil for 6 months has no detrimental effects on semen characteristics or reproductive hormones in men with normal baseline levels. J Urol. 2008;179:1060–5.

23. Purvis K, Muirhead GJ, Harness JA. The effects of sildenafil on human sperm function in healthy volunteers. Br J Clin Pharmacol. 2002;53:53S.
24. Hellstrom WJ, Overstreet JW, Yu A, Saikali K, Shen W, Beasley Jr CM, Watkins VS. Tadalafil has no detrimental effect on human spermatogenesis or reproductive hormones. J Urol. 2003;170(3):887–91.
25. Hellstrom WJ, Gittelman M, Jarow J, Steidle C, McMurray J, Talley D, Watts S, Mitchell CL, McGill JM. An evaluation of semen characteristics in men 45 years of age or older after daily dosing with tadalafil 20 mg: results of a multicenter, randomized, double-blind, placebo-controlled, 9-month study. Eur Urol. 2008;53(5):1058–65.
26. Khalaf MA, Abbas MF, El-Fakahany HM. Effects of chronic tadalafil use on the testes and sperm parameters of old albino rats. Andrologia. 2012;44 Suppl 1:370–5.
27. Dimitriadis F, Tsambalas S, Tsounapi P, Kawamura H, Vlachopoulou E, Haliasos N, Gratsias S, Watanabe T, Saito M, Miyagawa I, Sofikitis N. Effects of phosphodiesterase-5 inhibitors on Leydig cell secretory function in oligoasthenospermic infertile men: a randomized trial. BJU Int. 2010;106(8):1181–5.
28. Baxendale RW, Fraser LR. Mammalian sperm phosphodiesterases and their involvement in receptor-mediated cell signaling important for capacitation. Mol Reprod Dev. 2005;71:495–508.
29. Fournier V, Leclerc P, Cormier N, Bailey JL. Implication of calmodulin-dependent phosphodiesterase type 1 during bovine sperm capacitation. J Androl. 2003;24:104–12.
30. De Lefievre L, Lamirande E, Gagnon C. The cyclic GMP-specific phosphodiesterase inhibitor, sildenafil, stimulates human sperm motility and capacitation but not acrosome reaction. J Androl. 2000;21:929–37.
31. Biel M, Sautter A, Ludwig A, Hofmann F, Zong X. Cyclic nucleotide-gated channels—mediators of NO: cGMP-regulated processes. Naunyn Schmiedebergs Arch Pharmcol. 1998;358:140–4.
32. Scipioni A, Stefanini S, Santone R, Giorgi M. Immunohistochemical localization of PDE% in Leydig and myoid cells of prepuberal an adult rat testis. Histochem Cell Biol. 2005;124:401–7.
33. Cuadra DL, Chan PJ, Patton WC, Stewart SC, King A. Type 5 phosphodiesterase regulation of human sperm motility. Am J Obstet Gynecol. 2000;182:1013–5.
34. Setchell BP, Maddocks S, Brooks DE, Knobil E, Neill JD, editors. The physiology of reproduction. New York: Raven Press; 1994. p. 1063–175.
35. Francis SH. Phosphodiesterase 11: is it a player in human testicular function? Int J Impot Res. 2005;17:216–23.
36. Wayman C, Phillips S, Lunny C, Webb T, Fawcett L, Baxendale R, et al. Phosphodiesterase 11 regulation of spermatozoa physiology. Int J Impot Res. 2005;17:216–23.
37. Middendorff R, Muller D, Mewe M, Mukhopadhyay AK, Holstein AF, Davidoff MS. The tunica albuginea of the human testis is characterized by complex contraction and relaxation activities regulated by cyclic GMP. J Clin Endocrinol Metab. 2002;87:3486–99.
38. Middendorff R, Muller D, Wichers S, Holstein AF, Davidoff MS, Holstein AF, Muller D. Generation of cyclic guanosine monophosphate by heme oxygenases in the human testis—a regulatory role for carbon monoxide in sertoli cells? Biol Reprod. 2000;63:651–7.
39. Sundkvist E, Jaeger R, Sager G. Pharmacological characterization of the ATP-dependent low K(m) guanosine 3′,5′-cyclic mono- phosphate (cGMP) transporter in human erythrocytes. Biochem Pharmacol. 2002;63:945–9.
40. Mewe M, Bauer CK, Muller D, Middendorff R. Regulation of spontaneous contractile activity in the bovine epididymal duct by cyclic guanosine 5'-monophosphate-dependent pathways. Endocrinology. 2006;147:2051–62.
41. Chen J, Mabjeesh NJ, Matzkin H, Greenstein A. Efficacy of sildenafil as adjuvant therapy to selective serotonin reuptake inhibitor in alleviating premature ejaculation. Urology. 2003;61:197–200.
42. Bilge SS, Kesim Y, Kurt M, Aksoz E, Celik S. Possible role of sildenafil in inhibiting rat vas deferens contractions by influencing the purinergic system. Int J Urol. 2005;12:829–34.

43. Medina P, Segarra G, Torondel B, Chuan P, Domenech C, Vila JM, et al. Inhibition of neuroeffector transmission in human vas deferens by sildenafil. Br J Pharmacol. 2000;131:871–4.
44. Wang L, Chopp M, Szalad A, Liu Z, Bolz M, Alvarez FM, et al. Phosphodiesterase-5 is a therapeutic target for peripheral neuropathy in diabetic mice. Neuroscience. 2011;193:399–410.
45. Patil CS, Singh VP, Singh S, Kulkarni SK. Modulatory effect of the PDE-5 inhibitor sildenafil in diabetic neuropathy. Pharmacology. 2004;72:190–5.
46. Ali ST, Rakkah NI. Neurophysiological role of sildenafil citrate (Viagra) on seminal parameters in diabetic males with and without neuropathy. Pak J Pharm Sci. 2007;20:36–42.
47. Kamenov ZA. Comparison of the first intake of vardenafil and tadalafil in patients with diabetic neuropathy and diabetic erectile dysfunction. J Sex Med. 2011;8:851–64.
48. La Vignera S. Seminal vesicles of infertile patients with male accessory gland infection: ultrasound evaluation after prolonged treatment with tadalafil, a selective phosphodiesterase-5 inhibitor. Andrologia. 2012.
49. Dimitriadis F, Tsounapi P, Saito M, Watanabe T, Sylakos A, Tsabalas S. Is there a role for PDE5 inhibitors in the management of male infertility due to defects in testicular or epididymal function? Curr Pharm Des. 2009;15:3506–20.

94. Medina P, Segarra G, [illegible] C, Vila JM, et al. Inhibition of [illegible] by sildenafil. Br J Pharmacol. [illegible]
95. [illegible]
96. [illegible] Int J [illegible]
97. [illegible]
98. Patil CS, Singh VP, [illegible] 2004. Sildenafil [illegible] in diabetic neuropathy. Pharmacology. 2004;[illegible].
99. [illegible] ST, Kakkar NT. [illegible] of [illegible] in diabetic [illegible] J Pharm Sci. 2009;[illegible]
100. Kamenov ZA. [illegible] of the [illegible] diabetic neuropathy [illegible] diabetic erectile dysfunction. J Sex Med. 2008;[illegible]
101. La Vignera S. Seminal vesicles of infertile patients with [illegible] and [illegible] after prolonged treatment with tadalafil, a selective [illegible] Andrologia. 2013;[illegible]
102. [illegible] Wambach [illegible]

Chapter 14
Circumcision and Vasectomy: Do They Affect Sexual Function?

E. Charles Osterberg, Richard K. Lee, and Philip S. Li

Abbreviations

AIDS	Acquired immunodeficiency syndrome
HIV	Human immunodeficiency virus
ED	Erectile dysfunction
HPV	Human papilloma virus
IIEF	International Index of Erectile Function
MC	Male circumcision

Circumcision

Introduction

Male circumcision (MC) has been described since antiquity. Many anthropologists do not agree on the origins of circumcision, but some suggest the practice began over 15,000 years ago [1]. The earliest reports of the practice come from Egyptian mummies. Hieroglyphics can be found in many historic relics from multiple cultures [1]. While the religious or cultural forces that drove this practice in the past remain unknown, it remains the most commonly performed surgical procedure worldwide [2]. Currently, over 70 % of the male population born in the USA has been circumcised, mostly during the neonatal period [3]. No other surgical

P.S. Li (✉)
Department of Urology, Center for Male Reproductive Medicine and Microsurgery, Weill Cornell Medical College of Cornell University, 525 E. 68th Street, Box 269, New York, NY 10065, USA
e-mail: psli@med.cornell.edu

J.P. Mulhall and W. Hsiao (eds.), *Men's Sexual Health and Fertility*,
DOI 10.1007/978-1-4939-0425-9_14,

procedure however has generated as much controversy in the era of modern medicine. One of the controversies surrounding male circumcision lies with its impact on sexuality. In this chapter, we describe this relationship, highlighting the past and present literature examining how circumcision may impact physical and psychological factors in men and their sexual partners.

Circumcision and Sexually Transmitted Infections

From a global health perspective, there are currently three prospective, randomized clinical trials that have reported epidemiological data supporting the notion that adult male circumcisions significantly reduces the risk of HIV acquisition in African men by 51–76 % [4–6]. The possible mechanisms behind this include penile cornification, lower rates of penile injury during intercourse, fewer HIV receptors, and lower rates of inflammation/sexually transmitted infections. These trials documented acceptable surgical risks/adverse events. Furthermore, MC has been shown to significantly reduce the incidence of HSV-2 infection by 28–34 % and its prevalence by 32–35 % [7, 8]. Among female partners of neonatally circumcised men, there has been over a 40 % reduction in bacterial vaginosis and 48 % *Trichomonas vaginalis* [9]. A recent study from Uganda by Wawer et al. indicated that wives and girlfriends of circumcised men had a 28 % lower rate of infection with HPV (human papilloma virus) in 24 months [10]. While the impact of circumcision on disease prevention is beyond the scope of this chapter, the data is positive. Male circumcision reduces the risk of several sexually transmitted infections in both men and women.

Circumcision and Its Effect on Sexual Domains

Circumcision and Ejaculatory Latency, Sexual Sensitivity, and Sexual Satisfaction

It has long been postulated that the foreskin has an important role in sexual performance or satisfaction due to the thousands of erogenous nerve endings that lie within the inner mucosa layer of the foreskin [11]. Several studies have in fact reported an increased ejaculatory latency time following circumcision. Senkul and colleagues found that the mean ejaculatory latency time increased from 2.9 ± 0.4 min to 4.6 ± 0.7 min ($p = 0.02$) [12]. This phenomenon may be related to the keratinization or cornification process that occurs on the surface of the glans and shaft skin near to coronal sulcus after circumcision which may lower the sensitivity or alter the sexual excitability of the circumcised male. Taylor et al. provided anatomical and histological support of this theory by suggesting an irreplaceable loss of erogenous mucosa after circumcision [13]. Furthermore, some authors have suggested that neural reorganization and atrophy of the brain circuitry of sensory nerves supplying the distal glans occurs following circumcision [14]. While increased ejaculatory latency time after circumcision has been reported throughout the literature, some suggest that this is a potential benefit for sexual performance or satisfaction. In men with premature ejaculation, circumcision may improve sexual performance by affecting ejaculatory latency times; however, Gallo found that the majority of men do not go through with the procedure for refractory premature ejaculation [15].

Others have reported contrary findings in terms of sensitivity. Bleustein et al. reported a lack of difference in sensation on the glans of circumcised and uncircumcised men [16]. The authors evaluated approximately 60 neonatally circumcised and uncircumcised men with quantitative somatosensory testing on the dorsal midline glans using vibration, pressure, spatial perception, and warm/cold thermal thresholds. When controlling for sexual dysfunction as reported by the International Index of Erectile Function (IIEF) questionnaire, age, hypertension, and diabetes, there was no difference between cohorts of neonatally circumcised men versus uncircumcised men on somatosensory testing. Krieger et al. reported on a study of over 2,500 Kenyan men randomized to either immediate circumcision or delayed circumcision after 2 years. While 64 % of men reported increased penile sensitivity following circumcision, 6 % reported a decrease in sensitivity [17]. Masood, et al. found that 38 % of men reported increased penile sensation after circumcision, although 18 % of men reported decreased sensation ($p = 0.01$) [18]. Although penile sensation may be improved or changed after circumcision, there is a large variation in the use of the terms sexual sensitivity, sexual function, and sexual satisfaction in this literature, and it is often difficult to compare results across studies due to the variations in terminology.

Circumcision and Sexual Dysfunction

Sexual function has been classically described by Masters and Johnson who pioneered research into the nature of the human sexual response. Their model for sexual function incorporated four stages: excitement, plateau, orgasm, and resolution [19–21]. Any perceived subjective or objective interference with in any of these stages is broadly defined as sexual dysfunction.

The impact of circumcision on global sexual function beyond ejaculation has also been widely debated. Many studies have used validated questionnaires like the International Index of Erectile Function (IIEF) [22] to evaluate sexual dysfunction following circumcision. While such questionnaires have been externally validated [23, 24] it is often difficult to exclude confounding factors like the influence of the male psyche.

Aydur et al. prospectively examined 107 Caucasian men aged 22–44 years who underwent circumcision at varying ages (0–2 years, 3–5 years, and 6–12 years) but subsequently underwent evaluation of sexual function with the Golombok-Rust

Inventory of Sexual Satisfaction scale [25]. The authors found no relationship between childhood circumcision age and overall sexual function.

When comparing adult sexual function before circumcision done after puberty and postoperatively, Senkul et al. reported no difference in sexual function outcomes as assessed by the Brief Male Sexual Function Inventory (BMFSI) [12]. A similar study was performed by Collins et al., showing no differences in BMFSI scores preoperatively or 12 weeks postoperatively [26]. Masood et al. used the IIEF scores of 88 men to show that there was no difference in sexual function between those who were circumcised after puberty and controls [18].

Another unusual indication for circumcision was erectile dysfunction. In fact, in the early nineteenth century, erectile dysfunction or impotence was "treated" with circumcision [1]. Senkul et al. examined this question with a prospective study encompassing 42 men aged 19–28 years referred for circumcision for religious or cosmetic reasons. BMFSI scores preoperatively and postoperatively 12 weeks were equivalent [12].

In Uganda, Kigozi et al. prospectively randomized over 4,000 men to undergo circumcision versus control as part of a HIV prevention trial. In a subgroup analysis, the authors examined sexual satisfaction and sexual dysfunction between cohorts. They found no differences between the study arms in reported sexual desire, erectile function, and/or ejaculation based on IIEF scores [27].

Similarly, Krieger et al. performed a similar analysis in 2,500 Kenyan men undergoing circumcision as part of a prospective, randomized controlled trial (RCT) for HIV risk reduction. As with the Kigozi et al. study, the authors found no significant difference between cohorts with respect to the frequency of erectile dysfunction, inability to ejaculate, pain during intercourse, and/or lack of pleasure with intercourse [17].

In addition, male circumcision does not seem to affect a homosexual man's sexual function. Mao et al. examined a large cohort of homosexual men. While men who were circumcised later in life tended to engage in receptive anal intercourse, there were no differences in reported sexual dysfunction rates [28].

More broadly, Laumann et al. examined the sexual practices of a cross-section of American men aged 18–59 years using data from the National Health and Social Life Survey (NHSLS) [3]. The authors found that after controlling for age, men who were uncircumcised were more likely to complain of sexual dysfunction. In particular, the likelihood of having difficulty achieving or maintaining an erection was lower for circumcised men (OR = 0.66, CI 0.42–1.03) [3]. Furthermore, the authors also found that circumcised men reported 50 % less anxiety about sexual performance. Interestingly, it was noted that circumcised men performed a greater variety of sexual practices, reported more lifetime sexual partners, as well as more frequent masturbation. Taken together, the authors concluded that a clear benefit of circumcision with respect to sexual dysfunction could be seen, especially among those aged 45–59 years.

One study does report a negative association between circumcision and sexual function Frisch, et al. reported a negative association between circumcision and orgasm (OR = 3.25, CI 1.42–7.47) after adjusting for confounders (i.e., age, cultural background, religion, marital status, and frequency of sexual activity) in a large Danish cohort of men [29]. The authors hypothesized that this was secondary to decreased sensitivity of the penis after circumcision.

Circumcision and Its Effect on Female Partners

The impact of male circumcision on female sexual dysfunction has been reported, but confounders, questionable methodology, or biased data collection often limits these data. For example, in one US survey, 139 women who reported having sexual intercourse with both circumcised and uncircumcised men claimed to achieve orgasm more often with uncircumcised men (OR = 4.62 CI 3.7–5.8) [30]. Furthermore, the spouses of circumcised partners complained of increased vaginal discomfort, decreased vaginal secretions, and more negative postcoital feelings. Similarly, in a large Danish national health survey, the spouses of circumcised men report more incomplete sexual fulfillment (OR = 2.09, CI 1.05–4.16), orgasmic difficulties (OR 2.66, CI 1.07–6.66), and dyspareunia (OR = 8.45, CI 3.01–23.75) [29]. In contrast to these studies, Kigozi recently reported that Ugandan female partners reported superior sexual satisfaction after their spouses underwent circumcision [27]. Taken together, the current data are conflicting in terms of how male circumcision impacts female sexual function.

Conclusions on Male Circumcision

The impact of circumcision on sexual function is unclear given the heterogeneity in the studies that have been reported. The majority of studies report an equivocal effect on sexual function, with only one study demonstrating an improvement in sexual outcomes [3]. Although many have speculated about the effect of circumcision on sexual function, no prospective, randomized trials exist to confirm or refute this association.

The American Academy of Pediatrics with endorsement of the American College of Obstetricians and Gynecologists believe that current evidence indicates the health benefits of newborn male circumcision outweigh the risks and that the procedure's benefits justify access to this procedure for families who choose it [31]. The American Urologic Association believes that neonatal circumcision also has potential medical benefits and advantages but associated risks with the decision to perform the procedure resting with the parent or legal guardian [32].

Vasectomy

Introduction

Today, it is estimated that 6 % of couples worldwide rely solely on vasectomy for their contraception [33]. In the USA, this number increases to 7–10 % of American couples with a prevalence of 18 % of men by age 45 [34]. With more than 500,000 vasectomies performed every year, it is only second to circumcision as one of the most common surgical procedures performed [35]. As such, patients are electing for vasectomy most commonly between the ages of 30–50 years, with decades of life expectancy after their vasectomy [35]. With a prolonged life expectancy after vasectomy, its impact and consequences on a man's health has become a concern. Initially fueled by the fact that a large proportion of men develop anti-sperm antibodies after vasectomy, some authors postulate that vasectomy may have a negative effect on sexual health and long-term disease development [36, 37].

Vasectomy and Its Affect on Sexuality and Sexual Function

The incidence of psychological or sexual problems following vasectomy has been reported between 1 and 3 % [38]. An early study by Finkbeiner et al. reported that 0.3 % of men demonstrated new-onset erectile dysfunction following vasectomy with 2.5 % of men reporting worsening sexual desire [39].

Arratia-Maqueo et al. examined the effect of a vasectomy on one's perception of sexual satisfaction using IIEF scores. The authors examined 29 males who completed the questionnaires preoperatively and 12 weeks postoperatively. The authors found that vasectomy had no significant global influence on a man's sexual satisfaction [40]. Moreover, Bertero et al. found that vasectomy actually increased the mean total IIEF scores of 64 men from a total of 64–66 ($p < 0.001$) [41]. Overall, 67 % of their cohort experienced some improvement in IIEF scores postoperatively, with only 17 % reporting a worse score. Specifically, the sexual domains of desire and sexual satisfaction were most improved.

In one of the largest studies, Dias examined the long-term effects of 200 army soldiers following vasectomy [42]. The author found that 92 % of men reported sexual satisfaction following vasectomy with minimal effect on libido. This study however did not use validated questionnaires for sexual function.

The current literature suggests that vasectomy largely does not impact sexual function [43]. In a large review of the peer-reviewed literature, Philliber showed the majority of studies report no change in erectile function, duration of erections, time to orgasm, ability to control climax, volume of the ejaculate, and/or quality of the orgasm [44].

Vasectomy and Its Effect on Male Psyche

Early documentation of the impact of vasectomy on the male psyche has been reported since the 1970s [45]. Wolfers suggested that the concept of permanent sterilization may result in profound emotional setbacks, especially in a patriarchal society [46]. Rodgers and Sandlow reported a 40 % increase in psychological disturbances following vasectomy [47, 48]. In addition, several case studies have reported that a higher proportion of vasectomized men present in psychiatric clinic, although this did not necessarily imply a causal relationship between vasectomy and psychiatric disease [46]. One study suggests that the risk of hospitalization for mental disorders is lower in vasectomized men [49], yet American history demonstrates the many negative effects of forced sterilization eugenics on the male psyche [50]. In general, it is difficult to prove a direct causal relationship between vasectomy and any impact on the male psyche. Simple questionnaire surveys are an unreliable method to examine such a complex relationship.

Vasectomy and Its Effect on Female Sexual Partners

Couples have many options including both surgical and medical intervention when it comes to permanent sterilization. Some authors report improved marital relations and communication among partners who mutually decide on vasectomy over tubal ligation [51].

Hofmeyr et al. conducted a survey of 33 men and their spouses before and after vasectomy using the Index of Sexual Satisfaction (ISS) questionnaire, which measures behavior, attitudes, occurrences, and affection associated with marriage. The authors found that vasectomy did not impact one's marital satisfaction nor does it impact the communication within the marriage [52]. A similar study by Maschhoff et al. however demonstrated that vasectomy may improve marital stability. The authors found that women reported an improvement in marital communication, while men reported a 20 % decrease in thoughts of separation and divorce; overall, couples reported an improvement in sexual satisfaction [53]. A vasectomy's positive impact on female relations stems mainly from reduced anxiety of fertilization and increased frequency of coital relations leading to a global improvement in communication. This theory has been termed "re-affiliation syndrome." [53]

In summary, fewer than three studies have reported a negative impact on marital relations after vasectomy, while the majority of studies have reported no significant change. It is important to note, however, that most studies have been retrospective in nature, using non-validated questionnaires in different cultures with discordant follow-up intervals [44].

Vasectomy and Its Effect on Hormonal Function

Early prospective studies have suggested that vasectomy may impact the functioning of the hypothalamic–pituitary axis. Mo et al. found that men who underwent vasectomy 10–19 years previously had higher dihydrotestosterone levels, while men who underwent a vasectomy greater than 20 years ago had higher testosterone levels versus age-matched controls [54]. However in all other longitudinal studies, there has been no significant association of vasectomy with changes in the concentrations testosterone, luteinizing hormone, or follicle-stimulating hormone up to 25 years after the operation [55, 56].

Conclusions on Vasectomy

Although an abundance of studies exist on the positive or negative effects of vasectomy on sexual function, there remain no level I data to change current practice patterns. Similar to circumcision, the impact of vasectomy on sexual dysfunction is difficult to assess purely based on surveys or questionnaires. The studies presented are predominately descriptive and lack controls so the data presented must be taken cautiously with their inherent limitations. Nonetheless, vasectomy does not appear to negatively impact sexuality.

Beyond the scope of this chapter, an association between vasectomized men and the development of chronic disease states may exist. Initial concerns were raised in the 1970s when vasectomized Rhesus monkeys were found to have an increased risk of atherosclerotic disease [57]. Disease states that may be implicated include cardiovascular disease [58], thrombophlebitis [59], prostate cancer [60], testicular cancer [61], and urolithiasis [62]. However, other literature suggests that vasectomized men have a lower incidence of chronic disease [36]. The result of four large-scale, retrospective cohort studies has shown that vasectomy was not significantly associated with an increased risk of hospitalization and that the procedure does not increase adverse health outcomes in any of the aforementioned disease states [49, 63–65].

Taken together, vasectomy should continue to be offered to patients after informing them of the risks and/or benefits of the procedure. It remains the gold standard surgical alternative for sterilization that is proven to be safe and efficacious.

References

1. Dunsmuir WD, Gordon EM. The history of circumcision. BJU Int. 1999;83 Suppl 1:1–12.
2. Yegane RA, et al. Late complications of circumcision in Iran. Pediatr Surg Int. 2006;22 (5):442–5.

3. Laumann EO, Masi CM, Zuckerman EW. Circumcision in the United States. Prevalence, prophylactic effects, and sexual practice. JAMA. 1997;277(13):1052–7.
4. Auvert B, et al. Randomized, controlled intervention trial of male circumcision for reduction of HIV infection risk: the ANRS 1265 Trial. PLoS Med. 2005;2(11):e298.
5. Bailey RC, et al. Male circumcision for HIV prevention in young men in Kisumu, Kenya: a randomised controlled trial. Lancet. 2007;369(9562):643–56.
6. Gray RH, et al. Male circumcision for HIV prevention in men in Rakai, Uganda: a randomised trial. Lancet. 2007;369(9562):657–66.
7. Tobian AA, et al. Male circumcision for the prevention of HSV-2 and HPV infections and syphilis. N Engl J Med. 2009;360(13):1298–309.
8. Auvert B, et al. Effect of male circumcision on the prevalence of high-risk human papillomavirus in young men: results of a randomized controlled trial conducted in Orange Farm, South Africa. J Infect Dis. 2009;199(1):14–9.
9. Tobian AA, Gray RH, Quinn TC. Male circumcision for the prevention of acquisition and transmission of sexually transmitted infections: the case for neonatal circumcision. Arch Pediatr Adolesc Med. 2010;164(1):78–84.
10. Wawer MJ, et al. Effect of circumcision of HIV-negative men on transmission of human papillomavirus to HIV-negative women: a randomised trial in Rakai, Uganda. Lancet. 2011;377(9761):209–18.
11. Cold CJ, Taylor JR. The prepuce. BJU Int. 1999;83 Suppl 1:34–44.
12. Senkul T, et al. Circumcision in adults: effect on sexual function. Urology. 2004;63(1):155–8.
13. Taylor JR, Lockwood AP, Taylor AJ. The prepuce: specialized mucosa of the penis and its loss to circumcision. Br J Urol. 1996;77(2):291–5.
14. Halata Z, Munger BL. The neuroanatomical basis for the protopathic sensibility of the human glans penis. Brain Res. 1986;371(2):205–30.
15. Gallo L. Patients affected by premature ejaculation due to glans hypersensitivity refuse circumcision as a potential definite treatment for their problem. Andrologia. 2013
16. Bleustein CB, et al. Effect of neonatal circumcision on penile neurologic sensation. Urology. 2005;65(4):773–7.
17. Krieger JN, et al. Adult male circumcision: effects on sexual function and sexual satisfaction in Kisumu, Kenya. J Sex Med. 2008;5(11):2610–22.
18. Masood S, et al. Penile sensitivity and sexual satisfaction after circumcision: are we informing men correctly? Urol Int. 2005;75(1):62–6.
19. Pines M. "Human Sexual Response"—a discussion of the work of Masters and Johnson. J Psychosom Res. 1968;12(1):39–49.
20. Strassman HD. Sex and the work of Masters and Johnson. GP. 1968;38(4):109–14.
21. Pines M. Human sexual response: discussion of the work of Masters and Johnson. Rev Med Psychosom Psychol Med. 1969;11(4):459–71.
22. Rosen RC, et al. The international index of erectile function (IIEF): a multidimensional scale for assessment of erectile dysfunction. Urology. 1997;49(6):822–30.
23. Mahmood MA, et al. Translation, cross-cultural adaptation, and psychometric validation of the 5-item International Index of Erectile Function (IIEF-5) into Urdu. J Sex Med. 2012;9(7):1883–6.
24. Zegarra L, Loza C, Perez V. Psychometric validation of the International Index of Erectile Function in patients with erectile dysfunction in Peru. Rev Peru Med Exp Salud Publica. 2011;28(3):477–83.
25. Aydur E, et al. Effects of childhood circumcision age on adult male sexual functions. Int J Impot Res. 2007;19(4):424–31.
26. Collins S, et al. Effects of circumcision on male sexual function: debunking a myth? J Urol. 2002;167(5):2111–2.
27. Kigozi G, et al. The effect of male circumcision on sexual satisfaction and function, results from a randomized trial of male circumcision for human immunodeficiency virus prevention, Rakai, Uganda. BJU Int. 2008;101(1):65–70.

28. Mao L, et al. Does circumcision make a difference to the sexual experience of gay men? Findings from the Health in Men (HIM) cohort. J Sex Med. 2008;5(11):2557–61.
29. Frisch M, Lindholm M, Gronbaek M. Male circumcision and sexual function in men and women: a survey-based, cross-sectional study in Denmark. Int J Epidemiol. 2011;40(5):1367–81.
30. O'Hara K, O'Hara J. The effect of male circumcision on the sexual enjoyment of the female partner. BJU Int. 1999;83 Suppl 1:79–84.
31. Circumcision policy statement. Pediatrics. 2012; 130(3): 585–6.
32. Directors BO. Policy statement on neonatal circumcision. 2007. http://www.auanet.org/content/guidelines-and-quality-care/policy-statements/c/circumcision.cfm. Cited 12 Dec 2012.
33. Lee R, et al. A decision analysis of treatments for obstructive azoospermia. Hum Reprod. 2008;23(9):2043–9.
34. Monoski MA, et al. No-scalpel, no-needle vasectomy. Urology. 2006;68(1):9–14.
35. Barone MA, et al. Vasectomy in the United States, 2002. J Urol. 2006;176(1):232–6. discussion 236.
36. Massey Jr FJ, et al. Vasectomy and health. Results from a large cohort study. JAMA. 1984;252 (8):1023–9.
37. Schuman LM, et al. Health Status of American Men—a study of post-vasectomy sequelae. J Clin Epidemiol. 1993;46(8):697–958.
38. Jones E. Vasectomy sequelae: empirical studies. J Reprod Med. 1977;19(5):254–8.
39. Finkbeiner AE, Bissada NK, Redman JF. Complications of vasectomies. Am Fam Physician. 1977;15(3):86–9.
40. Arratia-Maqueo JA, et al. Evaluation of male sexual satisfaction after vasectomy. Actas Urol Esp. 2010;34(10):870–3.
41. Bertero E, et al. Assessment of sexual function in patients undergoing vasectomy using the international index of erectile function. Int Braz J Urol. 2005;31(5):452–8.
42. Dias PL. The long-term effects of vasectomy on sexual behaviour. Acta Psychiatr Scand. 1983;67(5):333–8.
43. Freund M, Davis JE. A follow-up study of the effects of vasectomy on sexual behavior. J Sex Res. 1973;9(3):241–68.
44. Philliber SG, Philliber WW. Social and psychological perspectives on voluntary sterilization: a review. Stud Fam Plann. 1985;16(1):1–29.
45. Ziegler FJ. Vasectomy and adverse psychological reactions. Ann Intern Med. 1970;73(5):853.
46. Wolfers H. Psychological aspects of vasectomy. Br Med J. 1970;4(5730):297–300.
47. Rodgers DA, Ziegler FJ, Levy N. Prevailing cultural attitudes about vasectomy: a possible explanation of postoperative psychological response. Psychosom Med. 1967;29(4):367–75.
48. Sandlow JI, et al. Psychological correlates of vasectomy. Fertil Steril. 2001;75(3):544–8.
49. Walker AM, et al. Hospitalization rates in vasectomized men. JAMA. 1981;245(22):2315–7.
50. Stern AM. Sterilized in the name of public health: race, immigration, and reproductive control in modern California. Am J Public Health. 2005;95(7):1128–38.
51. Shain RN, Miller WB, Holden AE. Factors associated with married women's selection of tubal sterilization and vasectomy. Fertil Steril. 1985;43(2):234–44.
52. Hofmeyr DG, Greeff AP. The influence of a vasectomy on the marital relationship and sexual satisfaction of the married man. J Sex Marital Ther. 2002;28(4):339–51.
53. Maschhoff TA, Fanshier WE, Hansen DJ. Vasectomy: its effect upon marital stability. J Sex Res. 1976;12(4):295–314.
54. Mo ZN, et al. Early and late long-term effects of vasectomy on serum testosterone, dihydrotestosterone, luteinizing hormone and follicle-stimulating hormone levels. J Urol. 1995;154 (6):2065–9.
55. Fisch H, et al. Detection of testicular endocrine abnormalities and their correlation with serum antisperm antibodies in men following vasectomy. J Urol. 1989;141(5):1129–32.
56. de la Torre B, et al. Lack of effect of vasectomy on peripheral gonadotrophin and steroid levels. Int J Androl. 1983;6(2):125–34.

57. Alexander NJ, Clarkson TB. Vasectomy increases the severity of diet-induced atherosclerosis in Macaca fascicularis. Science. 1978;201(4355):538–41.
58. Clarkson TB, Alexander NJ. Long-term vasectomy: effects on the occurrence and extent of atherosclerosis in rhesus monkeys. J Clin Invest. 1980;65(1):15–25.
59. Roberts HJ. Thrombophlebitis after vasectomy. N Engl J Med. 1971;284(23):1330.
60. Mettlin C, Natarajan N, Huben R. Vasectomy and prostate cancer risk. Am J Epidemiol. 1990;132(6):1056–61. discussion 1062–5.
61. Cale AR, et al. Does vasectomy accelerate testicular tumour? Importance of testicular examinations before and after vasectomy. BMJ. 1990;300(6721):370.
62. Kronmal RA, et al. Vasectomy and urolithiasis. Lancet. 1988;1(8575–6):22–3.
63. Petitti DB, et al. Vasectomy and the incidence of hospitalized illness. J Urol. 1983;129(4):760–2.
64. Nienhuis H, et al. Incidence of disease after vasectomy: a record linkage retrospective cohort study. BMJ. 1992;304(6829):743–6.
65. Goldacre MJ, et al. Follow-up of vasectomy using medical record linkage. Am J Epidemiol. 1978;108(3):176–80.

Index

J.P. Mulhall and W. Hsiao (eds.), *Men's Sexual Health and Fertility*,
DOI 10.1007/978-1-4939-0425-9, © Springer Science+Business Media New York 2014

N

MIX
Papier aus verantwortungsvollen Quellen
Paper from responsible sources
FSC® C105338

FSC
www.fsc.org

If you have any concerns about our products,
you can contact us on
ProductSafety@springernature.com

In case Publisher is established outside the EU,
the EU authorized representative is:
Springer Nature Customer Service Center GmbH
Europaplatz 3, 69115 Heidelberg, Germany

Printed by Libri Plureos GmbH
in Hamburg, Germany